A Practitioner's Guide to Clinical Occupational Therapy

Moya Kinnealey, Ph.D., OTR/L, FAOTA

Donna Weiss, Ph.D., OTR/L, FAOTA

Marlene J. Morgan, Ed.D., OTR/L

pro·ed
An International Publisher
8700 Shoal Creek Boulevard
Austin, Texas 78757-6897
800/897-3202 Fax 800/397-7633
www.proedinc.com

pro·ed
An International Publisher

8700 Shoal Creek Boulevard
Austin, Texas 78757-6897
800/897-3202 Fax 800/397-7633
www.proedinc.com

Tables 10.1 and 10.2: Adapted with prmission by Occupational Therapy Programs (2002).

ISBN-13: 978-141640312-8
ISBN-10: 1-4164-0312-4

Previously published by Harcourt Assessment, Inc. under ISBN 0761615024.

Printed in the United States of America

2 3 4 5 11 10 09 08 07

Acknowledgements

We gratefully acknowledge the community of academic and clinical scholars who through their willingness to collaborate and share their expertise have, in this book, created a nexus for a client-centered integration of theory and practice.

Moya Kinnealey
Donna Weiss
Marlene J. Morgan

Temple University
June 2004

Contributors

Nancy L. Beck, MA, OTR/L
Director of Rehabilitation Services
Belmont Center for Comprehensive Treatment
Philadelphia, PA

Janene Benson, OTR/L Senior Occupational Therapist
Occupational Therapy Section
Physical Medicine and Rehabilitation Department
Temple University Hospital
Philadelphia, PA

Cindy Brillman, OTR/L
President, CGB Rehab Inc.
Bryn Mawr, PA

Roberta Ciocco, OTR/L
Kinetic Rehabilitation Services
New Britton, PA

Meryl Cooperman, MS, OTR/L
Kinetic Rehabilitation Services
New Britton, PA

Kendall Daly, MBA, OTR/L
Moss Rehabilitation Hospital
Philadelphia, PA

James Foster, MS, OTR/L
Assistant Chief
Occupational Therapy Section
Physical Medicine and Rehabilitation Department
Temple University Hospital
Philadelphia, PA

Gail E. Huecker, MS, OTR/L
Director/Owner O.T. 4 kids, Inc.
Crystal River, FL

Arley Johnson, OTR/L
Senior Occupational Therapist
Occupational Therapy Section
Physical Medicine and Rehabilitation Department
Temple University Hospital
Philadelphia, PA

Nancy Allen Kauffman, EdM, OTR/L
Director, Occupational Therapy Programs
Newtown Square, PA

Moya Kinnealey, PhD, OTR/L, FAOTA, BCP
Chair, Department of Occupational Therapy
College of Health Professions
Temple University
Philadelphia, PA

Kristie P. Koenig, PhD, OTR/L
Assistant Professor, Department of Occupational Therapy
College of Health Professions
Temple University
Philadelphia, PA

Rozalyn Lipsitt, MHL, OTR/L
Assistant Professor, Department of Occupational Therapy
College of Health Professions
Temple University
Philadelphia, PA

Josette Merkl, MBA, OTR/L
Chief, Occupational Therapy Section
Physical Medicine and Rehabilitation Department
Temple University Hospital
Philadelphia, PA

Marlene J. Morgan, EdD, OTR/L
Assistant Professor, Department of Occupational Therapy
College of Health Professions
Temple University
Philadelphia, PA

Johnathan Niszczak, MS, OTR/L
Senior Occupational Therapist
Occupational Therapy Section
Physical Medicine and Rehabilitation Department
Temple University Hospital
Philadelphia, PA

C. Thomas North, PhD, OTR/L
Associate Professor
Department of Occupational Therapy
College of Health Professions
Temple University
Philadelphia, PA

Abu Panackal, OTR/L
Senior Occupational Therapist
Occupational Therapy Section
Physical Medicine and Rehabilitation Department
Temple University Hospital
Philadelphia, PA

Beth Pfeiffer, PhD, OTR/L
Assistant Professor and Program Coordinator of Certificate in Pediatrics
College Miseracordia
Dallas, PA

Ellen Rosenberg Potonyak, MS, OTR/L
Moss Rehabilitation Hospital
Philadelphia, PA

Michelle Schleicher, MS, OTR/L
General Health Care Resources, Inc.
North Wales, PA

Donna Weiss, PhD, OTR/L, FAOTA
Associate Dean
College of Health Professions
Temple University
Philadelphia, PA

Table of Contents

Introduction 1

Donna Weiss, Ph.D., OTR/L, FAOTA
Moya Kinnealey, Ph.D., OTR/L, FAOTA

How to Use This Book

Occupational therapists are concerned with the anatomical and physiological substrate of human behavior, the in-depth analysis of human occupation throughout the life span, and the effects of disabling conditions on functional behavior. Whether they are engaged in institutionally- or community-based practice, occupational therapists must analyze, synthesize, and relate complex arrays of observational and evaluative data, and design intervention strategies which facilitate their clients' meaningful participation in the tasks of life. Experienced clinicians have learned that attention to the client's personal context facilitates clinical problem solving and the development of relevant and effective intervention strategies.

This book is based on an ecological approach to the practice of occupational therapy, in which the therapist's knowledge of theory and clinical conditions is interwoven with the client's personal experience and aspirations. The evaluation, interventions, and related outcomes of treatment are viewed as interacting determinants of one another. Successful application of theory to practice requires that occupational therapists use abstract skills, such as critical thinking, clinical reasoning, and clinical problem solving.

The manner in which practitioners engage in the clinical reasoning process has been described and operationalized in the literature (Mattingly & Fleming, 1994; Schell, 1998). The simultaneous employment of procedural, conditional, narrative, and ethical aspects of the clinical reasoning process requires the therapist to interweave theoretical knowledge of disabling conditions with the individual client's aspirations and personal experience, in order to create a relevant and viable treatment program (Mattingly & Fleming, 1994; Schell, 1998).

Critical thinking, clinical reasoning, and clinical problem solving are complex processes that are central to the practice of occupational therapy, but are not readily visible to the learner. The hallmark of the progression from novice to expert is an increase in the efficiency of the clinical reasoning process—the speed, flexibility, and accuracy with which contextual data, clinical problem definition, evaluation, and the design of the treatment plan is integrated and implemented. The keys to expert performance are experience, organization of knowledge, efficiency in gathering and organizing data, and reflectivity (Johnson, 1988; Mattingly & Fleming, 1994). The primary task as one progresses toward expertise is not only to amass knowledge, but also to develop increasingly more efficient strategies for organizing and manipulating that knowledge for problem solving (Bruer, 1993; Lave & Wenger, 1991).

The traditional method of trans-generational transmission of professional information has been based on an apprenticeship model, in which the expert clinician "makes thinking visible" (Collins, Brown, & Holum, 1991, p. 6). Modeling, scaffolding, fading, and coaching are the components of apprenticeship and represent a progression from demonstrated problem solving, to guided problem solving, and then to independent problem solving.

First, the expert models the target process, often showing the novice what to do. Then, the expert provides a scaffold or support as the novice carries out a task. The level of support can vary from carrying out a task with the novice to giving occasional hints as to what to do next. Fading refers to the gradual removal of support as the novice assumes more and more responsibility. Coaching is an ongoing effort by the expert to oversee the novice's learning by choosing and structuring tasks, providing hints, diagnosing problems, offering encouragement, and giving feedback (Collins et al., 1991).

Metacognitive strategies, such as conceptual frameworks, help to reify expert thought processes and provide a tangible model of expert thinking for the novice (Bruer, 1993; West, Farmer, & Wolff, 1991). Reification of thought processes facilitates teacher and student interaction, and can help the student to become more cognizant of efficient methods for ordering and using information for clinical reasoning and independent problem solving (Lave & Wenger, 1991; Resnick, 1987; West et al., 1991).

The trend away from institutional to community-based services and toward administrative downsizing in all arenas, including healthcare, leaves novice occupational therapists with diminished access to expert on-site supervisors. As a result, there is less opportunity for the interactions described above, which are inherent to a progressive, interactive apprenticeship.

Purpose and Format

Although the written word cannot replace the interactive relationship between a novice and an expert practitioner, it is hoped that this book will provide the reader with the opportunity to see how some expert occupational therapists think. Each chapter is divided into five sections:

Synopsis of Clinical Condition

- Prevalence
- Etiology
- Identifying characteristics
- Target areas for intervention

Contextual Considerations

- Clinical
- Family
- Practice setting
- Sociopolitical
- Lifespan/lifestyle

Clinical Decision Making Process

- How to define focus
- How to establish goals for treatment
- How to design theory-based intervention
- How to evaluate progress
- How and when to determine change or termination of treatment

Case Study

- Case description
- Long-term goal
- Therapist goals and strategies
- Activity description
- Treatment session objective

Resources

- List of Web sites and other related sources

The structure of the book is consistent with the multimodal nature of the clinical reasoning process (Mattingly & Fleming, 1994). The synopsis of the clinical condition reflects the procedural aspects of clinical reasoning, and the contextual considerations comprise the narrative or conditional aspects. Through answers to a series of guided questions in the clinical decision making process section, the experts "make their thinking visible" (Collins et al., 1991, p. 6) and model how they relate theory to practice. Just as when the master craftsperson introduces an apprentice to the rubrics of a craft by providing an example of a completed product, the experts provide a reification of their thought processes by providing a case study that includes and assessment and interpretation of contextual data, an action plan, and expected outcomes.

The book encourages readers to structure their thinking and become more efficient—more expert—in data gathering and analysis, and in designing intervention that is grounded in theory and relevant to the context of the client.

Theoretical Concepts: Definitions

The following concepts are inherent to the philosophical and theoretical bases that inform the clinical decision making process of occupational therapy as put forth in this book. Conceptual definitions, followed by a diagram of the relationship between these concepts, appear below.

Occupation is defined as personally and culturally relevant activity that fosters meaningful societal participation.

Occupational Science is the study of human occupation, which incorporates aspects of the biological, anthropological, and social sciences. It recognizes the primacy of occupation to human existence, and the achievement of life goals with meaning and dignity.

The ***Philosophy of Occupational Therapy*** purports that human beings are intrinsically motivated to influence and be influenced by their environment through engagement in continuously adaptive purposeful activity or meaningful occupation. The adaptation process may be interrupted by biological, psychological, or environmental factors. Occupational therapy is rooted in the belief that purposeful activity or occupation may be used to prevent and mediate dysfunction caused by impairment of the adaptive process.

A ***Model for the Profession*** is an ordering and prioritization of the profession's philosophical components. It provides a unified method for describing domains of concern, ethical considerations, and legitimate tools for intervention. There are several models within the field of occupational therapy that provide this type of conceptual organization. Examples include the model of human occupation (Keilhofner, 2002), the Mosey performance model (Ludwig, 1993), the occupation adaptation framework (Dunn, 2000), and the person-environment-occupation framework (Dunn, 2000).

OT Theories and Frames of Reference are sets of constructs, concepts, and statements that attempt to explain observed phenomena. The purpose of theories is to guide science toward explaining, understanding, predicting, and potentially controlling the world around us. If models are likened to aerial photographs that provide gross geographic boundaries, then theories and frames of reference can be compared to road maps that facilitate navigation to specific locations.

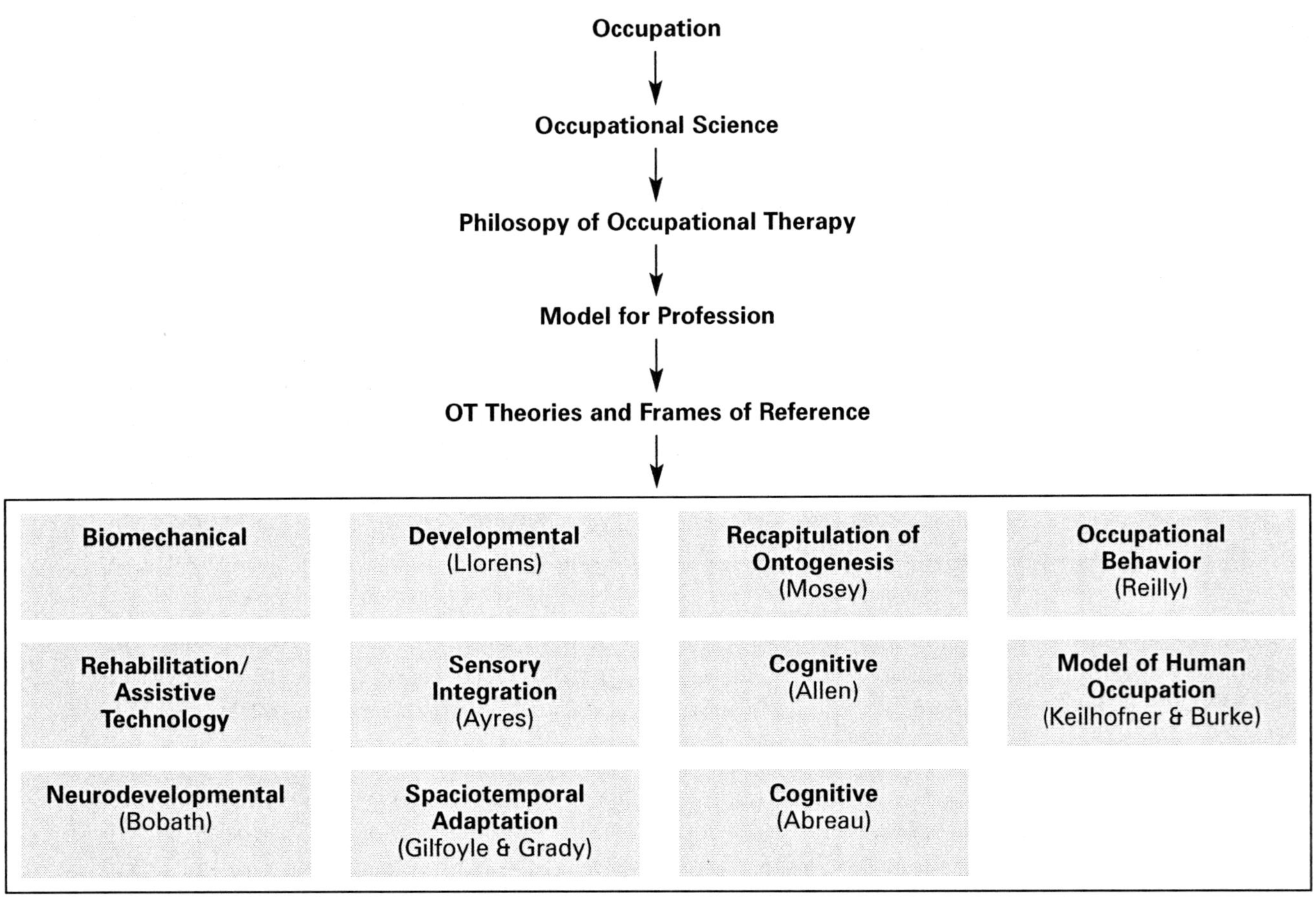

Figure 1.1 Relationships Among Theoretical Concepts

Theories of occupational therapy are neither right nor wrong, but are more or less useful given the context within which they are applied. Occupational therapy theories that were initially developed for specific populations or settings have been found useful when applied more broadly. There are a few true and fully developed theories of occupational therapy, such as sensory integration, and the model of human occupation. Others are useful but have not been fully developed or tested.

Still others are not truly theories, but rather frames of reference employed by a number of professions. The neurodevelopmental, rehabilitation, and biomechanical frames of reference could be considered in this latter category. These frames of reference help to define a problem, provide guidance for problem solving, and suggest outcome possibilities. (The outcome possibilities vary with the disciplinary orientation.) The contributing authors identify the theories and/or frames of reference that inform their decision making processes. They also indicate what frames of reference may be employed, either alone or in combination, depending on the clinical, family, practice setting, and lifespan/lifestyle context.

Structured Reflectivity: The Relationship of Research to Practice

As noted earlier, reflectivity is an important component of expert practice. Evidence-based practice and outcomes research are the functional manifestations of reflectivity, and are necessary for the vitality of the occupational therapy profession (Holm, 2000). Reflectivity requires both the critical analysis of existing literature to inform practice decisions, and the structured examination of the outcomes of treatment methodologies to assess their efficacy. Both practices simultaneously edify the individual clinician and the profession as a whole by evaluating and expanding the compendium of literature that informs and supports practice.

Clinicians who systematically cultivate their clinical curiosity by asking questions regarding the variables that affect and are affected by treatment are more likely to develop an evidence-based practice (Holm, 2000). The availability of electronic databases (such as MEDLINE, CINAHL, Cochrane Database of Systematic Reviews, ACP Journal Club, Evidence-Based Medicine, ERIC, PsychLit, and OT Search) facilitates the search for evidence regarding the relationship of variables such as populations, frequency, and duration of intervention and treatment outcomes. This curiosity, in tandem with clinical expertise, contributes to the development and maintenance of expert practice.

The perspectives shared in this book are based on the clinical expertise of the contributors and current supporting literature. Since practice is contextual and evolutionary, it is expected that there will be myriad viable treatment methodologies applicable in each of the presented clinical situations.

The challenge to the practitioner is to evaluate these methods through literature review, systematically examine the outcomes of evidence-based practice, and contribute their findings to the knowledge base of the profession. With that in mind, it would be prudent for the reader to consider this book the beginning of a professional dialogue about treatment, rather than the last word.

References

Bruer, J. (1993). The mind's journey from novice to expert: If we know the route, we can help students negotiate their way. *American Educator, 17(2),* pp. 6–15, 38–46, Summer, 1993.

Collins, A., Brown, J., & Holum, A. (1991). Cognitive apprenticeship: Making thinking visible. *American Educator, 15(3), pp. 6–11, 38–46, Winter, 1991.*

Dunn, W. (2000). *Best practice occupational therapy.* Thorofare, NJ: Slack.

Holm, M. (2000). Our mandate for the new millennium: Evidence-based practice. *The American Journal of Occupational Therapy, 54(6),* pp. 575–584.

Johnson, S. (1988). Cognitive analysis of expert and novice troubleshooting performance. *Performance Improvement Quarterly, 1(3),* pp. 38–54.

Keilhofner, G. (2002) *Model of human occupation.* Baltimore: Lippincott.

Lave, J. & Wenger, E. (1991). *Situated learning: Legitimate peripheral participation.* New York: Cambridge University Press.

Ludwig, F. M. (1993) Anne Cronin Mosey. In R. J. Miller & K. F. Walker (Eds.), *Perspectives on theory for the practice of occupational therapy* (pp. 41–64). New York: Aspen Publishers, Inc.

Mattingly, C., & Fleming, M. (1994). *Clinical Reasoning: Forms of inquiry in a therapeutic practice.* Philadelphia: FA Davis.

Resnick, L. (1987). *Education and learning to think.* Washington, DC: National Academy Press.

Schell, B. (1998). Clinical reasoning: The basis of practice. In E. Crepeau & M. Neistadt (Eds.), *Willard & Spackman's occupational therapy* (9th ed.). Philadelphia: Lippincott.

West, C., Farmer, J., & Wolff, P. (1991). *Instructional design: Implications from cognitive science.* Boston: Allyn and Bacon.

Prematurity 2

Janene P. Benson, OTR/L

Synopsis of Clinical Condition

Prevalence and Etiology

The length of a normal pregnancy is considered to be 40 weeks from the date of conception. Infants born before 37 weeks gestation are considered premature; almost 12% of babies in the United States are born prematurely. Of those born prematurely, about 83% are born between 32 and 36 weeks of gestation, about 10% are born between 28 and 31 weeks of gestation, and about 6% are born at less than 28 weeks of gestation (www.modimes.org, 2003). Although the underlying etiology is usually unknown, premature labor can be brought on by several different conditions. These include placental abruption, in which the placenta detaches from the uterus; placenta previa, in which the placenta grows too low in the uterus; premature rupture of membranes, in which the amniotic sac is torn; incompetent cervix, in which the cervix opens too soon; and maternal toxemia or infection. Premature labor is more common with a multiple pregnancy (i.e., twins, triplets, etc.) and for mothers with a history of past premature births or miscarriages. Social and behavioral issues may also contribute to the onset of preterm labor. One identifiable cause of prematurity is maternal drug abuse, particularly cocaine abuse (Edgren, 1998).

Common Characteristics and Symptoms

Premature infants are typically classified in two ways: by gestational age and by birth weight. Gestational age (GA) is the number of weeks an infant is born post conception. Classification by gestational age is as follows:

- Full term = 37–42 weeks
- Pre-term = 28–<37 weeks
- Extremely pre-term = <28 weeks
- Post-term = >42 weeks

Classification by birth weight is as average or low. Low birth weight is broken down into three additional subcategories:

- Average = >2500 grams
- Low birth weight (LBW) = 1500–2500 grams
- Very low birth weight (VLBW) = 1000–1499 grams

- Extremely low birth weight (ELBW) = <1000 grams
- Micro-preemies = <800 grams

Additionally, newborn infants can be classified by the relationship of birth weight to postconceptual age. This is determined by plotting the birth weight by gestational age on a standardized graph. Newborn age/weight classifications are as follows:

- AGA = appropriate for gestational age (between the 10th and 90th percentiles)
- SGA = small for gestational age (below the 10th percentile)
- LGA = large for gestational age (above the 90th percentile)

These classifications can be used in combination.

Common Characteristics and Symptoms

Characteristics of the premature infant at birth will vary based on gestational age. Physical characteristics may include the presence of lanugo, which is lost inutero at approximately 38 weeks gestation. The skin may appear red, mottled, and/or translucent with the vessels close to the surface. Little fat or muscle is present below the skin, and the infant may lack mature breast buds and ear cartilage, which appear at approximately 34 weeks gestation. Extremely premature infants may have eyelids that are still fused shut. The plantar creases of the feet that develop in utero at approximately 32 weeks gestation may be absent (Dubowitz & Dubowitz, 1981).

Neurological characteristics include hypotonia and lack of active flexor tone. The flexor muscles begin to develop in utero at approximately 32 weeks gestation when the infant begins to grow and the confined space of the uterus requires the infant to flex in the fetal position. Premature infants are typically very hyper-extensible and may lack full flexor range of motion (ROM). Many primitive reflexes do not begin to appear until after 28 weeks gestation and therefore may not be present in the premature infant. As the reflexes emerge, they are usually weaker than those found in a healthy, full term infant. Active movement of the premature infant is usually dominated by extensor patterns and appears disorganized, jerky and/or tremulous.

Neurobehavioral characteristics refer to an infant's level of awareness and interactive behavior. State behavior will influence response to the environment and can help determine when interaction with the infant is appropriate. Brazelton (1984) identified the following six neurobehavioral states in infants:

Sleep states

- Deep sleep
- Light sleep
- Drowsy

Awake states

- Quiet alert
- Active awake
- Crying

Young premature infants spend much of their time in the light sleep and drowsy states.

In addition to sleep-wake states, premature infants also exhibit behavioral cues or signals, which indicate responses to stimulation or stress. These cues reflect the infant's readiness to interact, tolerance of handling, and tolerance of the environment. Self-regulatory signals (approach signals) suggest that the premature infant is able to interact and tolerate stimulation. Stress signals (avoid signals) suggest that the premature infant is unable to cope with interaction or tolerate stimulation. Common behavioral cues identified in premature infants are listed below.

Stress (avoid) signals

- Oxygen desaturation
- Color changes
- Change in heart rate
- Change in respiration
- Vomiting or spitting up
- Seizures
- Arching
- Limb extension
- Twitching
- Finger or toe splaying
- Saluting
- Sitting on air
- Grimacing
- Frowning
- Gaze aversion
- Yawning
- Sneezing
- Hiccups
- Generalized hypotonia
- Glassy eyes
- Irritability

Self-regulatory (approach) signals

- Stable heart rate
- Stable respiratory rate
- Stable color
- Relaxed limbs
- "Ooh" face
- Leg bracing
- Hand or foot clasp

- Grasping
- Sucking on fingers
- Hands to mouth
- Minimal motor activity
- Alertness
- Relaxed facial expression (Als, Lester, Tronick, & Brazelton, 1982)

Prematurity now surpasses birth defects as the leading cause of death in neonates, accounting for 23% of deaths in the first month of life (Smith, 2003). Due to advances in medical technology and care for the neonate, babies born as early as 23 weeks gestation and 500 grams are now surviving. Babies born prematurely face a greater risk of serious health problems, generally proportionate to gestational age. This is due, in part, to low birth weight, less developed organs, and decreased ability to fight infection. Extremely premature infants have the highest risk for complications and long-term disabilities, including cerebral palsy, mental retardation, lung and gastrointestinal disorders, and vision and hearing loss. The following are common complications frequently seen in premature infants.

Respiratory distress syndrome (RDS) is the most common problem seen in premature infants. Most infants born before 34 weeks gestation will suffer from RDS. The likelihood and severity of the disease are proportionate to gestational age—the more premature the infant, the more likely and more severe RDS will occur. RDS is caused by immaturity of the infant's lungs, which lack the protein surfactant. Surfactant creates a protective film that prevents the alveoli in the lungs from collapsing. Lack of surfactant results in ineffective breathing, which is referred to as RDS. Infants with RDS are treated with artificial surfactant at birth. Depending on the severity of the RDS, many premature infants require additional respiratory support in the form of mechanical ventilation, nasal continuous positive airway pressure (CPAP), or nasal canula.

Bronchiopulmonary dysplasia (BPD) is a chronic lung disorder that primarily affects premature infants who require prolonged mechanical ventilation for treatment of respiratory distress syndrome. These infants develop lung damage as a result of fluid in the lungs and the development of scar tissue. The presence of scar tissue causes small areas of the lungs to collapse and other areas to over-expand leading to spasms and constrictions, which create breathing difficulties. Depending on the severity of the BPD, treatment ranges from supplemental oxygen to a tracheotomy with continued ventilator support. These infants' lungs usually heal over the first two years of life, however, some severely affected infants will develop a chronic lung disease similar to asthma.

Intraventricular hemorrhage (IVH), commonly referred to as a "bleed," is a serious and fairly common complication of prematurity. IVH is characterized by ruptured blood vessels, resulting in bleeding in the brain near or into the ventricles. While this bleeding can occur before birth or later, it usually occurs within the first four days of life, when the more premature infant is at higher risk. IVH is diagnosed via ultrasound and graded for severity on a scale of I–IV, characterized as follows:

- Grade I—small amount of bleeding limited to the area around the ruptured blood vessels near the ventricle.
- Grade II—bleeding that extends into the ventricle but no ventricle enlargement occurs.

- Grade III—bleeding that extends into the ventricle with resulting enlargement of the ventricle.
- Grade IV—large amount of bleeding that extends into the ventricle with resulting enlargement of the ventricle and bleeding into the surrounding brain tissue.

The most common IVHs are mild (Grades I and II). Most of these resolve on their own and do not cause identifiable brain damage. These infants have no or few long-term deficits related to their IVH. More severe IVHs (Grades III and IV) can cause the ventricles to expand rapidly, creating pressure on the surrounding brain tissue which can lead to brain damage. In some cases the ventricle continues to enlarge, causing a condition known as posthemorrhagic hydrocephalus, which may require surgical placement of a shunt system to redirect excess fluid collecting in the ventricle. Infants with severe IVH are at high risk for long-term deficits, including cerebral palsy, motor and coordination deficits, seizures, hearing loss, vision deficits, and learning disabilities.

Periventricular leukomalacia (PVL) is a condition in premature infants in which there is softening of the brain tissue due to cell death of the white matter around the ventricles. PVL is caused by decreased blood flow to the brain and decreased oxygen in the blood. PVL can occur alone or in conjunction with severe IVH. In severe cases of PVL, porencephalic cyst formation, ventricle scarring and cerebral atrophy can occur. Because PVL usually affects the motor tracts of the brain, these infants are at high risk for long-term motor deficits and cerebral palsy. They may also have hearing loss, vision deficits, learning disabilities, and seizures.

Retinopathy of prematurity (ROP) occurs primarily in infants born before 32 weeks gestation with the more premature infants at higher risk. ROP is an abnormal development of the blood vessels in the eyes, which can lead to bleeding and scar formation that can damage the retina. Most cases heal on their own with little or no vision loss. More severe cases require intervention and can result in vision loss or blindness. ROP has been associated with high oxygen concentrations delivered during mechanical ventilation.

Necrotizing entercolitis (NEC) is a potentially dangerous condition that can develop in premature infants in which a portion of the infant's intestines becomes necrotic and is destroyed. NEC occurs when blood supply to the intestines is decreased or interrupted, allowing bacteria that are normally present to invade the area, causing further damage. Depending on the severity of the disease, bowel damage can range from minimal to extensive. Treatment also depends on severity. Some cases can be treated by allowing the infant to eat nothing by mouth, possibly for several weeks, to give the bowel complete rest and time to heal. More severe cases may require surgery to remove the necrotic bowel and create a temporary ostomy to allow the bowel to heal. In the most severe cases, the infant may develop short gut syndrome. Short gut occurs when there is not enough healthy bowel remaining to adequately absorb nutrition. As a result, the infant will require intravenous nutrition for a prolonged period and may eventually require special formula. Feeding problems, both physiologic and behavioral in nature, can occur in infants with NEC. Infants who require multiple surgeries as a result of NEC may also experience weakening of the abdominal muscles, which can affect later acquisition of motor skills.

Due to premature infants' immature immune systems, infections are common and include pneumonia, sepsis, and meningitis. Infections occur three ways: intrauterine/congenital, perinatal, and acquired. Intrauterine infections occur during pregnancy.

They are not common but can be serious. If the infection occurs early in gestation, it can result in nervous system or tissue abnormalities and even brain damage. These infections include toxoplasmosis, rubella, cytomegalovirus, herpes simplex, and HIV. Perinatal infections occur during delivery through the birth canal. These include group B streptococcus, E. coli, chlamydia, and hepatitis B. Acquired infections occur after birth through contact. These include staph epi, staph aureus, pseudomonas, and respiratory syndrome. Infections are typically treated with antibiotics or antiviral drugs. The problems resulting from infection depend primarily on the severity and type of infection. One problem commonly related to infection is hearing loss.

Target Areas for Intervention

Precautions associated with premature infants depend greatly on gestational age, post-conceptional age, medical stability, complications, and the infant's state and interactive behaviors. It is important to have an understanding of the equipment used frequently in the neonatal intensive care unit (NICU.) Knowledge of physiological parameters for premature infants is essential. Understanding the meaning of premature infants' neurobehavioral states and cues is also essential. Universal precautions and strict hand washing practices should always be observed to prevent infection in these fragile infants.

Although premature infants may require occupational therapy intervention at various stages of their lives, this chapter will focus on intervention during the initial acute hospitalization in the NICU. The primary goal for intervention with the premature infant is to enhance and optimize development. The occupational therapist in the NICU can assume many roles while working with the premature infant, including that of developmental specialist, educator, and advocate. There are five typical areas of focus for intervention with the premature infant in the NICU. They are:

- Positioning
- Caregiver-infant interaction/caregiver education
- Sensory intervention/environmental adaptations
- Developmental/motor intervention
- Feeding

Positioning intervention with the premature infant is an important and often early focus of the occupational therapist in the NICU. Goals for positioning are to minimize motor disorganization, promote physiologic flexion, discourage arching and rigidity, prevent cranial molding, and counteract emerging stereotypical postures. Other goals for positioning are to encourage midline orientation and provide boundaries and containment to promote self-regulation. Such interventions support development by providing the infant with positive input without prolonged direct handling or undo stress.

Promoting caregiver-infant interaction and caregiver education is another important and early focus of the occupational therapist in the NICU. The birth of an infant with special needs can be a trying experience for any parent. A range of reactions and emotions including fear, denial, anger, guilt, loss, frustration, and powerlessness are common. In addition, the NICU can be a very overwhelming environment for parents. Parents can often feel like "secondary caregivers" in this acute setting. These feelings, coupled with the medical condition of the infant, can create barriers to parent-infant bonding. Early identification and remediation of parent-infant interaction difficulties are important to maximizing the infant's developmental outcome. By educating the parents on their infant's states and behavioral cues as well as general development, and by assisting parents in interactions with their infant, occupational therapists can have a positive impact on parent-infant bonding and developmental outcomes.

Premature infants do not have mature neural systems and therefore have difficulty synthesizing all of the sensory input they receive (Peterson-DeGroff, 1996). A focus of the occupational therapist in the NICU is frequently on sensory intervention and environmental adaptation. The NICU environment can be very over-stimulating to a premature infant's immature sensory system, and can elicit stress behaviors. Therefore, early sensory intervention focuses more on adapting the infant's environment to reduce stimulation rather than on providing stimulation. When the infant becomes more physiologically stable and the neural system matures, the focus of sensory intervention includes providing carefully graded stimulation to enhance the infant's auditory, visual, tactile/proprioceptive, and vestibular skill development (Vergara, 1993). Sensory stimulation should be offered based on the infant's level of stress and the infant's reaction to stimulation.

Premature infants are at risk for developing abnormal motor patterns and developmental delay. Another important area of focus for the occupational therapist in the NICU is on preventing the development of abnormal posture and movement patterns, while facilitating normal development through handling and therapeutic exercise appropriate to the infant's developmental level. The primary goals for intervention are to facilitate flexion, decrease extension of the neck, trunk, and extremities, decrease shoulder elevation and retraction, and promote weight bearing and weight shifting.

The evaluation and treatment of feeding problems in premature infants is another essential focus of the occupational therapist in the NICU. Infants rely on sucking as their primary source of feeding. This is a very complex task, especially for the premature infant. In addition to needing adequate oral-motor control to suck, the infant must also be able to coordinate sucking, swallowing, and breathing, be able to tolerate the stimulation involved with feeding, and have adequate endurance to sustain feeding. Most premature infants do not exhibit all of the characteristics of optimal oral-motor readiness for feeding until approximately 36 weeks gestation (Long, 1997). The primary goals for intervention are to promote the appropriate tactile responses, state control, motor control, oral-motor control, physiologic control, coordination of suck-swallow-breathe, and endurance necessary for safe and efficient feeding. Caregiver education is also an important aspect of feeding intervention in the NICU.

Contextual Considerations

Clinical

The purpose of the clinical occupational therapy assessment of the premature infant in the NICU is to delineate the infant's strengths, weaknesses, and needs in order to plan a program. The clinical evaluation must include information on neurobehavioral organization, neuromuscular status, and developmental status (including sensory processing). When indicated, the evaluation should also include information on feeding.

The neurobehavioral evaluation includes information on the infant's state behavior, self-regulatory abilities (including approach signals), tolerance for stimuli and handling (including stress signals), temperament, and interactive abilities. Collection of this information is primarily through observation and may require several sessions to gain an accurate picture. There are several assessment tools available, including the *Neonatal Behavioral Assessment Scale* (Brazelton, 1984), *Neonatal Neurobehavioral Examination* (NNE: Dubowitz & Dubowitz 1981), *Neurobehavioral Assessment of Pre-term Infant* (NAPI; Dubowitz & Dubowitz, 1981), *Assessment of Pre-term Infant Behavior* (APIB; Als, Lester, Tronick, & Brazelton, 1982), and *Naturalistic Observation of Newborn Behavior* (Als, 1986), which provide information regarding the neurobehavioral status of the premature infant.

The neuromuscular evaluation includes information regarding the infant's muscle tone, ROM, posture, reflex development, and motor activity. This information is collected through handling and observation. Assessment tools available include the *Neonatal Neurological Examination* (Dubowitz and Dubowitz, 1981) and *INFANIB* (Ellison, 1994) which will provide neuromuscular information including movement, tone, and reflexes.

The developmental evaluation includes information regarding the infant's visual, auditory, tactile, vestibular, proprioceptive, and motor development, and the developmental achieved within each area. This information is also collected through handling and observation. Assessment tools available include the *Bayley Scales of Infant Development–II*™ (Bayley, 1993), *Peabody Developmental Motor Scales–2* (PDM-2; Folio & Fewell, 2000), and *Alberta Infant Motor Scale* (AIMS; Piper & Darrah, 1994) which will provide information on general development of the infant.

The feeding evaluation includes information regarding oral-motor reflexes, muscle tone and strength, postural stability, oral-motor coordination, coordination of suck-swallow-breathe, response to tactile input, physiologic control, and endurance. Most therapists evaluate feeding with self-developed criterion-referenced evaluations that include the aforementioned basic feeding components (Vergara, 1993). It is important to note that many assessment tools require specialized training and/or certification.

Family

It is important to remember that the parents of premature infants have had the responsibility of parenting thrust upon them earlier than expected. While denied the expected preparation time, parents are also faced with an infant who is physically and behaviorally different from the full-term infant they anticipated. The occupational therapist can play a key role in helping the parents adapt to the NICU environment and understand their infant's unique behaviors in order to interact effectively, promote bonding, and optimize development.

Since the mid-late 1980s there has been a philosophical shift from child-centered to family-centered provision of services. Although it can be difficult to shift focus from the critically ill infant to the family as a whole, family-centered care principles should be employed by a therapist dealing with families of premature infants. The key elements of family-centered care include:

- Recognizing that the family is a constant in the infant's life.
- Facilitating parent/professional collaboration at all levels of healthcare.
- Honoring the racial, ethnic, cultural, religious, and socioeconomic diversity of families.
- Recognizing family strengths and individuality, and respecting different methods of coping.

- Sharing complete and unbiased information with parents on a continuing basis and in a supportive manner.
- Encouraging family-to-family support and networking.

A major goal of family-centered care is to support parents in the caregiver role (Long, 1997). The manner in which medical and nursing care is given often sets up barriers to providing family-centered care in the NICU. Valuing parent-professional collaboration and incorporating it into NICU care can assist professionals in meeting the needs of both the infant and parents by removing some of these barriers (Kreibel, Munsick-Bruno, & Lowe, 1991). Although changing the dynamics of providing care in the NICU may be difficult, establishing collaborative relationships with parents should be a primary focus of the occupational therapist (Holloway, 1994).

In preparing for discharge from the NICU, the occupational therapist can educate the family in ways to promote their infant's development at home. Referral to a NICU follow-up clinic, early intervention, and/or outpatient occupational therapy services is often also warranted.

Practice Setting

Although this chapter focuses on the NICU as the primary practice setting, occupational therapists may also encounter premature infants in a variety of other settings at various stages in the infant's life. Home-based early intervention services to promote developmental milestones and later, school-based services to promote academically related skills are often required. Some infants may benefit from inpatient and/or outpatient rehabilitation. Occupational therapists working in home care often provide intervention to former premature infants. When disabilities related to prematurity are severe, some infants may eventually require care in a long-term care facility.

Sociopolitical

Two primary laws apply to premature infants and their families. The Family and Medical Leave Act of 1993 mandates that most employers provide up to twelve weeks of unpaid leave for the birth of a child or the care of a seriously ill family member with continuation of the employee's health benefits (Zaichkin, 1996). Under the Individuals with Disabilities Education Act, or IDEA, programs were developed for disabled infants and toddlers (from birth to three years) and their families. All 50 states and Puerto Rico have statewide early intervention programs to address the needs of infants and toddlers who are developmentally delayed or at risk for delay, and their families.

In addition, premature infants and their families may qualify for benefits under other government programs. They include Social Security, Medicaid, and Women, Infants, and Children (WIC) programs. These programs provide financial, medical, and nutritional assistance to qualifying persons.

Lifestyle/Lifespan

It is important to assist parents in understanding the possible short-term and long-term issues related to their premature infant. Issues may be medical, developmental, financial, and familial.

The premature infant's gestational age and hospital course will greatly influence medical issues after discharge. Needs can include tube feeding, medications, monitors, tracheostomy care, and ostomy care. Some families may require cardiopulmonary resuscitation (CPR) training. Some infants may require follow-up with any number of medical specialists including neurology, ophthalmology, cardiology, and surgery. Infants who are discharged with complex medical needs may qualify for nursing services in the home to assist the parents.

Gestational age and medical complications also influence developmental issues. Premature infants are at higher risk for developmental delay than are healthy, full-term infants. Severe IVH and PVL can greatly affect the motor tracts of the brain and are red flags to possible future motor and speech delays. Former preemies account for approximately one-third of children with cerebral palsy. Approximately 60% are considered "normal," 24% have mild disabilities (i.e., learning disabilities, attention deficit disorder, vision deficits, mild cerebral palsy, etc.), and 16% have severe disabilities (i.e., spastic quad cerebral palsy, mental retardation, etc. (Long, 1997). Although it is impossible to accurately predict outcomes, it is important to make the parents aware of the developmental issues for which their premature infant may be at risk.

The family's economic resources and the infant's medical needs will influence financial issues. Sicker infants may require a longer NICU stay and infants with chronic illnesses may require frequent hospitalizations after NICU discharge. Some families' employment or financial situations may not allow time off from work during these times. The medical needs of the infant may require 24-hour care, which may make it necessary for one parent to leave his or her job. Some equipment and nursing care may not be covered under medical insurance. Daycare for an infant or child with medical needs or a disability can be expensive and difficult to find, if available at all. All of these issues have the potential to cause financial strain on a family.

The birth of a premature child can be devastating to families. The stress of having a sick infant can strain familial relationships and can cause feelings of both physical and emotional separation. Parents, as well as other family members, may be employing all their resources to cope with the situation personally and may not have any energy left to support one another (Zaichkin, 1996). Siblings may feel neglected if the infant's care requires an excessive amount of a parent's time.

Clinical Decision Making Process

Defining Focus for Intervention

The focus for occupational therapy intervention will depend on a variety of factors, including timing of the referral, gestational and post-conceptual ages, and medical stability. If an infant is very premature, very sick, and in the first few weeks of life, occupational therapy focus will be on environmental adaptations to reduce stress, positioning to promote physiologic flexion and provide containment, developmentally supportive care, and parent education. A complete evaluation is often too stressful for the infant at this early stage. Observation and screening are often the best methods to determine the needs for the aforementioned focus areas. Though educating the parents should always be a focus of intervention, it is particularly important at this time. Most parents of preemies will be overwhelmed by the NICU and will need thorough orientation to the unit, equipment, staff, and their baby's unique issues.

As the infant grows and becomes more medically stable, a more complete evaluation will be possible. Areas of focus for evaluation will be on neurobehavioral status (stress signals, state behavior, self-regulatory skills, etc.), neuromuscular status ROM, tone, quality of active movements, reflexes, etc.), and developmental status (visual skills, auditory skills, etc.). Focus for intervention includes promotion of state control and self-regulatory skills, improving tolerance for handling, promotion of normal muscle tone and movement patterns, and promotion of developmentally appropriate skills. Another important focus is on parent-infant interaction. Getting a parent involved with kangaroo care (providing skin-to-skin contact by placing the infant on the parent's chest) of the infant is a good way to promote bonding, and studies have shown it to be physiologically beneficial for the infant as well (Luddington-Hoe, Thompson, Swinth, Hadeed, & Anderson, 1994).

When medically and developmentally appropriate, feeding is often a main focus for intervention with premature infants. Typically these infants need to work on sucking, coordination of suck-swallow-breathe, and endurance. Environment, positioning, nipple selection, oral-motor stimulation, and oral-motor skills are focuses within feeding intervention. Since it is impossible for the occupational therapist to be present during all feedings, education of parents and nursing staff on guidelines for safe and efficient feeding of the infant is essential.

When the infant is ready to leave the hospital, discharge planning is the final focus of the occupational therapist working in the NICU. It may be necessary to provide the family with a home program for ROM, feeding, and/or developmental stimulation. A referral to early intervention or outpatient services may be required.

Lastly, it may be necessary to adapt the infant's car seat for safe transport home. More often than not, even the smallest of infant car seats are too large for preemies. It may be necessary to provide a commercially available car seat insert or use blanket rolls around the infant's head, along the sides, and between the legs to prevent the infant from sliding down or to the side in the seat, which could potentially restrict breathing.

Establishing Goals for Intervention

Goals for intervention will also be dictated by timing of referral, gestational and post-conceptual ages, and medical stability. For example, nippling would not be a goal for a 2-week-old, 24-week gestation preemie, but could be for a 9-week-old, 28-week gestation preemie. It is important to consider the infant's neurobehavioral strengths and weaknesses when establishing goals. State control, self-regulatory skills, and tolerance for handling will usually be initial goals as these skills are the foundation for addressing other goals. It would be impossible to work on a goal of visual tracking for example if the infant screams uncontrollably when handled.

Designing Theory-Based Intervention

There are many different frames of reference applicable to this population. These may include syntactic theory of development/developmental care, biomechanical, developmental, neurodevelopmental treatment, and sensory integration.

Intervention with premature infants should be based on the theory of developmental care. The premise of developmental care is based on the synactive theory of development, pioneered by psychologist Heidelise Als and associates after extensive research with premature infants (Als, 1986). This theory is much too complex to address in detail within the confines of this chapter. In short, the synactive theory of development outlines how infants interact with the environment through various hierarchically organized behavioral subsystems: physiologic (autonomic), motor, state, interactive/attentional, and self-regulation. Stability in the lower subsystems is necessary for higher level functioning (Vergara, 1993). From this theory emerged the approach known as individualized developmental care. The theory indicates that assessing the infant's ability to cope with the environment and stimulation will provide the caregiver with information to modify each infant's environment, and form treatment strategies to maximize positive outcomes. Developmental care should encompass all disciplines, including occupational therapy. The occupational therapist is often the person to assess and design each infant's individualized developmental care program and adapt/modify the environment accordingly. This plan then becomes the foundation for all intervention, including therapeutic, nursing, and medical intervention.

The biomechanical frame of reference is used with premature infants who frequently have neuromuscular or musculoskeletal issues, since they typically lack physiologic flexion and exhibit low muscle tone and abnormal movement patterns. For example, knowledge and understanding of biomechanical neurodevelopmental and developmental principles are necessary for intervention with a preemie whose lack of flexion and predominant extensor movement patterns and resulting structural changes make it difficult for the infant to get his or her hands to his or her face or mouth for self-calming.

The developmental frame of reference is used in this population as in any other pediatric population. It is necessary to have a good understanding of normal development in order to identify emerging atypical development and promote achievement of developmental milestones. For example, does a 14-week-old, 28-week gestation preemie who is able to hold his head up for extended periods truly have good head control? Or is increased extensor tone allowing him to hold his head up? Knowledge of developmental principles suggests that a 2-week-old infant (the infant's corrected age) does not have enough head control to maintain an erect head and neck, therefore extensor tone is likely the underlying cause. Premature infants are at high risk for developmental delay and early identification and intervention are key to improving developmental outcomes.

Neurodevelopmental treatment principles are often used to treat the older preemie population. Positioning principles and handling techniques of this approach can be beneficial in treating infants who demonstrate neurological and motor problems. Keep in mind that neurodevelopmental treatment (NDT) is frequently used with children with cerebral palsy, and many premature infants who are later diagnosed with CP show early neuromuscular problems.

Use of the sensory integration approach with premature infants can be beneficial, but sensory input must be carefully graded and monitored. Although these techniques are not appropriate for use with the young preemie, they can be applied to the older preemie whose neural system is more mature and able to tolerate the stimulation. For example, sensory integration principles and techniques may be useful when working on feeding with an infant who demonstrates tactile defensiveness of the face and mouth after prolonged intubation.

Evaluating Progress

Progress is evaluated by achievement of established goals. Because preemies can change and develop so rapidly, evaluation and reevaluation of progress is an ongoing process. Improved physiologic status, decreased ventilator requirements, weight gain, decreased medication requirements, and increased awake/alert time can be less obvious signs of progress.

Determining Change in or Termination of Treatment

Change in or termination of treatment is warranted when the infant fails to progress, or has met all of the goals established.

Case Study

Description

Billy is a 2-week-old infant born at 26 weeks gestation, weighing 775 grams, to a 32-year-old mother with good prenatal care. Billy's parents have a 4-year-old daughter at home, which makes frequent visitation difficult. Billy was intubated at delivery due to poor respiratory effort and continues to require mechanical ventilation for RDS. A head ultrasound revealed a right Grade II IVH. Billy had an intravenous line in his right arm. Episodes of apnea, bradycardia, and oxygen desaturation have been documented.

Occupational therapy evaluation found Billy to have poor state control and poor tolerance for environmental stimulation. Billy demonstrated significant stress signs with care giving and poor self-calming skills. Supine resting position was with legs in slight flexion, arms extended at the sides, and neck rotated to the right and extended. Active movements were disorganized, jerky, and predominated by extension. Billy was able to open his eyes for brief periods when the lights were dimmed. Goals for Billy are as follows:

Long- and Short-Term Goals

The long-term goal of intervention for Billy is to enable him to improve his state control, increase his tolerance for environment, and develop self-calming skills.

These goals will be reached in part through successfully achieving the following short-term goals:

1. Transition smoothly from sleep state to quiet alert state.
2. Tolerate diaper change with minimum signs of stress.
3. Calm with moderate therapist assistance.
4. Maintain an optimally flexed position with assistive devices.

Therapist Goals and Strategies

The therapist's goals include:

1. Promote physiologic flexion and midline orientation.
2. Promote state control and self-calming.
3. Minimize positional deformities, abnormal tone, and abnormal movement patterns.
4. Provide an environment that reduces infant stress and promotes self-regulatory behaviors.
5. Educate family and caregivers on infant's abilities and weaknesses and how to optimally interact with the infant.
6. Promote infant-parent bonding.

The therapist's strategies include:

1. Utilize positioning aids to facilitate flexion and midline orientation, to provide containment and boundaries, and to reduce cranial molding.
2. Take pictures and leave bedside instructions to promote carryover of optimal positioning with caregivers.
3. Employ four-handed care techniques whenever possible during care giving and routine procedures.
4. Adapt the infant's environment to reduce stressful stimuli (i.e., provide an isolette cover to shield the infant from light and visual stimuli, dim lights, and reduce noise, etc.).
5. Explore calming techniques that work best with the infant.
6. Provide parents with opportunities to observe their infant's various states and signals to promote understanding of behaviors.
7. Provide parents with opportunities for positive interactions with their infant.

Activity

Kangaroo Care

Billy's mother will hold him skin to skin on her chest in a private, quiet, and dimly lit area of the nursery (since Billy is still intubated, a screen will be provided around his warmer bed and the tube taped to Mom to prevent accidental extubation). Mom will be guided in holding Billy in a flexed position with opportunities for hands to face and hands to mouth, skills important for self-calming in infants. Initially, this therapeutic holding would be for a short period with close supervision giving mom the opportunity to identify Billy's stress and approach signals, assist him in self-calming, and gain confidence in her ability to interact with her infant. As the infant becomes more able to tolerate sensation and self regulate, and Mom becomes more confident and comfortable, the activity can be graded to increase time, handling, and stimulation.

Treatment Objectives

1. Billy will tolerate handling and his environment for 10 minutes.
2. Mom will correctly identify Billy's stress and approach signals and respond appropriately.

Resources

The following resources can be helpful for gathering clinical data:

Neuro-behavioral data:

- Observation
- *Neonatal Behavioral Assessment Scale* (NBAS)
- *Neonatal Neuro-Behavioral Exam* (NNE)
- *Neuro-Behavioral Assessment of Pre-term Infant* (NAPI)
- *Assessment of Pre-Term Infant Behavior* (APIB)

Neuromuscular Data:

- Active/passive ROM
- Manual muscle test
- Reflex testing
- Neonatal neurological exam
- *Movement Assessment of Infants* (MAI)

Developmental data:

- *Bayley Scales of Infant Development–II*
- *Peabody Developmental Motor Scales–2* (PDMS–2)
- *Alberta Infant Motor Scale* (AIMS)

Feeding data:

- Clinical evaluation
- *Neonatal Oral-Motor Assessment Scale* (NOMAS)

The following resources can be helpful for gathering family data:

- Informal interview of parents
- Awareness of cultural, ethnic, and/or religious issues and concerns

The following are common practice settings:

- NICU
- Early intervention, school system, inpatient/outpatient rehab, home care, long-term care facility

The following resources can be helpful for gathering sociopolitical data:

- Medicaid legislation
- Individuals with Disabilities Education Act (IDEA)
- Family Medical Leave Act (FMLA)
- Social Security Income Benefits (SSI)
- Women, Infants, and Children (WIC)

The following can be helpful in understanding and managing specific lifestyle/lifespan issues:

Medical:

- Medications
- Tube-feeding
- Monitor training
- CPR training
- Trach care
- Ostomy care
- Follow-up appointments
- Home nursing

Developmental:

- At risk for delay
- Cerebral palsy
- Learning disability

- Mental retardation
- Vision deficits

Financial:

- Equipment costs
- Home nursing costs
- Daycare costs
- Time off from work
- Need for 24 hour care

Family:

- Coping skills
- Interpersonal relationships
- Sibling relationships

Internet Resources

American Association of Premature Infants:
www.aapi-online.org

Association for Retinopathy of Prematurity & Related Diseases:
www.ropard.org

Institute for Family Centered Care:
www.familycenteredcare.org

Miscellaneous:
www.comeunity.com/premature /preemiepgs.html
www.preemie.org
www.preemies.com
www.premature-infant.com

Published Resources

Klein, A. (1998). Caring for your premature baby. New York: HarperResources.

Ludington-Hoe, S. (1993). Kangaroo care: The best you can do to help your pre-term infant. New York, NY, Bantam Books.

Wyly, V. (1995). Premature infants and their families: Developmental interventions. San Diego, CA, Bantam BooksR. Gross, R., Spiker, D., & Haynes, C. (1997). Helping low birthweight, premature babies: The infant health and development program. Stanford, CA: Stanford University Press.

Zaichkin, J. (1996). Newborn intensive care—what every parent needs to know. Santa Rosa, CA: NICU.

References

Als, H. (1986). A synactive model of neonatal behavioral organization: Framework for the assessment of neurobehavioral development in the premature infant and for support of infants and parents in the neonatal intensive care environment. In J. K. Sweeney (Ed.), *High risk neonate: Developmental therapy perspectives* (pp. 1–55). New York: Hawthorn Press.

Als, H., Lester, B. M., Tronick, E. Z., & Brazelton, T. B. (1982). Toward a research instrument for the assessment of pre-term infants' behavior (APIB). In H. Fitzgerald, B. M. Lester, & M. S. Yogman (Eds.), *Theory and research in behavioral pediatrics* (Vol. 1; pp. 35–132). New York: Plenum.

Bayley, N. (1993). *Bayley scales of infant development* (2nd ed.). San Antonio, TX: The Psychological Corporation.

Brazelton, T. B. (1984). *Neonatal behavioral assessment scale.* Philadelphia: Lippincott.

Dubowitz, L., & Dubowitz , V. (1981). *The neurological assessment of the pre-term and full-term newborn infant.* Philadelphia: Lippincott.

Edgren, A. (1998). Prematurity. In *Gale Encyclopedia of Medicine.* Detroit, MI: Gale Group.

Ellison, P. H. (1994). *The INFANIB.* San Antonio, TX: Therapy Skill Builders.

Folio, M. R., & Fewell, R. R. (2000). *Peabody Developmental Motors Scales,* (2nd ed.). Austin, TX: Pro-Ed.

Holloway, E. (1994). Parent and occupational therapist–collaboration in the neonatal intensive care unit. *American Journal of Occupational Therapy, 48,* 535–538.

Individuals with Disabilities Act (IDEA) Amendments of 1997, Pub. L. No. 105–17.

Kreibel, R., Munsick-Bruno, G., & Lowe, R. (1991). NICU infants born at developmental risk and the individualized family service plan/process. *Children's Health Care, 20(1),* 26–33.

Long, T. (1997, September). *Therapeutic intervention in the neonatal intensive care unit.* Workshop presented by Pacific Coast Seminars, San Francisco.

Luddington-Hoe, S. M., Thompson, C., Swinth, J., Hadeed, A. J., & Anderson, G. C. (1994). Kangaroo care: Research results and practice implications and guidelines. *Neonatal Network, 13,* 19–27.

Peterson-DeGroff, M. (1996). *Developmental care: Over stimulation and your premature baby.* Retrieved February 10, 2003 from http://www.prematurity.org/overstimulation.html

Piper M.C., & Darrah, J (1994). *Alberta infant motor scale* (AIMS). *Motor Assessment of the Developing Infant.* Philadelphia: Saunders.

Smith, C. (2003). *Premature birth rates rising in state, U.S.* Retrieved February 10, 2003 from http://www.seattlepi.com/local/106628_preemie31.shtml

Vergara, E. (1993). *Foundations for practice in the neonatal intensive care unit and early intervention: A self-guided practice manual.* Rockville, MD: American Occupational Therapy Association.

www.modimes.org/prematurity/prematurity.asp. Retrieved February 10, 2003.

Zaichkin, J. (1996). *Newborn intensive care—what every parent needs to know.* Santa Rosa, CA: NICU.

Regulatory Disorders 3

Moya Kinnealey, Ph.D., OTR/L, FAOTA

Synopsis of Clinical Condition

Prevalence and Etiology

Regulatory disorders are presumed to be constitutionally or biologically-based. Although some cases may have a genetic link, many cases have no clear precipitating factor. Negative temperamental predispositions are often exacerbated by caregiver patterns and early maturational factors such as prematurity, drug exposure in utero, difficult births, and low birth weight.

Common Characteristics and Symptoms

Regulatory disorder is a diagnosis of children in infancy and early childhood (National Center for Clinical Infant Programs [NCCIP], 1994). It is characterized by difficulties in regulating physiological, sensory, attentional, motor or affective processes, and maintaining a calm, alert, and emotionally positive state. Presenting problems include sleep disturbances, behavioral lethargy or hyperactivity, feeding difficulties, fearfulness of changes in routine or environment, and impaired ability to play alone or with others. The diagnosis involves distinct behavioral patterns and sensory, sensorimotor, or organizational processing difficulty. Some of the sensorimotor processing difficulties include over or under sensitivity to auditory or visual stimuli, temperature, or odors. Modulation difficulties include hypersensitivity to tactile stimulation, food textures and tastes, and under-reactivity to pain. Motoric difficulties include diminished ability to coordinate oral musculature and tolerate movement challenges due to poor muscle tone and decreased postural stability. Consequentially, deficits appear in the modulation of motor activity, the performance of fine motor skills, verbal articulation, and the use of visual spatial cues. There are qualitative difficulties in attending, relating, and interacting with people other than the primary caregiver (NCCIP, 1994).

Regulatory disorders impact arousal, attention, affect, and action in early childhood (Williamson & Anzalone, 2001). In later childhood, they may be identified as dysfunction in sensory integration (DSI) or dysfunction in sensory modulation (*DSM*) which can be further categorized as sensory sensitivity, sensory avoidance, sensory seeking (Dunn, 1997) and language, somatosensory, or vestibular-based dyspraxia.

There are four types of regulatory disorders based on predominant characteristics. They include Type I Hypersensitive, Type II Under-Reactive, Type III Motorically Disorganized, and Type IV Other.

Type I: Hypersensitive

The two distinct behavioral patterns that are typical of Type I Hypersensitive are (1) fearful and cautious or (2) negative and defiant. The fearful and cautious child is sensitive to sensory stimuli, and sensory input may have a cumulative effect. The child is easily upset, unable to sooth himself, and cannot quickly recover from frustration. Although auditory verbal processing abilities are intact, the child overreacts to touch, movement, light, and noises. The negative and defiant child is often fearful and cautious, and over-reactive to touch and sound. The child also tends to be stubborn and controlling, but not necessarily aggressive. The child has great difficulty with change or making transitions, may be compulsive and perfectionist, and may be slow to engage. Auditory processing and fine motor control may be problematic, but visual spatial orientation and postural control is usually good (NCCIP, 1994).

Type II: Under-Reactive

Children in the Type II: Under-Reactive category are typically withdrawn and difficult to engage, and self-absorbed. Characteristic behaviors of the withdrawn child include disinterest in exploring relationships or the environment, and the appearance of apathy or exhaustion. The child is often under-reactive to sound and movement, but either over- or under-reactive to touch. Visual spatial processing, motor planning, and explorative abilities may be compromised (NCCIP, 1994). The self-absorbed child may be creative and imaginative, and tend to focus on personal sensations, thoughts, and emotions rather than attend to or communicate with other people. The child may demonstrate a fantasy life with enormous imagination and creativity, and use it to avoid challenges or competition. Auditory-verbal processing and other sensory and motor capacities may be diminished.

Type III: Motorically Disorganized

The motorically disorganized child demonstrates poor control of behavior coupled with a craving for sensory input. The child may appear disorganized, fearless, aggressive, or impulsive. Motor and sensory patterns are characterized by sensory under-reactivity to touch and sound, and decreased ability to modulate movement. As a result, auditory or visual-spatial processing is disorganized and motor performance is often unfocused and diffused (NCCIP, 1994).

Type IV: Other

This category is for children who have motor and sensory processing difficulty but whose behavioral patterns are not adequately described by one of the other three types.

Target Areas for Intervention

The foci for occupational therapy intervention is the (1) normalization of the infant's response to sensory stimulation, (2) improvement in motor organization and development, and (3) establishment of positive sensory, emotional and social interactions between infant and caregiver. Some conditions such as eczema and food allergies may cause symptoms similar to regulatory disorders. It is also important to rule out maternal mental illness, as this may impact behavior and regulation. Medical causes of irritability and eating problems such as reflux and cleft pallet need to be considered separately.

Note that if an infant is medically fragile and has regulatory disorders, time and care must be taken in handling so the infant can maintain self-regulation. Regulatory disorders can interfere with mother-infant bonding and parental attachment in the infant. In many cases, the child's irritability, behavioral difficulties, and eating and sleeping disorders may impact the functioning of the entire family.

Contextual Considerations

Clinical

The child with regulatory disorders may be referred to community- or home-based early intervention programs because of developmental delay and/or behavioral problems. Failure to thrive due to feeding difficulties may necessitate referral to a medical facility, and behavioral and emotional difficulties may prompt referral to a mental health facility. The diagnosis is relatively new, and its root sensory and regulatory basis is not readily apparent. The therapist must pay special attention to the presenting symptomatology and referral complaints.

A hypersensitive child may be identified as requiring intervention due to extreme irritability, including poor eating and sleeping routines and delayed motor and/or play and social development. The child may be easily startled, upset by movement, arch and pull away when held or handled, and react strongly to sounds and noise in the environment. Eating and sleeping are frequently of concern when the infant, disliking the feeling of being held or the oral stimulation of the nipple, may suck briefly but not enough to be satiated. The resultant sensation of hunger may impede the ability to fall asleep and stay asleep for predictable periods of time.

A child who is gravitationally insecure and wary of movement may experience gastrointestinal upset when moved, and may not move from one position to the next to explore his or her environment. The aversion to movement may result in family members being concerned and cautious about physical interactions and inadvertently limiting opportunities for movement. The paucity of movement experience fosters tonal abnormalities which hamper motor development. Of equal concern is the under-reactive child who may be described as very good, sleeps a great deal, but is difficult to engage. This child may not be developing as expected because more than the usual amount of sensorimotor stimulation is required to achieve an alert state. On the other hand, the motorically disorganized child may not appear delayed until he or she is walking and is expected to explore his or her environment.

Evaluation is done primarily through parent and/or caretaker interview, observation, and handling of the child. Assessing responses to touch, movement, and other environmental stimuli is essential. Several published tests, including the *Infant/Toddler Sensory Profile* (Dunn, 2002), the *Test of Sensory Functions in Infants* (DeGangi & Greenspan, 1989), and the *Hawaii Early Learning Profile*™ (HELP; Furuno, S., O'Reilly, K., Hosaka, C.M., Zeisloft, B., & Altman, T., 1984) can assist in the examination and identification of the sensory bases of behavioral response patterns that emerge.

Family

The goodness of fit between the caretaker and the child is one of the most important factors affecting positive developmental outcomes. It is important to help family members understand and interpret the child's responses to the sensory environment and learn techniques to help foster self-regulation in the child.

Practice Setting

Since children from birth to age three are expected to have early intervention services provided to them in their natural environments, they are most frequently seen by the occupational therapist at home with their parent or caretaker. They may also be seen in daycare centers, medical settings, and mental health centers.

Sociopolitical

The Public Law 105–17, Individuals with Disabilities Education Act (IDEA, 1997), mandates that children from birth to age three are seen in their natural settings, most typically at home with parents or caretakers, or in daycare centers. Early intervention services are coordinated and provided at state and local levels through Interagency Coordinating Councils and the designated lead agency for the state. Depending on the state, this may be the Department of Education or the Department of Human Services. There are federal guidelines with which all states must comply, which emphasize interagency coordination of early identification. Additionally, intervention should be family centered, community-based in natural environments, and culturally sensitive. Some states may have additional state requirements and regulations, and may have adopted specific models for intervention. For example, New Jersey and some other states use a transdisciplinary model.

According to federal regulations, occupational therapy is considered a primary service for children from birth to age three. It may be either the only service provided, or one of several services. Other mandated services include service coordination, special instruction, speech and language therapy, physical therapy, nursing, nutrition, and family training (IDEA, 1997).

Lifestyle/Lifespan

After the age of three, children are no longer diagnosed as having regulatory disorders. Effective intervention by the parents and professionals may mitigate the disorder and the child may be developing normally by age three. If the disorder persists into early childhood and adolescence, a variety of diagnoses may be rendered by medical, psychological, or educational personnel depending on the symptoms and the age of the child. These diagnoses include autistic spectrum disorder, attention deficit hyperactivity disorder, behavior problems or social skill deficits, psychological diagnosis, and learning disabilities. These diagnoses may have underlying sensory integration or sensory processing problems, and many children respond well to occupational therapy-based on a sensory integration approach. The literature supports the notion that regulatory disorders and disrupted patterns of attachment in early childhood can contribute to mental health issues requiring psychotherapy in adulthood (DeGangi, 2000).

Dysfunction in sensory integration (DSI) and sensory modulation disorders (SMD) are not presently medical or psychological diagnoses, although awareness regarding the cause, identification, and treatment for these disorders is growing among health and educational professionals.

Clinical Decision Making Process

Defining Focus for Intervention

The chief complaint of the parent or referral source should be the focus of intervention, but insight into the child's constitutional needs, the interactive patterns between the child and the human and non-human environment, and sensory processing issues are crucial. The most effective intervention strategies are designed by the therapist to be home-based and reflective of the values, beliefs, and resources of the family. Intervention strategies for other settings such as hospital or daycare settings will be reflective of institutional programs and resources, but should always include follow-up activities that are relevant to the abilities and needs of the primary caregivers in those settings.

Establishing Goals for Intervention

The following should be kept in mind when establishing goals for intervention:

- Assess the "goodness of fit" between the child and caregiver by examining the sensory, emotional, and social interaction between caregiver and child.
- Help the family read and interpret the child's behavior in terms of sensory systems and self-regulatory ability.
- Establish whether the child is hypersensitive or under-responsive to environmental stimuli.

Designing Theory-Based Intervention

A family centered intervention based on a sensory integration frame of reference is the most appropriate for addressing regulatory disorders. Sensory integration treatment involves desensitizing sensory hypersensitivities, enhancing the sensory responsiveness of under-reactive children, facilitating a calm, alert state through self-regulation, and enhancing purposeful activity through play. The child's interest, motivation and abilities develop in a playful atmosphere that promotes self-direction and mastery. For example, activities such as swaddling and rocking that provide deep-pressure touch and graded movement are effective ways to calm a child who is hypersensitive to touch, sound, and movement. Light touch, unpredictable movement, and loud noise should be avoided. Intervention outcomes are enhanced by extending therapy goals and techniques into daily activities and family routines.

Evaluating Progress

Progress can be tracked by identifying improvements in the child's overall mood and adaptability. The child is happier, less irritable, more amenable to interaction with family, better able to sustain a calm, alert state, and more engaged in environmental exploration and play behaviors.

Determining Change in or Termination of Treatment

Changing the goals of treatment is warranted when the child appears bored or unmotivated. After self-regulation and a calm alert state is achieved, the child's goals should address developmentally appropriate motor, play, and social skills. Termination of service is appropriate either when the above goals are achieved or the environmental supports are such that they continuously foster the child's development. For example, some families intuitively and accurately interpret the child's signals and behaviors, and provide ongoing appropriate stimulation through play, self-care, and eating and sleeping routines. Family outings become possible as regulation is achieved, thereby providing additional opportunities for integration of new skills at playgrounds, in playgroups, and with other children.

Case Study

Description

Bria was referred at one month of age to the early intervention system because of delayed development. She was discharged to home weighing 3.8 pounds, in the 3rd percentile of weight for her age. She was hearing impaired and was irritable most of the time. Any movement or touch exacerbated her irritability. Bria would fuss unless she was held against her mother's chest, neck, or stomach. Bria ate small amounts of formula at a time along with medication for reflux. Bathing was extremely difficult because Bria was very stressed by getting undressed to get in and out of the bath. However, once she was in the bath, it was one of the few times that she seemed to relax.

Long- and Short-Term Goals

The long-term goal of intervention for Bria is to enable her to increase food intake and gain weight.

The short-term goal of intervention for Bria is to help her achieve a calm alert state and foster stress free parent/infant interaction.

Therapist Goals and Strategies

The therapist's goals include:

1. Reduce Bria's negative response to touch and movement.
2. Promote self-regulation.
3. Reduce family stress resulting from care of Bria.

The therapist's strategies include:

1. Teach parent to read and respond appropriately and effectively to Bria's behavioral signals.
2. Encourage deep pressure touch, skin to skin contact, and gentle up and down movement to reduce negative response to the sensory environment.
3. Limit stimulation to one modality at a time to reduce sensory overload.

Activity

Encourage holding by the mother, swaddling to reduce hypersensitivity to touch, and gentle up and down movements that Bria can tolerate. Place Bria under a warm baby blanket before dressing and undressing. To reduce agitation, perform an infant massage with warm baby oil under a warm baby blanket.

Treatment Objectives

1. Bria will become increasingly tolerant of touch and movement.
2. Bria will be able to tolerate position changes.

Resources

The following resources can be helpful for gathering clinical data:

- History: developmental, medical, behavioral, and state regulation
- Observation of child's behavior in response to environmental stimuli and handling (i.e., over- or under-responsiveness to environmental stimuli)
- *Infant/Toddler Sensory Profile*
- *Test of Sensory Functions in Infants*
- Hawaii Early Learning Profile Assessment and Activity Guide (HELP strands)

The following resources can be helpful for gathering family data:

- Interaction with caregivers (selective and restrictive)
- Parental reports regarding eating, sleeping, and play patterns and ability to adjust to transitions which affects the entire family

The following are common practice settings:

- Home environment
- Daycare center
- Hospital
- Behavioral clinic

The following resource can be helpful for gathering sociopolitical data:

- PL 99–457 OT, (birth to age three) that is family centered, culturally sensitive, and community-based

The following can be helpful in understanding and managing lifestyle/lifespan issues:

- Inability to self-regulate may result in a variety of diagnosis in later childhood, such as persistent anxiety and social skill deficits

References

DeGangi, G. (2000). *Pediatric disorders of regulation in affect and behavior.* New York: Academic Press.

DeGangi, G. A., & Greenspan, S. I. (1989). *Test of sensory functions in infants.* Los Angeles: Western Psychological Services.

Dunn, W. (2002). *Infant/toddler sensory profile manual.* San Antonio, TX: The Psychological Corporation.

Furunos, O'Reilly, K., Hosaka, C.M., Zeisloft, B, & Altman, T. (1984).) *Hawaii early learning profile.* Palo Alto, CA: VORT.

National Center for Clinical Infant Programs. (1994). *Diagnostic classification 0–3: Diagnostic classification of mental health and developmental disorders of infancy and early childhood.* Arlington, VA: Zero to Three.

Williamson, G. G., & Anzalone, M. E. (2001). *Sensory integration and self regulation in infants and toddlers: Helping very young children interact with their environment.* Arlington, VA: Zero to Three.

Pervasive Developmental Disorders 4

Beth Pfeiffer, Ph.D., OTR/L

Synopsis of Clinical Condition

According to the fourth edition of the *Diagnostic and Statistical Manual of Mental Disorders* (*DSM–IV*), pervasive developmental disorders include autism, pervasive developmental disorder—not otherwise specified (PDD–NOS), Asperger's disorder, Rett's disorder, and childhood disintegrative disorder (American Psychiatric Association [APA], 1994). These disorders have similar diagnostic criteria, but certain characteristics vary and symptoms range from mild to severe. The varying degrees of symptoms have led to the use of the term autistic spectrum disorder (ASD). This chapter will focus on the three most common ASD conditions: autistic disorder, PDD–NOS, and Asperger's disorder. These three have commonalities in their diagnostic criteria and share many clinical features and interventions.

Prevalence and Etiology

The rate of ASD has been growing in recent years. The Centers for Disease Control (2003) recently estimated that autism affects 2 to 6 per 1,000 individuals. It is estimated that the rate of autism is growing 10% to 17% per year, making it a common developmental childhood condition. An earlier study identified the prevalence of all autism spectrum disorders at a rate of at least 22 per 10,000 (Bryson, 1996). Autism spectrum disorder is three to four times more common in boys than in girls.

Co-morbidity is the co-occurrence of conditions that may or may not be causally related (Ghaziuddin, 2002). Individuals with ASD commonly develop co-morbid conditions throughout the course of a lifetime. The most common of these include attention deficit hyperactivity disorder, obsessive compulsive disorder, anxiety and mood disorders, tic disorders, seizure disorders, and sleep disorders (Tsai, 2000).

There is no known single cause for ASD, although there are well-documented associations with abnormalities in brain structure or function. Many studies identify neuropathologies in both the temporal lobe and limbic system (Bauman & Kemper, 1985; Bauman & Kemper, 1994). These two systems work together to mediate social-emotional functioning, a primary area of concern for individuals with pervasive developmental disorders. Specifically, abnormalities were found in the size and density of tissue in the temporal lobe and limbic system. The limbic system includes the structures of the amygdala and hippocampus (Lundy-Ekman, 1998), both located within the temporal region. Abnormalities in the amygdala are of particular interest and importance in individuals with ASD. It is strongly believed that the amygdala "plays a critical role in emotional arousal, assigning behavioral significance to environmental stimuli, and attaching emotional relevance to stimuli" (Schultz, Romanski, & Tsatsanis, 2000, p. 187). Social and emotional problems and abnormal responses to environmental stimuli are all characteristics of ASD.

The cortical and subcortical frontal lobe region is also associated with ASD. Two studies have identified decreased frontal lobe perfusion in individuals with autistic disorder (George, Costa, Houris, Rang, & Ell, 1992; Zilbovicus et al., 1995). One section of the frontal lobe, the orbital-medial pre-frontal cortex (PFC) has a key role in social and emotional functions. This section is interconnected with limbic areas, such as the amygdala. It is speculated that a faulty connection between the amygdala and the orbital-medial pre-frontal cortex could contribute to the inappropriate emotional and social behavior associated with ASD (Schultz et al., 2000).

It has been theorized that ASD etiologies are genetic and environmental. Research has indicated that ASD aggregates in families. There is an extremely high rate of concordance of ASD in identical versus fraternal twins, and a higher rate of siblings with the condition (Miller-Kuhaneck & Glennon, 2001). Chromosomal studies have identified further support for genetic links. Chromosomal alterations are present in a fairly large number of individuals with ASD, although the alterations are not consistent.

There are varying speculations about the environmental etiology of ASD and further research is warranted. Some believe that pre-natal exposure to toxins is the cause of abnormal brain development in children with ASD. In particular, toxins such as pesticides and polychlorinated biphenyls (PCBS) have been identified. Others have speculated relationships with vaccinations and autoimmune disorders and ASD. Symptoms of autism and PDD–NOS often present around ages two to three, with a regression in skills. Researchers have explored the possibility that an abnormal immune system response to vaccinations, or the possible exposure to mercury in vaccinations, leads to the regression (Miller-Kuhaneck & Glennon, 2001).

Autoimmune disorders are more common in family members of children who have ASD (Comi, Zimmerman, Frye, Law, & Peedan, 1999). There also are documented autoimmune abnormalities in certain individuals with ASD (Miller-Kuhaneck & Glennon, 2001). Much of the research in these areas is inconclusive, and therefore the etiologies of ASD continue to be speculative in nature.

Common Characteristics and Symptoms

In order for a child to be diagnosed with autistic disorder, he or she must present with delays in social interactions, social communications, or symbolic or pretend play prior to three years of age. The child must meet a total of six or more items from three main areas in the *DSM–IV,* with at least two from Category 1 and one each from Category 2 and 3 (APA, 1994). The three main areas include a qualitative impairment in social interactions; a qualitative impairment in communication; and restricted, repetitive or stereotyped patterns of behavior, interests, and activities.

Qualitative impairments in social interactions include impairments in the use of nonverbal behaviors, limitations in peer relationships, a lack of social or emotional reciprocity, and a lack of spontaneous initiative to share enjoyment, interests, or achievements with others.

Qualitative impairment in communication includes a delay or lack of development of spoken language, impairment in the ability to initiate or sustain conversations with others (for those that do speak), stereotyped and repetitive use of language, and limitations in pretend or social imitative play for their age.

Restricted, repetitive, or stereotyped patterns of behavior, etc., include a preoccupation in a restricted interest of abnormal intensity and focus, inflexibility in certain rituals or routines, motor patterns that are stereotypical or repetitive, and a preoccupation with parts of objects.

In order for a child to meet the criteria for PDD–NOS, certain criteria for autistic disorder are met, but not the full criteria (APA, 1994). These children have features of autistic disorder that are not due to other disorders. Asperger's disorder also has many features of high-functioning autistic disorder, but such children differ in cognitive and language functions. An individual with Asperger's disorder has average to above average cognitive abilities, and often develops expressive language within normal developmental ranges (Attwood, 1998). Social interactions and functioning are significantly impaired in all three disorders. There is ongoing controversy in diagnosing ASD due to the overlap and the high rate of co-morbidity with other childhood conditions.

A child with an ASD may or may not have verbal language delays, but non-verbal language delays are almost always present (Attwood, 1998). Individuals with autistic disorder or PDD–NOS frequently experience delays in expressive language development, although this characteristic is absent in Asperger's disorder. Social development does occur but is often qualitatively different. Deficits in communication contribute to delays in social development. Eye contact and responsiveness to another person may be decreased, as well as an understanding of the pragmatics (i.e., the practical ability to use language in social situations). Children with ASD have a decreased interest in interacting with others and prefer isolated activities. They often have limited range of representational play activities and often have restricted interests (Miller-Kuhaneck & Glennon, 2001). For example, they may be resistant to change and insist on certain routines and rituals. They may also engage in stereotypical or self-stimulatory behaviors.

It has been estimated that 75% of individuals with autism demonstrate some level of mental retardation (Huebner & Dunn, 2001). This often differentiates autism and Asperger's disorder, as there are no cognitive deficits associated with Asperger's disorder.

Although not yet part of the diagnostic criteria for ASD according to the *DSM–IV*, sensory processing and integration issues are identified as common (Mayes & Calhoun, 1999; Ornitz, 1974). Kientz and Dunn (1997) compared sensory processing in children with autism to children without autism, and identified significant differences in their patterns of processing sensory information. The children with autism demonstrated significant tactile sensitivity compared with the control group. Other researchers have also supported these findings. In one study, as many as 70% of children diagnosed with pervasive developmental disorders demonstrated disturbances in sensory modulation (Ornitz, 1974). Another study showed that 100% of children diagnosed with pervasive developmental disorders demonstrated somatosensory (tactile, vestibular, and proprioceptive) disturbances, and 50% demonstrated hyper- or hyposensitivity to sensory input (Mayes & Calhoun, 1999).

Motor problems vary in individuals with ASD. Clumsiness and incoordination are identified as common characteristics in individuals with Asperger's disorder (Volkmar et al., 1994) and issues in motor planning can be found across the autistic spectrum. It is important to note that characteristics and degree of symptoms can vary significantly among individuals.

Target Areas for Intervention

The role of an occupational therapist working with an individual with ASD varies depending on contextual factors such as age, intervention setting, and the primary reason for referral. Pervasive developmental disorders suggest multiple areas of focus. It is likely that over the course of a person's lifetime, an occupational therapist may focus interventions on almost all areas of occupation, including activities of daily living, instrumental activities of daily living, education, work, play, leisure, and social participation. For the person with ASD, treatment interventions may focus on sensory processing and integration, sensorimotor function, and social-emotional development.

One of the most widely used interventions by occupational therapists in the treatment of ASD is sensory integration (Watling, Deitz, Kanny and McLaughlin, 1999). Used in combination with other interventions, including behavioral and developmental approaches, a primary focus is frequently on the modulation of sensory input, as many individuals with ASD tend to under- or over-respond to sensory input, or demonstrate a mixed reactivity. This, in turn, affects behavior, communication, and functional skills. Other areas of specific occupational therapy interventions include improving the motor planning necessary for play and daily living activities, as well as interventions focused on promoting social skills.

Contextual Considerations

Clinical

Autistic spectrum disorders are pervasive developmental disorders that frequently affect many areas of functioning. An evaluation must address the primary concerns of the referral source and the family, and could include many domains of occupational therapy practice. A top-down evaluation process promotes occupationally-based interventions. Using this approach, evaluation must initially collect information on the occupational profile of the individual through interviews and observations (Fisher, 1998). Along with identifying relevant and meaningful occupations, this involves collecting information about the individual or family's concerns, problems, and priorities. Observing the individual engaging in targeted occupations is important to identify the discrepancies between the demands of the task and the skills of the individual. After identifying the primary problems and priorities, the next stage involves using assessment tools that focus more specifically on areas of occupation, performance skills, and client factors. Pervasive developmental disorders affect many areas of function and there are a variety of assessment tools that are appropriate for individuals with ASD. Since many individuals are not able to complete standardized assessments, caregiver interviews or questionnaires and clinical observation are sometimes the most appropriate assessment measures for people with ASD. A number of individuals with ASD can complete more formalized assessment procedures and therefore both kinds are discussed.

Adaptive behavior measures provide a method for evaluating many areas of occupational function. Frequently, the general areas of social, self-help, motor, and communication skills are assessed.

The *Vineland Adaptive Behavior Scales* (Sparrow, Balla, & Cicchetti, 1984) specifically measure the areas of communication, daily living skills, socialization, motor skills, and maladaptive behaviors. It is appropriate for use with individuals from birth to 18 years 11 months, and for low-functioning adults. There are norms based on all of these age groups. The scales are completed through an interview with the parent or caregiver.

The *Adaptive Behavior Assessment System* (ABAS; Harrison & Oakland, 2000) assesses the areas of communication, community use, functional academics, school living, health and safety, leisure, self-care, self-direction, social skills, and work through the completion of a rating form. There are parent, teacher, and adult versions of the ABAS. Caregivers or the adults themselves can complete the adult rating scale. It is a norm-referenced test for individuals from school age through adulthood. Adaptive behaviors are highly correlated with cognitive deficits although these scales also provide important information regarding the function of individuals with ASD that do not have cognitive deficits.

There are general developmental scales such as the *Hawaii Early Learning Profile*™ (*HELP;* Furuno, O'Reilly, Hosaka, Zeisloft, & Allman, 1984) and the *Early Learning Accomplishment Profile* (ELAP; Glover, Preminger, & Sanford, 1988) that are helpful in assessing overall development in young children from birth to five years of age. Often these types of general developmental scales are used to determine eligibility in for early intervention services.

There are documented differences in play in children with ASD. Restricted representation play is a common characteristic of ASD. As play is the main occupation of preschool children, the *Revised Knox Preschool Play Scale* (Knox, 1997) provides an observational measure assessing the space and material management, pretense/symbolic aspects of play, and participation in play. This is a tool that has a history of use with preschool children diagnosed with ASD.

If a child is referred for a school-based assessment, the *School Function Assessment* (SFA; Coster, Deeney, Haltiwanger & Haley, 1998) can guide in intervention planning for those children with ASD who are in elementary school. The SFA has three main parts assessing participation in school related settings, the task supports needed for participation, and activity performance. Activity performance has 21 separate scales measuring a variety of functions necessary for optimal school performance. Some of these include functional communication, written work, clothing management, school travel, and behavioral regulation—to name only a few. This is a questionnaire that can be completed in sections, or by one individual who is familiar with the child, or by a team of professionals. Social and emotional measures are particularly relevant to the ASD population due to the nature of the condition.

The *Function Emotional Assessment Scale* (FEAS; Greenspan, DeGangi, & Weider, 1996) is an observation assessment looking at the infant's or young child's emotional and social functioning with parents or caregivers. It also provides information on the related motor, sensory, language, and cognitive capabilities.

The *Social Skills Rating Scale* (SSRS; Gresham & Elliott, 1990) assesses more specifically the social skills of a child or adolescent, and is standardized for kindergarten through twelve grades. There are teacher, child, and parent versions of the SSRS.

Dysfunction in sensory processing and integration is prevalent in individuals with ASD. Some of the most helpful tools in providing insight into sensory processing in relationship to everyday functioning and behavior are the *Infant/Toddler Sensory Profile* (Dunn, 2002), *Sensory Profile* (Dunn, 1999), and *Adolescent/Adult Sensory Profile* (Brown & Dunn, 2002). The three profiles cover the ages from birth to adulthood. The caregiver or parent completes standardized questionnaires, with the exception of the *Adolescent/Adult Sensory Profile.* The individual completes this unless he or she is unable to do so, in which case a caregiver can do so.

The *Test of Sensory Function in Infants* (TSFI; DeGangi & Greenspan, 1981), the *DeGangi-Berk Test of Sensory Integration* (TSI; Berk & DeGangi, 1983), and the *Sensory Integration and Praxis Tests* (SIPT; Ayres, 1998) are all standardized tests assessing sensory integration. These require the child to participate in more formal testing procedures. The TSFI is a criterion-referenced rating scale intended to be a screening tool for sensory integration dysfunction in infants between 4 and 18 months of age. The TSI is a norm-referenced test designed to assess sensory integration dysfunction in preschoolers. The SIPT is a battery of 17 tests specifically assessing sensory integration and praxis for children between the ages of 4 years to 8 years 11 months. Administration and interpretation requires specialized training and certification.

The *Peabody Motor Scales, Second Edition* (Folio & Fewell, 2000) and *Bruininks-Oseretsky Test of Motor Proficiency* (Bruininks, 1978) are helpful tools to assess overall motor function. The *Quick Neurological Screening Test, Second Edition* (Mutti, Sterling, & Spalding, 1978) assesses certain motor and perceptual functions related to neurological integration.

The *Developmental Test of Visual Perception, Second Edition* (Hammill, Pearson, & Voress, 1998) and the *Beery Developmental Test of Visual Motor Integration* (Beery, 1997) may also help determine underlying performance deficits in the areas of visual motor and perceptual skills. Finally, clinical observations are an essential part of the evaluation process.

Family

Intervention strategies for the child need to be supplemented with ongoing family education. Parents, siblings, and other caregivers require information regarding the nature of the child's conditions, the ramifications of the condition on functional behavior, the scope and purpose of occupational therapy, and other components of the intervention program. They also require guidance regarding additional supportive services and resources that are available in the local community (Galvin, 2001). This could include referrals for other services, including speech and language therapy, physical therapy, psychologists, developmental pediatricians, nutritionists, and neurologists. ASD support groups frequently meet in community settings and serve as both a support system and a place for families to acquire knowledge.

Collaboration with a multidisciplinary team that includes families is essential for the most effective interventions. Recent law and policies promote the involvement of the parents in the intervention process. For example, laws guiding early intervention services mandate family-focused interventions. Due in part to these laws, parents are becoming more educated in the service delivery systems and often serve as advocates for their children. Providing resources and education allows parents to be more successful advocates. With education, families can also implement important interventions in the context of the home and other community settings. For example, a child with a sensory processing dysfunction often benefits from a sensory diet implemented into daily routines. Education is essential in helping the family successfully integrate and modify these interventions.

As mentioned previously, many children with ASD are unable to attend or participate fully in formalized assessment procedures, and therefore families serve as important informants for their children. Inclusion of the family in all evaluation procedures encourages an understanding of the family's priorities, culture, and dynamics, plus the development of viable and relevant intervention plans.

Practice Settings

Individuals with ASD can receive occupational therapy services in a variety of settings, including early intervention services in the home or community, school-based services, outpatient rehabilitation or private practice facilities, and community living centers or adult day programs. They may receive services in more than one setting at a time.

Early intervention services are for children primarily between the ages of birth through five. Children who qualify for occupational therapy from birth to age three typically receive these services in their homes or other community settings such as daycare centers. The occupational therapist's role is to provide family-focused intervention, which often involves family education. Occupational therapy is considered a primary service for the birth to three population, and is most commonly provided directly and individually. In many states, intervention funding switches to the school system when a child turns three. Typically a child will enter into a preschool program. The family continues to be an important component of the service delivery process, which focuses on the development of school readiness skills and the facilitation of school participation. Direct services can be individual or within a group setting. Consultation may also be provided to the classroom teacher or other professional working with the child. Typically, a developmental model focused on sensorimotor development, play skills, social and emotional development, and self-help skills guides the treatment of children with ASD.

School-based occupational therapy (OT) is one of the largest practice areas in the profession. Many children and adolescents with ASD will receive OT services in the school system in order to support successful performance and participation. Services can be provided in varying forms, including consultation, monitoring, and direct intervention, both in groups or individually. The occupational therapist, in consultation with other professionals such as teachers, physical therapists and speech therapists, may provide suggestions on how to improve a child's writing, attention span, and/or social skills.

Children and adults with ASD can receive private therapy through outpatient pediatric rehabilitation facilities or private practice therapy clinics. Certain clinics may specialize in an area of practice, such as providing sensory integration therapy specifically for individuals with ASD. Adults with ASD sometimes receive services within community living centers or adult day programs. These services often focus on helping the individual develop the ability to modulate and regulate sensory input, in order to improve attention and decrease secondary behaviors, and engage successfully in self-maintenance and vocational training.

Sociopolitical

Legislation significantly influences intervention funding for children with ASD. The Individuals with Disabilities Education Act (IDEA) is probably the most influential legislation regarding the provision of services for children and adolescents with ASD (Stephens & Tauber, 2001). Part C of IDEA defines services for children between the ages of birth to 2 years 11 months. Part B defines services for children and adolescents in special education from 3 to 21 years of age. Part B of IDEA stipulates that a child must fall under one of the categories of disability identified in IDEA. Autism is included as a category of disability.

The legislation further identifies services as either primary or related. A service that is considered primary may be provided in the absence of other services. Occupational therapy is a primary service under Part C of IDEA, but it is a related service under Part B. In the latter case, the child must be receiving special education with an Individual

Education Plan in order to be eligible for occupational therapy. Funding is provided from both federal and state governments in order to implement programs under IDEA.

Other legislation influencing the provision of services for individuals with ASD include the Rehabilitation Act of 1973 and the Americans with Disabilities Act of 1990. The Rehabilitation Act identifies that reasonable accommodations must be made in schools so that the needs of individuals with disabilities can be meet as adequately as those without disabilities (Case-Smith, 1996). Children with ASD who do not qualify for services under IDEA can sometimes qualify for occupational therapy services under the Rehabilitation Act. Under this law, a child does not need to receive special education services in order to qualify for occupational therapy.

Funding for outpatient rehabilitation or private practice settings often comes from family resources or medical insurance. Certain medical insurance providers identify ASD as a developmental disorder and therefore will not cover occupational therapy interventions for it. Although this is not the case for all medical insurance, education continues to be necessary when working with insurance providers concerning the roles and scope of occupational therapy.

Lifestyle/Lifespan

ASD is considered a lifelong condition, but intensive services provided in childhood and adolescence appear to have resulted in a large population of individuals with ASD integrating into their communities and living productive and functional lives (Howlin, 2000). Occupational therapists are often involved in the development of programs that assist the transition of a child with ASD from early intervention to school and finally to the world of work. Transitions can be particularly challenging for both the child and the family, and consistent professional support and ongoing education is paramount. As the child progresses from early intervention settings to adulthood, the focus of service and intervention changes from the home or community environment into a school and community-based environment. It also often changes from direct and individual treatment to primarily indirect or group treatment.

The role of the occupational therapist is to prepare and educate the family and the child and to promote those skills necessary for optimal performance, and make the transition into each setting. For instance, parental separation issues may emerge as the child moves from early intervention to preschool, while the move to elementary school requires a transition from a part-time to a full-time program. Another major school transition is into the junior high or high school environment, where the student nay be expected to function more independently and often with less structure. Preparations for transitions from the school setting to adult life in the community start as early as elementary school in terms of preparation for future adult roles. For example, a focus on independent daily living activities provides an individual with ASD a foundation for participation in future adult roles. Encouraging families to have children participate in household chores and other responsibilities are important for future transitions (Miller-Kuhaneck & Glennon, 2001).

By law, formal post school transition planning starts at age 14. IDEA requires that each student's Individual Education Plan include annual statements addressing transition services. These often include goals focused specifically on life after high school and services required to assist in the transitional process. The student is involved in setting goals and identifying priorities along with professionals and the family. Community involvement, social skills, behavioral concerns, and vocational skills are often the primary focus of occupational therapy in the high school years. Occupational therapy interventions may continue into adulthood, addressing similar issues in order to further promote independence.

Along with transition planning, it is important to understand family dynamics and supports across the life span of the individual. The sibling of a child with ASD can face certain challenges. Families may have difficulty managing the balance of care between the child with ASD and siblings. In certain communities, support groups are available for siblings of children with disabilities, or more specifically of children with ASD. Obtaining necessary services and resources for a child with ASD can pose financial stress on the family.

Interventions often involve complementary approaches. Along with occupational therapy, individuals with ASD may benefit from speech and language therapy, physical therapy, special education, psychological services, behavioral interventions, and dietary interventions. A list of alternative and complementary approaches (Lerner, 2001) is identified in Table 4.1. Some of these approaches are considered controversial due to limited research, while others have solid effectiveness research.

Table 4.1
Common and Alternative Treatment Interventions for Individuals With Autistic Spectrum Disorders

Intervention	Types or Methods
Structural Therapy	Osteopathy
	Cranial-Sacral Therapy
	Chiropractic
Treatments to Boost Immune System	Dietary Modifications
	Feingold Diet
	Gluten and Casein Free Diet
	Yeast Decreasing Diets
	Nutritional Supplements
	Vitamins and Minerals
	Amino Acids
	Essential Fatty Acids
	Probiotics and Antifungals
	Immunotherapy
	IVIG—Intravenous immune globulin therapy—often used when children have high titers believed to be related to vaccines
	Secretin
Treatments Addressing Sensory Processing	Sensory Integration
	Vision Therapy
	Auditory Integration Training
Facilitated Communication	A facilitator provides physical support to the hand, arm, or wrist while the child or adolescent points to a picture or letter or types

(*Continued*)

Table 4.1 (*Continued*)

Intervention	Types or Methods
Medication	Psycho-stimulants Antidepressants Hypertensives Anticonvulsants Antipsychotics
Applied Behavioral Analysis/ Discrete Trial Training	Repetitive teaching trials based on providing a stimulus and reinforcing the response; structured curriculum of skilled-based tasks
Floortime/Development, Individual and Relationship-Based Intervention	Focused on affective and relationship-based interventions to address social, communication, cognitive, play, sensory, and motor planning issues
Miller Method	Teaches communication and cognition while focusing on physical organization
Treatment of Education of Autistic and Related Communication Handicapped Children (TEACHH)	Structured teaching approach focused on providing environmental modifications, concrete visual presentation of information, and use of routine to teach skills

Clinical Decision Making Process

Defining Focus for Intervention

The focus for home-based treatment may include promoting optimal interactions with family members, modulating responses to sensory stimulation, and fostering developmentally appropriate skills. For example, treatment interventions may focus on feeding and eating issues related to oral hypersensitivity or decreasing self-stimulatory behaviors interfering with play and interactions. In the school environment, treatment interventions might focus on the development of social skills for peer interaction and sensorimotor skills for computer usage, handwriting, and physical education.

In adolescence and adulthood, treatment interventions often focus on promoting independence in activities of daily living, vocational skills, and the social skills necessary to live in the community.

In general, treatment interventions can vary greatly and must be determined by individual needs, the family priorities, and cultural beliefs. As pervasive developmental disorders occur on a spectrum, children can vary greatly in their individual needs.

Establishing Goals for Intervention

Goals are established based on the results of the evaluation and reason for referral. It is also important to consider the priorities of the individual and the family. Including the individual and family in the goal writing process can promote successful outcomes. The service delivery model has a significant impact on the goal writing process. Goals for a child receiving services through early intervention are developed by the family or caregivers during the Individual Family Service Plan meeting. The parents or caregivers identify the goals toward which they would like to see their child work, and these are documented in the exact language presented. The role of the occupational therapist in this process is to educate the family in goal development and identify strategies and objectives that support the goals identified by the family.

In contrast, goals established in the school setting are developed by the occupational therapist with input from the family and educational professionals. These goals need to be measurable and relate to school performance.

ASD can affect many areas of functioning, including social skills, communication, motor skills, cognition, sensory processing, and activities of daily living. These may all be areas of concern identified during the evaluation process, but the goal writing process needs to focus on the most significant areas of concern and goals may have to be prioritized. Sociopolitical factors such as funding sources also impact the goal writing process. For example, insurance companies may require that goals be written in a specific format and that they only address those areas relevant to medical intervention, such as activities of daily living or motor skills. However, all goals should be functional and promote participation in occupation and roles of the individual.

Designing Theory-Based Intervention

In general, multiple theoretical frameworks are used to guide intervention planning. The developmental theory is particularly applicable to this population. It is based on the premise that individuals develop certain life skills in both a parallel and sequential fashion that promotes adaptive functioning (Shortridge & Walker, 1993). For example, children simultaneously develop motor and cognitive skills, but learn to sit before they learn to walk. ASD can delay the development of skills in many areas, including psychosocial, cognitive, language, motor, sensory processing, and daily living skills. Using developmental theory to inform treatment, an occupational therapist might structure situations that require parallel play, and progress to more active interaction with peers.

Sensory integration theory is also widely used to design interventions for the ASD population. It is well documented that individuals with ASD are more likely to experience dysfunctions in sensory integration and modulation (Kientz & Dunn, 1997; Mayes & Calhoun, 1999; Ornitz, 1974). This theory is based on the assumption that meaningful registration of sensory input must occur for an individual to make an adaptive response. Another assumption is that the brain has plasticity, and therefore intervention can change the way the brain responds to sensory input. Dysfunction in sensory integration and modulation is manifested in hypersensitivity to touch and/or sound, avoidance behaviors, sensory-seeking activities such as self-stimulation or self-injurious behaviors, attention disorders, and an inability to make effective adaptive responses. Modulation of sensory responses through structured sensory motor experiences is often the focus of intervention.

The acquisitional frame of reference is used to teach functional skills. It assumes that the learning of functional skills is based on reinforcement (Royeen & Duncan, 1999). Another assumption is that learning a skill results in the belief that one has competence and can influence the environment. This approach is often used in skill-based learning programs, and in programs to modify behavior. Applied behavioral analysis (ABA) and discrete trial training (DTT) are popular approaches with this population.

The psychosocial frame of reference has its theoretical base in developmental theories related to temperament, attachment, social skills, play, and coping abilities (Olson, 1999). It focuses on peer and family interactions. By addressing and understanding those areas (such as temperamental qualities, attachment relationships, interactional patterns, and play skills) intervention focuses on promoting optimal interactions between peers and family members. This is particularly relevant to the ASD population, as communication and social abilities are frequently areas of concern.

Evaluating Progress

Observations and interviews are very important aspects of identifying progress in the ASD population. In some instances, progress may occur that cannot be measured by more formal assessment procedures but only observed or identified by caregivers. For example, after treating an individual with ASD for sensory modulation dysfunction, there may be changes in flexibility and less of a need for control. Such changes involve the overall quality of life, and are not typically addressed in formal assessment procedures.

Evaluation of progress is ongoing, and based on established goals and the treatment plan. In most practice settings, anecdotal records are kept along with more formal documentation methods. For example, three-, six-, and nine-month progress notes are often required, as well as formal annual reviews, for the early intervention population. The service delivery model (along with funding sources) determines the specific guidelines for documenting progress.

Determining Change in or Termination of Treatment

Change in treatment is warranted if the primary concerns for the individual have deviated, if there is minimal progress towards goals, or if goals have been achieved. For example, a transition to a community living arrangement may signal the achievement of goals for self-care independence, but may also signal the need for new goals such as the use of public transportation.

Termination of treatment occurs when the individual has met his or her goals, or there has been a plateau of progress over time. It is also important to identify when there is a plateau in progress and re-evaluate whether a continuation of occupational therapy services are warranted. At this point, a referral to other professionals for alternate interventions may be appropriate. Once again, both the service delivery model and funding sources help to determine termination or changes. For example, a family may need to discontinue services after 30 treatment sessions if that is all that is covered by the insurance company, and there are financial constraints.

Case Study

Description

Jonathan is a four-year-old boy who is diagnosed with PPD–NOS. He lives with his mother, an older sister, and a younger brother. Jonathan currently attends a special education program five days a week for half-days where he receives one hour of speech therapy a week in the classroom setting. He received occupational therapy in his home at the age of two through an early intervention program, but no longer qualified when he turned three and transitioned into a preschool setting. Jonathan's teacher is concerned with Jonathan's unusual responses to sensory activities, and his delayed play and motor skills, and recently referred him for an occupational therapy evaluation. She reported that he also has a difficult time attending to sit-down group activities. Jonathan was evaluated through clinical and classroom observations and interviews with his mother and classroom teacher. He also completed the *Peabody Motor Developmental Scales.*

Jonathan does not like to be touched by other people, and will often pull away when someone attempts to touch him. He prefers to play by himself away from the other children during free-play time, and engages in limited reciprocal play. Jonathan frequently cries during messy play times and insists on washing his hands immediately. During snack time, he will only eat crunchy or chewy foods and avoids all soft-textured foods or those with varying consistencies. Jonathan's mother reported that he has a very limited food repertoire at home, and is extremely fussy during grooming tasks such as brushing his teeth and hair. He refuses to have his hair cut by anyone other than his mother. Jonathan is easily distracted by sensory stimuli in the environment, and often is unable to attend for more than a few minutes during group activities due to sensory distractions. Sensory defensiveness appears to be influencing Jonathan's ability to participate fully in his classroom setting.

Along with this, motor planning difficulties appear to further impact Jonathan's play skills. He engages in very little symbolic play with other children and tends to use the same play schemes with most of his toys. Jonathan will imitate a simple symbolic play scheme when one is introduced by an adult, but he does not come up with these schemes on his own. He prefers to stack or line up objects. Motor planning deficits also impact Jonathan's overall motor skills. On the *Peabody Developmental Motor Scales,* Jonathan performed fine motor skills in the 25th percentile and gross motor skills in the 30th percentile for his age range.

Long- and Short-Term Goals

The long-term goal of intervention for Jonathan is to help him participate in circle time activities for a period of twenty minutes.

The short-term goals of intervention for Jonathan are:

1. Attend to group activities in the classroom setting 80% of the time.
2. Initiate and participate in reciprocal play activities with other children in the classroom during 70% of the freeplay time.
3. Expand play skills in order to sequence five or more ideas during symbolic play.
4. Eat and enjoy a variety of foods with varying textures during snack time 80% of the time.

Therapist Goals and Strategies

The therapist's goals include:

1. Decrease Jonathan's sensory defensiveness.
2. Increase Jonathan's body awareness for motor planning.
3. Educate the family and professionals on techniques to expand play skills.

The therapist's strategies include:

1. Engage in activities which provide calming and inhibitory sensory input, including deep pressure, proprioception, and slow linear vestibular sensory input to decrease hypersensitivity.
2. Provide home instruction and classroom in-service on floortime techniques to foster reciprocal and symbolic play skills.
3. Engage in activities that provide proprioceptive and vestibular feedback to increase body awareness necessary for motor planning.
4. Provide consultation on classroom modifications in order to decrease extraneous sensory stimuli.
5. Provide opportunities for play time initially with one other child in a safe and structured format and then in less structured play settings.
6. Model appropriate play schemes.
7. Implement an oral sensory stimulation program.

Activity

Jonathan will choose activities to complete in an obstacle course. The choices will include equipment that provides deep-pressure tactile, proprioceptive, or inhibitory vestibular sensory input. He will then help set up the course, in order to expand motor planning schemes and participate in the obstacle course on his own. Eventually, he will be asked to choose a doll or toy to maneuver through the course with him to expand pretend and symbolic play schemes with objects such as a doll, stuffed animal, or toy car/truck. He will also choose one other child to participate in the obstacle course with him and then expand this to a group of children. Suggestions will be made to parents and teachers on games that can be carried out at home and school as well as toys that foster symbolic and reciprocal play.

Treatment Objectives

1. Jonathan will complete a sequence of four new motor schemes with minimal assistance as needed.
2. Jonathan will participate in symbolic play requiring the sequence of at least two new play schemes.
3. Jonathan will interact with at least one other child to successfully guide that child through the obstacle course he developed.

Resources

The following resources can be helpful for gathering clinical data:

- Clinical and contextual observations
- Interviews with caregivers and professionals working with individual
- Adaptive/functional/developmental measures

    - *Vineland Adaptive Behavioral Scales*
    - *Adaptive Behavior Assessment System* (ABAS)
    - *Hawaii Early Learning Accomplishment Profile* (HELP)
    - *Early Learning Accomplishment Profile* (ELAP)
    - *School Function Assessment* (SFA)
- Play and social/emotional measures
    - *Functional Emotional Assessment Scale* (FEAS)
    - *Social Skills Rating System* (SSRS)
- Sensory processing and integration measures
    - *Infant/Toddler Sensory Profile*
    - *Sensory Profile*
    - *Adolescent/Adult Sensory Profile*
    - *Test of Sensory Function in Infants* (TSFI)
    - *DeGangi-Berk Test of Sensory Integration* (TSI)
    - *Sensory Integration and Praxis Tests* (SIPT)
- Motor and neurological measures
    - *Peabody Motor Scales–2*
    - *Bruininks-Oseretsky Test of Motor Proficiency*
    - *Quick Neurological Screening Test–2*
    - *Developmental Test of Visual Perception–2*
    - *Test of Visual Motor Integration*

The following resources can be helpful for gathering family data:

- Education and support systems
- Family history
- Advocacy groups

The following are common practice settings:

- Family interview for evaluation
- Early intervention programs (birth through three years)
- Preschool programs (three though five years)
- Special education programs
- Outpatient rehabilitation or private practice programs
- Adult community living arrangements and adult day programs

The following resources can be helpful for gathering sociopolitical data:

- IDEA
- Rehabilitation Act
- Americans with Disabilities Act
- Descriptions of coverage from medical insurance companies

Attention to the following can be helpful in understanding and managing understanding lifestyle/lifespan issues:

- Transitions
  - Early intervention to preschool
  - Preschool to school
  - School to adult community
- Family
  - Siblings
  - Financial stressors
  - Support groups
- Complementary approaches
  - Physical therapy
  - Speech and language therapy
  - Special education
  - Behavioral interventions
  - Dietary interventions

Internet Resources

The National Autism Society
www.autismsociety.org

Published Resources

Huebner, R. A. (2001). *Autism: A sensorimotor approach to management.* Gaithersburg, MD: Aspen Publishers, Inc.

Miller-Kuhaneck, H. (2001). *Autism: A comprehensive occupational therapy approach.* Bethesda, MD: American Occupation Therapy Association, Inc.

Murray-Slutsky, C. & Paris, B. A. (2000). *Exploring the spectrum of autism and pervasive developmental disorders: Intervention strategies.* San Antonio, TX.: Therapy Skill Builders.

Myles, B. S., Cook, K. T., Miller, N. E., Rinner, L. & Robbins L. A. (2001). *Asperger syndrome and sensory issues: Practical solutions for making sense of the world.* Shawnee Mission, KS: Autism Asperger Publishing Co.

References

American Psychiatric Association. (1994). *Diagnostic and statistical manual of mental disorders* (4th ed.). Washington DC: Author.

Attwood, T. (1998). *Asperger syndrome: A guide for parents and professionals.* London: Jessica Kingsley Publishers.

Ayres, A. J. (1989). *Sensory integration and praxis test.* Los Angeles: Western Psychological Services.

Bauman, M. L., & Kemper, T. L. (1985). Neuroanatomic observations of the brain in early infantile autism. *Neurology, 35,* 866–874.

Bauman, M. L., & Kemper, T. L. (1994). Neuroanatomic observations of the brain in autism. In M. L. Bauman & T. L. Kemper (Eds.), *The neurobiology of autism* (pp. 119–145). Baltimore: Johns Hopkins University Press.

Beery, K. (1997). *Beery-Buktenica developmental test of visual-motor integration* (VMI; 4th ed.). Parsippany, NJ: Modern Curriculum Press.

Berk, R., & DeGangi, G. (1983). *DeGangi-Berk test of sensory integration.* Los Angeles: Western Psychological Services.

Brown, C., & Dunn, W. (2002). *Adolescent/adult sensory profile.* San Antonio, TX: The Psychological Corporation.

Bruininks, R. H. (1978). *Bruininks-Oseretsky test of motor proficiency.* Circle Pines, MN: AGS.

Bryson, S. E. (1996). Brief report: Epidemiology of autism. *Journal of Autism and Developmental Disorders, 26,* 165–167.

Case-Smith, J. (1996). An overview of occupational therapy with children. In J. Case-Smith, A. S. Allen, & P. N. Pratt, *Occupational therapy for children,* (3rd ed.; pp. 3–17). St. Louis, MO: Mosby.

Centers for Disease Control. (2003). *Autism information center.* Retrieved on February 9, 2003 from http://www/cdc.gov/ncbddd/dd/aic/about/default.htm

Comi, A., Zimmerman, A., Frye, V., Law, P., & Peedan, J. (1999). Familiar clustering of autoimmune disorders and evaluation of medical risk factors. *Journal of Child Neurology, 14,* 388–394.

Coster, W., Deeney, T., Haltiwanger, J., & Haley, S. (1998). *School function assessment.* San Antonio, TX: The Psychological Corporation.

DeGangi, G., & Greenspan, S. (1981). *Test of sensory functions in infants.* Los Angeles: Western Psychological Services.

Dunn, W. (1999). *Sensory profile.* San Antonio, TX: The Psychological Corporation.

Dunn, W. (2002). *Infant/toddler sensory profile.* San Antonio, TX: The Psychological Corporation.

Fisher, A. G. (1998). Uniting practice and theory in an occupational framework. *American Journal of Occupational Therapy, 52,* 509–520.

Folio, R., & Fewell, R. (2000). *Peabody developmental motor scales* (2nd ed.). Austin, TX: Pro-Ed.

Furuno, S., O'Reilly, K., Hosaka, C. M., Zeisloft, B., & Allman, T. (1984). *The Hawaii early learning profile.* Palo Alto, CA: VORT.

Galvin, D. (2001). The family of a child with autism. In H. Miller-Kuhaneck (Ed.), *Autism: A comprehensive occupational therapy approach,* (4th ed.; pp. 43–53). Bethesda, MD: AOTA.

George, M. S., Costa, D. C., Houris, K., Rang, H. A., & Ell, P. J. (1992). Cerebral blood flow abnormalities in adults with infantile autism. *Journal of Nervous and Mental Disease, 180,* 413–417.

Ghaziuddin, M. (2002). Asperger syndrome: Associated psychiatric and medical conditions. *Focus on Autism and Other Developmental Disabilities, 17,* 138–144.

Glover, M. E., Preminger, J. L., & Sanford, A .R. (1988). *The early learning accomplishment profile (ELAP).* Winston-Salem, NC: Kaplan Press.

Greenspan, S., DeGangi, G., & Wieder, S. (1996). *Functional emotional assessment scale.* Bethesda, MD: The Interdisciplinary Council on Developmental and Learning Disorders.

Gresham, F. M., & Elliott, S. N. (1990). *Social skills rating system.* Circle Pines, MN: AGS.

Hammill, D., Pearson, N. A., & Voress, J. K. (1998). *Developmental test of visual perception* (2nd ed.). Austin, TX: Pro-Ed.

Harrison, P. L., & Oakland, T. (2000). *Adaptive behavioral assessment system.* San Antonio, TX: The Psychological Corporation.

Howlin, P. (2000). Outcome in individuals with autism or Asperger syndrome. *Autism, 4 (1),* 63–83.

Huebner, R. A., & Dunn, W. (2001). Introduction and basic concepts. In B. A. Huebner (Ed.), *Autism: A sensorimotor approach to management* (pp. 3–35). Gaithersburg, MD: Aspen.

Kientz, M. A., & Dunn, W. (1997). Comparison of the performance of children with and without autism on the sensory profile. *American Journal of Occupational Therapy, 51*, 530–537.

Knox, S. (1997). Development and current use of the Knox preschool play scale. In L. Parham & L. S. Fazio (Eds.), *Play in occupational therapy for children* (pp. 35–51). St. Louis, MO: Mosby.

Lerner, P. S. (2001). Alternative and complementary approaches in the treatment of autism. In H. Miller-Kuhaneck (Ed.), *Autism: A comprehensive occupational therapy approach* (pp. 237–268). Bethesda, MD: AOTA.

Lundy-Ekman, L. (1998). *Neuroscience fundamentals for rehabilitation.* Philadelphia: Saunders.

Mayes, S. D., & Calhoun, S. (1999). Symptoms of autism in young children and correspondence with *DSM. Infants and Young Children, 12(2)*, 90–97.

Miller-Kuhaneck, H., & Glennon, T. J. (2001). An introduction to autism and pervasive developmental disorders. In H. Miller-Kuhaneck (Ed.), *Autism: A comprehensive occupational therapy approach* (pp. 1–23). Bethesda, MD: AOTA.

Mutti, M., Sterling, H., & Spalding, N. V. (1978). *Quick neurological screening test* (Rev. ed.). Los Angeles: Western Psychological Services.

Olson, L. J. (1999). Psychosocial frame of reference. In P. Kramer & J. Hinohosa (Eds.), *Frames of reference for pediatric occupational therapy,* (2nd ed.; pp. 323–376). Philadelphia: Lippincott.

Ornitz, E. M. (1974). The modulation of sensory input and motor output in autistic children. *Journal of Autism and Childhood Schizophrenia, 4(3)*, 197–215.

Royeen, C. B., & Duncan, M. (1999). Acquisitional frame of reference. In P. Kramer & J. Hinohosa (Eds.), *Frames of reference for pediatric occupational therapy,* (2nd ed.; pp. 377–400). Philadelphia: Lippincott.

Schultz, R. T., Romanski, L. M., & Tsatsanis, K. D. (2000). Neurofunctional models of autistic disorder and Asperger syndrome: Clues from neuroimaging. In A. Kiln, F. R. Volkmar, & S. S. Sparrow (Eds.), *Asperger syndrome* (pp. 159–171). New York: Guilford Press.

Shortridge, S. D., & Walker, K. (1993). Lela A. Lorens. In R. J. Miller & K. F. Walker (Eds.), *Perspectives on theory for the practice of occupational therapy* (pp. 65–102). Gaithersburg, MD: Aspen.

Sparrow, S. S., Balla, D. A., & Cicchetti, D. V. (1984). *Vineland adaptive behavior scales: Interview edition survey form manual.* Circle Pines, MN: AGS.

Stephens, L. C., & Tauber, S. K. (2001). Early intervention. In J. Case-Smith (Ed.), *Occupational therapy for children* (pp. 708–730). St. Louis, MO: Mosby.

Tsai, L. (2000). Children with autism spectrum disorders: Medicine today and in the new millennium. *Focus on Autism and Other Developmental Disabilities, 15*, 138–145.

Volkmar, F. R., Klin, A., Siegel, B., Szatmari, P., Lord, C., Campbell, M., et al. (1994). *DSM–IV* autism/P.D.D. field trial. *American Journal of Psychiatry, 151*, 1361–1367.

Watling, R., Deitz, J., Kanny, E. M., & McLaughlin, J. F. (1999). Current practice of occupational therapy for children with autism. *American Journal of Occupational Therapy, 53*, 498–505.

Zilbovicius, M., Garreau, B., Samson, Y., Remy, P., Barthelemy, C., Syrota, A., et al. (1995). Delayed maturation of the frontal cortex in childhood autism. *American Journal of Psychiatry, 152*, 248–252.

Attention Deficit Hyperactivity Disorder

5

Gail E. Huecker, MS, OTR/L

Synopsis of Clinical Condition

Prevalence and Etiology

Attention deficit hyperactivity disorder (ADHD) is manifested by limitations in impulse control and attention span (Hempel, 2003). Commonly described as childhood hyperactivity, ADHD accounts for at least half of all referrals to child mental health clinics (Ingersoll, 1988). The fourth edition of the *Diagnostic and Statistical Manual of Mental Disorders (DSM–IV)* reports an ADHD prevalence of 3% to 5% in school-aged children (American Psychiatric Association [APA], 1994).

The *DSM–IV* also describes ADHD as occurring much more frequently in male children as compared to female children, with male-to-female ratios ranging from 4:1 to 9:1. Some researchers believe, however, that girls with ADHD may neither be as accurately identified by these statistics since the problems of hyperactive girls are not as visible, nor as troublesome to adults as the problems of hyperactive boys (Berry, Shaywitz, & Shaywitz, 1985; Ingersoll, 1988).

The exact etiology of ADHD is unknown. ADHD has been linked to body chemistry, the structure and function of nerve cells, maternal alcohol and drug use, or genetic and environmental factors (National Institute of Mental Health [NIMH], 1994).

Common Characteristics and Symptoms

The *DSM–IV* describes signs of inattention as: becoming easily distracted by irrelevant sights and sounds; failing to pay attention to details and making careless mistakes; rarely following instructions carefully and completely; and losing or forgetting things. Signs of hyperactivity and impulsivity are described as: feeling restless; often fidgeting with hands or feet; squirming, running, climbing, or leaving a seat in situations where sitting or quiet behavior is expected; blurting out answers before hearing the whole question; and having difficulty waiting in line for a turn.

In confirming the diagnosis of ADHD, the *DSM–IV* (p. 78) states that, "the essential feature of ADHD is a persistent pattern of inattention and/or hyperactivity-impulsivity that is more frequent and severe than is typically observed in individuals at a comparable level of development." The *DSM–IV* further classifies subtypes of ADHD into the following three categories: (1) ADHD, combined type, (2) ADHD, predominantly inattentive type, and (3) ADHD, predominantly hyperactive-impulsive type. The *DSM–IV* clearly specifies that to be accurately diagnosed with one of the above three subtypes; some symptoms have to be present before age seven, there must be impairment from the symptoms in two or more settings (i.e., school and home), and there must be clinically significant impairment in social, academic, or occupational functioning.

Target Areas for Intervention

When there is significant impairment in social, academic, or occupational functioning, some children with ADHD may be referred for occupational therapy (OT) intervention. The therapist must decipher the underlying sensorimotor and sensory integrative problems that may be contributing to the inability to attend. The primary areas to be addressed are: reaction to sensory stimuli and antigravity movement, motor planning, and social emotional responses. All of these areas impact social, academic, and/or occupational functioning.

The inattention, hyperactivity, and impulsivity most commonly associated with ADHD are related to abnormal sensory integrative and sensorimotor processing, and the consequent disorder in the ability to transmit, interpret, and respond appropriately to sensory stimulation from the environment (Ayres, 1979; Greenspan, 1992). Characteristic symptoms include: sensory hypo- or hypersensitivity, sensory defensiveness, unusual patterns of arousal, dyspraxia, and emotional and social difficulties (Oetter, 1986; Cermak, 1988; Burpee, 1994; Wilbarger & Wilbarger, 1991).

Ayres (1979) described a variety of behaviors which can result from increased sensory sensitivity. These behaviors include excess emotional reactions, hyperactivity, or other behavioral manifestations including excessive fighting, the inability to sit quietly at a school desk, and increased motor activity. The inability to enjoy "contact comfort" with a significant other has been described by Royeen (1985).

Sensory registration refers to an individual's ability to accurately perceive incoming sensory information. Sensory registration deficits occur when an individual exhibits significant delays in responding to sensory information, or when there is an apparent failure to notice sensory stimulation at all (Oetter, 1986; Bundy & Koomar, 1991).

Clinically, children with sensory registration deficits may appear to have a heightened pain tolerance, or may "brush off" bruises or scratches as if "nothing ever happened." They may also be described as the children who have poor safety awareness, and often seek out movement activities that can interfere with their personal safety (i.e., jumping from high places).

Another focus for OT intervention is the child's postural attention, or the ability to receive consistent information about the body and its relationship to the environment in terms of space, place, and time (Oetter, 1986).

Dyspraxia can result when a child has underlying difficulty processing somatosensory (tactile and proprioceptive) information, and when there is inadequate postural control to allow smooth, coordinated movement when executing a task (Cermak, 1988).

Other conditions that are present with ADHD and related to sensory processing disturbance are fluctuations in levels of alertness and arousal. These can be reflected by disorganized sleep patterns or by fluctuations in the individual's ability to attend during interactions with unfamiliar people, tasks, and environments which the individual perceives as over-stimulating (Oetter, 1986).

Vestibular-related disorders, specifically shortened duration of postrotary nystagmus (PRN), is another sensory integrative deficit which has been linked to resultant attentional deficits. Children with a shortened duration of PRN also demonstrate poor balance, difficulty maintaining antigravity postures, and low muscle tone (Cermak, 1988). Kimball (1986) proposed that a large percentage of children with ADHD have an under-responsive vestibular system, thus contributing to their attention deficits. Huecker and Kinnealey (1998) confirmed Kimball's research in a descriptive study, by reporting a vestibular processing disorder in more than 50% of children with ADHD, making them hyporesponsive to vestibular stimulation.

It has also been suggested that children with ADHD who demonstrate sensory integration deficits report a high incidence of social/emotional challenges, including poor frustration tolerance, difficulty making friends, rigid personalities, and feelings of anxiousness, anxiety, or depression (Huecker & Kinnealey, 1998).

Many children with attention disorders also exhibit auditory processing deficits, commonly diagnosed as a central auditory processing disorder (CAPD; Greenspan, 1992). Many children with auditory processing deficits are frequently accused of "not following directions" or "not listening," and they may fail to get their work completed on time.

It is estimated that 50% or more of children with ADHD have a learning disability (Stahl, 1995). Between 15% and 20% of children and adolescents with learning disabilities will have ADHD (Silver, 1990). Because ADHD can interfere with a child's ability to concentrate and pay attention, this diagnosis—in conjunction with the diagnosis of learning disability—can make it exceptionally difficult for a child to function in school (NIMH, 1994).

Another condition sometimes found in conjunction with ADHD is a rare disorder called Tourette's syndrome. Children diagnosed with Tourette's syndrome typically have tics and other uncontrolled movements, such as eye blinks, facial twitches, grimacing, shrugging, or sniffing. Typically, this syndrome is controlled with medications (NIMH, 1994).

It has been estimated that almost half of all children with ADHD are boys, and they are sometimes diagnosed as having an oppositional defiant disorder. Children with this disorder reportedly exhibit behaviors that include lashing out at others; acting stubborn, belligerent, or defiant; and having significant temper tantrums. If a child with ADHD and ODD does not receive proper medical treatment, he or she may progress to more serious behaviors, and may then be diagnosed with a conduct disorder. Children with this disorder typically take unsafe risks and break laws. They may steal, set fires, destroy property, or harm others (NIMH, 1994). Eventually, these children may become involved with the juvenile system due to their uncontrolled behavior.

Many children with ADHD may also be diagnosed with anxiety disorder or depression. An estimated one-fourth of children with ADHD feel anxious and/or depressed (NIMH, 1994).

Contextual Considerations

Clinical

The clinical evaluation of a child who has ADHD should assess sensory processing, motor control, praxis/cognition, developmental status, communication, activities of daily living (ADL), and social and emotional functioning. Through assessment in these areas, the OT should be able to determine if the child demonstrates soft neurological processing deficits, and if there is impairment in function at home and/or school. For children ages 4 years to 8 years 11 months, the *Sensory Integration and Praxis Test* (SIPT) (Ayers, 1989) is extremely helpful in determining if sensory integration and praxis/motor planning problems are present.

The SIPT has been described as a sophisticated and psychometrically sound assessment tool designed to provide diagnostic and descriptive information related to sensory integrative and pracic functions (Mailloux, 1990). The SIPT consists of 17 subtests that assess abilities related to praxia and various aspects of sensory processing including vestibular, proprioceptive, kinesthetic, tactile, and visual processing (Ayres, 1991). In addition to the 17 subtests of the SIPT, both a sensory history and clinical observations are necessary supplements for a complete assessment of sensory integrative dysfunction.

Other sensory processing deficits that children with ADHD may exhibit are assessed through clinical observations and a sensory history. Most standard clinical observations include general assessment of activity level, response to touch, visual control, coordination, praxis or motor planning, and postural responses including reflexes and balance reactions.

The most commonly used sensory history is the *Sensory Profile* (Dunn, 1999). It is most appropriate to use the *Sensory Profile* for children between the ages of 5 and 10 years. The *Sensory Profile* is completed by a parent/caregiver and includes information regarding sensory processing, modulation, and behavioral and emotional responses. The *Sensory Profile* is standardized and can be use to provide baseline data and assess progress.

The *Quick Neurological Screening Test* (QNST–II; Mutti, Sterling, & Spalding, 1978) is a quick and accurate instrument for detecting the soft neurological signs often associated with learning disabilities. It is designed for use with children as young as 5 years, but can also be used for older children, adolescents, and adults. Because it can be completed in 20 to 30 minutes, the QNST–II is easy to use in a variety of settings, including outpatient, private practice, school, or home.

Other assessments for the school-aged child may be needed to further evaluate visual motor skills, visual perception, and fine/gross motor coordination. Common examples include the *Beery Developmental Test of Visual Motor Integration* (Beery, 1997), the *Developmental Test of Visual Perception* (Hammill, Pearson, & Voress, 1993), the *Bruninks–Osteretsky Test of Motor Proficiency* (Bruninks, 1978), and the *Test of Visual Perceptual Skills–Revised.* The *Pediatric Examination of Educational Readiness–Revised* (Levine & Schneider, 1983), and the *Pediatric Examination of Educational Readiness at Middle Childhood–Revised* (Levine, 1985) are also beneficial in assessing soft neurological processing deficits and academic-related performance.

For the younger child with ADHD, a developmental assessment can be helpful to determine developmental levels in the areas of motor skills, cognition, language, self-help skills, and social/emotional functioning. Examples of general developmental assessments include the *Peabody Developmental Motor Scales–2* (PDMS–2) (Folio & Fewell, 2000), the *Learning Accomplishment Profile* (LAP), the *Hawaii Early Learning Profile*™ (HELP) (Furuno, O'Reilly, Hosaka, Zeisloft & Altman, 1984), or the *Pediatric Developmental Inventory* (PEDI) (Haley, Coster, Ludlow, Haltiwanger, & Andrellos, 1992).

Most of these developmental assessments are completed through use of both clinical observation and parent interview.

In assessing ADL skills, the OT should focus on areas most affected by regulation of sensory input, including sleep cycles, bowel and bladder control, and feeding/eating. Sensory processing deficits can significantly affect a child's ability for self-regulation within these areas. Children often have difficulty "winding down" to get to sleep, or awaken frequently throughout the night. Nightmares are also commonly reported. Disturbed sleep patterns can only add to their difficulty focusing and attending. Some children are delayed in bowel/bladder control, and bed-wetting can be a common occurrence. Feeding/eating issues often seen include children who are "picky" eaters, possibly secondary to oral hypersensitivity. These children can gag easily on foods, and therefore may limit their diet to only a few textures. It is also common for parents to report their child "over-stuffs" or "pockets" food in his or her mouth when eating. If a child exhibits hypo- or under-responsiveness to sensory input, it can be difficult to process when their mouth is full. This can create a choking hazard, and oral-motor intervention should be a definite focus of the treatment plan.

Other areas that should be assessed in reference to ADL skills include grooming, bathing, and dressing. Sensory defensiveness (SD) can significantly contribute to grooming issues, including difficulty tolerating haircuts, nail trimming, tooth brushing, or face washing. Bathing issues may include anxiety with water in the face or not wanting hair washed. SD can also affect dressing skills. Some children can be averse to certain clothing textures or tags in their clothes, or to the seams in their socks. Dyspraxia, fine motor deficits, and poor body awareness can all interfere with a child's ability to dress independently. Children may not notice if their clothing is on inside out or backward, or they may be unable to manipulate fasteners on clothing secondary to fine motor delays. All of these issues are typically frustrating for the parent and child.

Family

When interviewing the family of a child with ADHD who exhibits sensory processing deficits, an OT should be empathetic and sensitive. Parents are frequently frustrated, and believe their child is only being "difficult, stubborn, or lazy," and may be unaware that the behaviors their child exhibits may have a neurological base.

It can be difficult to discipline a child with ADHD, and some parents may ask for suggestions in this area. When providing suggestions, it is important for the OT to be sensitive to cultural issues regarding discipline. Parents may feel guilty that their child is having social or developmental delays, and may not set enough limits for behavior. This can be difficult for children with ADHD, who thrive on structure and routine to help organize themselves.

If parents feel guilty about their child, they may be fostering dependency without being aware of it. For example, if the child with ADHD is frustrated about difficulty dressing, a parent may do it for him or her and the child develops "learned helplessness." Therefore, it is important to model independent behaviors and empower the child for success. In addition, if a parent feels guilty, this can often lead to depression. It is important for the OT to recognize depression in parents and refer them to the appropriate professionals. If the parent is depressed to the point of being unable to function as a caregiver, this will not encourage the child to develop organizational skills.

Practice Setting

Occupational therapists working with children with ADHD may work in a variety of settings, including private practice, home, school, and early intervention centers or daycare centers. In a private practice, there should be a variety of specialized equipment available to meet the needs of the child. Direct/individualized treatment may be the most beneficial in the early stages of care, whereas treatment in small groups may be beneficial in the later stages to help address social/emotional concerns.

Specialized equipment may be less available for an OT working in the home. The therapist should help parents establish home activities that utilize equipment already available. Examples may include enhanced deep-pressure activities such as wheelbarrow walking, jumping on mattresses, swinging outdoors, rearranging furniture, or carrying in groceries.

The school-based OT must provide services that are educationally relevant in terms of the child's academic functioning. The Individuals with Disabilities Education Act (IDEA, 1997) mandates that all children have the right to a free, appropriate public education in the least restrictive environment. If the child with ADHD is having academic difficulty, the child may be referred to an OT as a supportive service. The OT's role may be to address the child's fine motor delays, handwriting problems, problems focusing and attending during seated work, poor organizational and sequencing skills, and sensory processing deficits as they relate to social interaction (i.e., interaction with other children on the playground).

The OT working with children ages three to five may also work in an early intervention center or daycare center. In these settings it is important for the therapist to be a team member and use a transdisciplinary approach while working with other professionals. Instead of pulling a child out of his or her classroom for therapy, an inclusion model is frequently helpful to integrate functional needs into the daily routine.

As noted above, since a diagnosis of ADHD is often associated with many conditions the occupational therapist should be cognizant of the role of the other members of the professional team, which can include psychologists, speech-language pathologists, teachers, social workers, and physicians.

Sociopolitical

As mentioned earlier, IDEA mandates a free, appropriate public education for children with disabilities (IDEA, 1997). Since children with ADHD may have learning disabilities, school-based occupational therapists may be involved in the development of legally required individual education plans (IEPs). Some children with ADHD may not qualify for services under IDEA but may qualify for classroom adaptations under the National Rehabilitation Act, section 504 which defines disability more broadly than IDEA (NIMH, 1994).

ADHD is viewed as a behavioral diagnosis, and, therefore, some insurance companies do not see treatment as medically necessary.

It is important for the OT in private practice to consult with pediatricians (and other physicians) who may refer the child with ADHD for therapy to discuss the possible neurological processing deficits that may be interfering with the child's function. The physician may be able to use other diagnosis codes such as motor apraxia to more accurately describe the neuromotor nature of the child's condition.

Lifestyle/Lifespan

Since ADHD has a genetic factor, some parents of children with ADHD may have the same diagnosis. Therefore, suggestions to parents about controlling behavior and how to better organize their child may be unnatural to them. Many children with ADHD function better in a set routine that is clearly structured. The OT may be able to educate parents on setting up a behavior plan to improve behavior such as modeling and rewards, or making a consistent schedule for the child. In some situations, it may also be helpful to refer the parent to other professionals or support groups that can help establish parenting skills.

Another important family consideration for helping the child with ADHD is establishing a home-based program for enhanced organization, improved behavior, and improved social/emotional functioning. When the child exhibits extreme regulatory and modulation difficulties, the occupational therapist should provide the family with sensory activities—consistent with family resources and routines—that are designed to enhance the child's ability to process tactile, proprioceptive, auditory, and vestibular input.

There is also growing information about prevention through allergy testing for specific food sensitivities that can contribute to hyperactivity and impulsivity (Zavik & Thompson, 2002). An OT should be familiar with nutritional concepts, such as food sensitivities and allergies, and refer parents to a nutritionist when appropriate.

Clinical Decision Making Process

Defining Focus for Intervention

The focus of OT treatment for the child with ADHD may vary depending on where services will be provided. Treatment will also vary depending on the frequency and duration of the service the funding source allows. For example, if the OT is working in a private practice setting in which Medicaid is the primary funding source, a child is allowed up to 14 fifteen-minute units of OT per week, as long as the therapy is deemed medically necessary and approved by a physician. In this type of setting, with 14 units allowed per week, a therapist will be able to complete a thorough evaluation of the child's functioning. The SIPT may be the most appropriate assessment tool to define the child's underlying sensory processing and praxis deficits. However, this assessment would have to be completed in hourly increments on separate days to meet Medicaid guidelines.

Throughout the evaluation, the OT should gain information about primary parental concerns. These concerns should become the main focus of OT intervention once treatment is initiated. For example, if a parent's primary concerns are related to self-grooming difficulties related to sensory defensiveness, then normalizing sensory processing should become the primary goal. If a child is referred for an occupational therapy evaluation but will not be able to attend therapy regularly because of funding issues, then establishing a home program is of primary importance.

The primary criterion for school-based occupational therapy is educational relevance. The focus of intervention might be fine motor control for handwriting, improving organizational skills for letter or number formation, improving postural control for better attention while seated in a desk, or self-regulation strategies for social interaction. In educational settings where inclusionary rather than pull-out services are preferred, occupational therapy services may be consultative, and intervention strategies may be group rather than individually oriented. In that case, activities programs such as *How Does Your Engine Run?* (Williams & Shellenberger, 1996) and *Handwriting without Tears*™ (Olsen, 2001) can be used to improve attention span and handwriting for a larger group.

Establishing Goals for Intervention

Primary parental concerns should become goals within the private practice setting, whereas primary teacher concerns should become goals within the school setting. Since goals need to be functional and measurable, they should be worded clearly, with only one objective to be met per goal. It is also important to establish short-term goals that will ultimately allow the child to achieve his or her long-term goal, regardless of the practice setting.

If a child with ADHD is also developmentally delayed, it will be important to take into account the child's developmental status in order to make the goals attainable. For example, if the child is five years old but functioning at a four-year-old level, it may not be appropriate to establish a goal that the child be able to tie his shoes independently. A child with ADHD frequently exhibits increased frustration. Therefore, goals should be broken down into small steps, giving the child several opportunities at success while working toward the major goal.

Designing Theory-Based Intervention

The sensory integration frame of reference may be the most commonly used when working with the child with ADHD. This frame of reference allows the therapist to evaluate the underlying neurological constructs that may be contributing to the child's developmental, social, or behavioral issues. Ayres (1991) defined sensory integration as the neurological process that organizes sensation from one's own body and from the environment and makes it possible to use the body effectively within the environment. According to this view, higher-level organizational and learning abilities are dependent upon the integrity of lower-level brain centers which govern arousal levels and attention span (Ayres, 1979; Fisher & Murray, 1991). The therapist using a sensory integration frame of reference will design activities to remediate deficits in muscle tone, postural control, sensory defensiveness, and oculomotor control in order to achieve specific behavioral goals. Such goals include improved attention span, increased frustration tolerance, and motor coordination.

Evaluating Progress

Formal evaluations such as the SIPT and the *Sensory Profile* can provide quantitative data that can be used to monitor changes in function and provide feedback regarding the efficacy of treatment. They can be used at the outset of treatment and periodically throughout treatment. Qualitative data from clinical observation and the anecdotal reports of caregivers can be used to monitor changes in function and provide feedback regarding the efficacy of treatment. Regulations regarding the frequency and form of progress documentation vary with the practice setting and funding source.

Determining Change in or Termination of Treatment

A therapist should be able to determine when a change in treatment is warranted as the child progresses in therapy. For example, the child may appear to have behavior under control and be less impulsive and more aware of safety. At that point, the child may be ready to join a peer group or a small group of children in treatment, to address more social interaction concerns. It is also helpful to guide treatment changes based on information the parent or teacher provides. If the parent or teacher reports that the child is more organized, less impulsive, and able to attend for longer periods of time, it may be an appropriate time to introduce higher-level intervention strategies, such as a handwriting group.

Termination of treatment is warranted once the child has met his or her established goals, or if it appears the child is not going to be able to meet the goals due to other circumstances (i.e., social concerns in the home). If the child has met his or her goals, the parent will likely appear much calmer concerning how the child is functioning. Before discharge, the family should be able to demonstrate proficiency in carrying through a home program. If transition to a new environment triggers additional organizational or behavioral challenges, the child may be referred to occupational therapy again. If the child appears unable to meet his or her expected goals secondary to other circumstances, then a referral to other professionals may be warranted. For example, family dynamics, or other social or emotional pressures may exacerbate anxiety and impulsivity. In this situation, it may be appropriate to recommend that the family seek psychological counseling or additional social services.

Case Study

Description

Vince is a six-year-old boy with ADHD. He was referred to OT secondary to his parents' primary concerns about his academic difficulties. Specifically, teachers had reported poor handwriting, difficulty focusing/attending, poor organizational skills, and inappropriate social/emotional functioning. Other concerns included stubborn and defiant behavior, poor oculomotor (eye tracking) skills, and negative behaviors during grooming tasks (i.e., nails trimmed, haircuts, etc.).

Vince lives at home with his parents and younger sister. He attends a private school where he is in a regular kindergarten classroom with eight children. Although he has exhibited other developmental delays, Vince has never received any therapy services. Stimulant medication had been used with no significant effect on his ability to attend/focus. He is currently on no medications. Medical history is significant for strabismus in his right eye, which was surgically corrected.

Results of Vince's SIPT indicated generalized sensory integrative dysfunction. Areas of severe dysfunction (−3.00 standard deviations [SD] below the norm) included standing and walking balance, localization of tactile stimuli, graphesthesia, praxis on verbal command, and postural praxis. His postrotary nystagmus score (PRN) was −2.82 SD below the norm, and the sequencing and oral praxis subtests indicated moderate dysfunction (between −2.0 and −2.5 SD below the norm). Visual perception scores (space visualization and figure ground) fell within the average range on the SIPT.

Results of the sensory profile indicated that Vince demonstrated definite differences (−3.0 SD below the norm) with tactile, auditory, multisensory, and vestibular processing, sensory modulation deficits related to endurance/tone, sensory sensitivity, poor modulation of movement affecting activity level, and emotional/social responses at −2.0 SD below the norm. Results of clinical observations indicated Vince was unable to assume or maintain either prone extension or supine flexion postures. He also appeared to have decreased oculomotor (eye tracking) control, poor convergence, difficulty planning smooth movements, decreased musculature contraction, and postural insecurity (i.e., fear of movement beyond his postural control).

Areas of strength reported during the evaluation include regular sleep patterns, good eating skills, independent toileting, and independent dressing. Vince is a quiet child who does not play interactively with other children or toys, and also seems fearful of many new tasks. His favorite activities include playing with books and cars. It has been recommended that Vince receive two hours of individual/direct therapy services per week in a private practice setting, in addition to a weekly consult with his kindergarten teacher.

Long- and Short-Term Goals

The long-term goal of intervention for Vince is to enable him to attend to a cognitive/fine motor activity for 15 minutes without requiring redirection.

The short-term goals for Vince are:

1. Maintain a supine-flexed posture on the floor or over a large therapy ball for 10 seconds without compensation.
2. Maintain a prone-extended posture for five minutes during a movement activity on suspended equipment.
3. Wheelbarrow walk for 10 feet with his feet held without falling to his elbows.
4. Allow his nails to be trimmed by a primary caregiver without an aversive response.
5. Follow a two-step motor command 80% of the time without directions repeated.

Therapist Goals and Strategies

The therapist's goals include:

1. Normalize sensory processing by reducing sensory defensiveness and enhancing body awareness.
2. Increase motor coordinative control through enhanced antigravity control and co-contraction.
3. Enhance motor planning through improved body awareness and vestibular processing.
4. Provide teacher education regarding strategies to enhance academic performance.

The therapist's strategies include:

1. Educate parents on implementing an intense tactile/pressure program with the use of therapy brushes and a large muscle vibrator; to be performed 3 to 5 times per day.

2. Visit the home to instruct parents on sensory activities to enhance self-regulation and attention.
3. Educate school staff on the "How Does Your Engine Run?" program.
4. Provide opportunities in the clinic for enhanced tactile, proprioceptive, and vestibular processing, as well as oral motor and eye-tracking activities.
5. Provide activities in the clinic incorporating play with peer and co-therapists, to enhance social functioning.
6. Educate parents on implementation of a therapeutic listening program one hour daily to enhance visual, vestibular, and auditory processing, and to improve postural control and motor planning.
7. Collaborate with other members of the professional team such as the speech language pathologist, teacher, and psychologist on goal setting and implementation of strategies.

Activity

Vince will straddle a tire swing that is 12 to 18 inches off the ground, and will pick up "fish" (stuffed beanbags) from the "ocean" (floor mats) without his feet touching the "water" while swinging. After a fish is successfully picked up, Vince will throw each fish into a "tub" with one hand without falling into the ocean.

Treatment Objectives

Vince will maintain adequate flexion posture on suspended equipment for 3 to 5 minutes while engaged in a dynamic upper extremity activity.

Resources

Internet Resources

Children and Adults with ADD largest ADD organization
www.chadd.org
www.attention.com
www.ConductDisorders.com
www.ADHDnews.com

The American Occupational Therapy Association
www. aota.org

Sensory Integration International
www.sensoryint.com

Published Resources

Anderson, E., & Emmons, P. (1996). *Unlocking the mysteries of sensory dysfunction.* Arlington, TX: Future Horizons.

Anderson, N., & Peiper, H. (1996). *A.D.D.—The natural approach*: Help for children with attention deficit disorder and hyperacivity. East Camaar, CT: Safe Goods.

Ayres, J. (1991). *Sensory integration and the child.* Los Angeles, CA: Western Psychological Services.

Frick, S. (2000). *Listening with the whole body.* Madison, WI: Vital Links.

Greenspan, S. (1992). *Infancy and early childhood.* Madison, CT: International Universities Press.

Greenspan, S., & Weider, S. (1998). *The child with special needs.* Reading, MA: Addison-Wesley.

Henry, D. (2001). *Tool chest: For teachers, parents & students.* Bethesda, MD: The American Occupational Therapy Association, Inc.

Kranowitz, C. (1989). *The out of sync child.* New York, NY: The Berkley Publishing Group.

Olsen, J. (2001). *Handwriting without tears.* Cabin John, MD: Handwriting Without Tears.

Williams, M., & Shellenberger, S. (1996). *How does your engine run? A leader's guide to the Alert Program for self-regulation, revised edition.* Albuquerque, NM: Therapy Works, Inc.

Zavik, J., & Thompson, J. (2002). *Toxic food syndrome.* Fort Lauderdale, FL: Fun Publishing.

References

American Psychiatric Association. (1994). *Diagnostic and statistical manual of mental disorders* (4th ed.). Washington, DC: Author.

Ayres, A. J. (1979). *Sensory integration and the child.* Los Angeles: Western Psychological Services.

Ayres, A. J. (1991). *Sensory integration and praxis tests.* Los Angeles: Western Psychological Services.

Berry, C. A., Shaywitz, S. E., & Shaywitz, B. A. (1985). Girls with attention deficit disorder: A silent minority? A report on behavioral and cognitive characteristics. *Pediatrics, 76,* 801–809.

Bundy, A. C., & Koomar, J. A. (1991). The art and science of creating direct intervention from theory. In A. G. Fisher, E. A. Murray, & A. C. Bundy (Eds.), *Sensory integration theory and practice* (pp. 251–317). Philadelphia: FA Davis.

Burpee, J. D. (1994, March). *Developmental disabilities, dyspraxia, and sensory integration: A treatment process for pediatric therapists.* Paper presented at conference, Langhorne, PA.

Cermak, S. A. (1988a). The relationship between attention deficit and sensory integration disorders (Part 1). *Sensory Integration Special Interest Section Newsletter, 11(2),* 1–4.

Cermak, S. A. (1988b). The relationship between attention deficit and sensory integration disorders (Part 2). *Sensory Integration Special Interest Section Newsletter, 11(3),* 3–4.

Dunn, W. (1999). *Sensory profile.* San Antonio, TX: The Psychological Corporation.

Fisher, A. G., & Murray, E. A. (1991). Introduction to sensory integration theory. In A. G. Fisher, E. A. Murray, & A. C. Bundy (Eds.), *Sensory integration theory and practice* (pp. 3–26). Philadelphia: FA Davis.

Greenspan, S. I. (1992). *Infancy and early childhood: The practice of clinical assessment and intervention with emotional and developmental challenges.* Madison, CT: International Universities Press.

Hempel, K. (2003). *The Health Gazette.* Attention Deficit Hyperactivity Disorder, 6-1-03. www.tfn.net/HG/adhd.html

Huecker, G., & Kinnealey, M. (1998). Prevalence of sensory integrative disorders in children with attention deficit hyperactivity disorder: A descriptive study. *The Journal of Developmental and Learning Disorders, 2(2),* 265–292.

Individuals with Disabilities Education Act (IDEA) Amendments of 1997 (P.L. No. 105-117). U.S.C., 1400.

Ingersoll, B. (1988). *Your hyperactive child: A parent's guide to coping with attention deficit disorder.* New York: Doubleday.

Kimball, J. G. (1986). Prediction of methylphenidate (Ritalin) responsiveness through sensory integrative testing. *The American Journal of Occupational Therapy, 40(4),* 241–248.

Levine, M.D. (1985). *Pediatric examination of educational readiness in middle childhood (PEERAMID).* Cambridge, MA: Educators Publishing Services, Inc.

Levine, M.D., & Schneider, E.A. (1983). *Pediatric examination of educational readiness (PEER).* Cambridge, MA: Educators Publishing Services, Inc.

Mailloux, Z. (1990). An overview of the sensory integration and praxis tests. *The American Journal of Occupational Therapy, 44(7),* 589–594.

Mutti, M., Sterling, H., & Spalding, N.V. (1978). Quick neurological screening test (QNST) (Rev. ed.). Los Angeles: Western Psychological Services.

Neuwirth, S. (1994). Attention Deficit Hyperactivity Disorder NIH Publication #96-3572. Reprinted 1996. 1–44.

Oetter, P. (1986a). A sensory integrative approach to the treatment of attention deficit disorders. *Sensory Integration Special Interest Section Newsletter, 9(2),* 1–2.

Oetter, P. (1986b). Assessment: The child with attention deficit disorder. *Sensory Integration Special Interest Section Newsletter, 9(1),* 6–7.

Olsen, J. (2001). *Handwriting without tears.* Cabin John, MD: Handwriting Without Tears.

Royeen, C. B. (1985). Domain specifications of the construct tactile defensiveness. *The American Journal of Occupational Therapy, 39(9),* 596–599.

Silver, L. (1990). Attention deficit hyperactivity disorder: Is it a learning disability or a related disorder? *Journal of Learning Disabilities, 23(7),* 394–397.

Stahl, C. (1995). Solving the riddle of ADHD. *Advance for Occupational Therapists, 11(7),* 15–50.

Wilbarger, P., & Wilbarger, J. L. (1991). *Sensory defensiveness in children aged two to twelve: An intervention guide for parents and other caretakers.* Santa Barbara, CA: Avante Educational Programs.

Williams, M., & Shellenberger, S. (1996). *How does your engine run? A leader's guide to the Alert Program for self-regulation* (Rev. ed.). Albuquerque, NM: Therapy Works, Inc.

Zavik, J., & Thompson, J. (2002). *Toxic food syndrome.* Fort Lauderdale, FL: Fun Publishing.

Cerebral Palsy

6

Meryl S. Cooperman, MS, OTR/L
Roberta T. Ciocco, OTR/L

Synopsis of Clinical Condition

Prevalence and Etiology

The term cerebral palsy is used to describe neuromuscular dysfunction associated with static encephalopathy. It occurs in 1.5 to 2 of every 1,000 births and is the leading cause of disability in children that affects function and development (Thorogood, 2001).

The etiology of cerebral palsy appears to be varied. It is often diagnosed after one year of age when the child does not meet expected motor milestones. The initial insult to the brain can occur up to two years of age and continue to be classified as cerebral palsy. The table below lists possible causes (Ratanawongsa, 2001; Thorogood, 2001).

Table 6.1
Possible Causes of Cerebral Palsy

Prenatal	Neonatal	Postnatal
Intrauterine infections	Prematurity (<32 weeks)	Trauma
Congenital malformations	Low birth weight (<2500 grams)	Infection
Toxic or teratogenic agents	Growth retardation	Intracranial hemorrhage
Multiple births	Periventricular-intracranial hemorrhage	Coagulopathies
Abdominal trauma (mother)	Trauma	
Maternal illness	Infection	
	Bradycardia and hypoxia	
	Seizures	
	Hyperbilirbinrmia	
	Abnormal birthing presentations	

Common Characteristics and Symptoms

The presentation of muscle tone in the extremities is used to classify the type, distribution, and severity of cerebral palsy. Muscle tone is the state of the muscle during rest and movement, and should vary according to activity. Children with cerebral palsy have difficulty with postural control and with modulating muscle tone during movement, problems that are also referred to as static and dynamic tone. The degree of the muscle activation at rest can be described as increased or decreased tone. In some forms, the muscle tone is variable and movement may be involuntary. The area of the lesion in the brain dictates the dysfunction in the muscle tone and the classification of the type of cerebral palsy.

The classification of cerebral palsy by type of motor dysfunction has been described in three or four main categories, with recognition that there are mixed types. The motor dysfunction is related to the area of insult in the brain. The three main categories are spastic, dyskinetic, and ataxia. The fourth is flaccid or hypotonia, but this presentation is believed to be transient or a part of other three categories. The distribution of the motor dysfunction and the degree of involvement are used to further delineate the presentation of cerebral palsy in the individual child (Ratanawongsa, 2001; Thorogood, 2001; Scherzer & Tscharnuter, 1982; Gordon, Schanzenbacher, Case-Smith, & Carrasco, 1996).

The distribution of the muscle tone ranges from involvement of the entire body to involvement of a single limb. Quadriplegia indicates involvement of the four extremities, trunk, and oral motor area. Diplegia refers to involvement of the lower extremities to a greater extent than the upper extremities. Hemiplegia is used to describe involvement in one side of the body, with the upper extremity typically involved more than the lower extremity. Involvement of only one limb is called monoplegia.

Cerebral palsy is further classified by the degree of involvement for each type. The terms mild, moderate, and severe are used to describe the amount of impairment. A child may be described as having severe spastic quadriplegia, mild ataxia, or moderate right hemiplegic athetosis. These descriptions help healthcare professionals target interventions appropriately, since the term cerebral palsy describes a broad array of conditions and functional levels.

Although cerebral palsy is defined based on motor dysfunction, a sensory impairment often co-exists. The sensory impairment can be loss of the sensation from the area of brain damage, altered functioning of a sensory system such as vision and hearing, sensory processing difficulties, and impaired sensory feedback from movement differences (Erhardt & Merrill, 1998).

Spastic cerebral palsy is the most common form and comprises 70% to 80% of the cases (Thorogood, 2001). The primary area of the lesion is in the cerebral cortex. The distribution can be quadriplegic, diplegic, hemiplegic, or monoplegic. Spastic cerebral palsy is characterized by increased tone in the extremities. The trunk can be either hypo- or hypertonic. The child has difficulty with the end ranges of movement, and consequently only moves in the midranges. Postural control and stability is often diminished, and the child does not have the sufficient proximal stability to maximize function of the extremities. Movements are slow, require effort, and incorporate synergistic movement patterns. The limited movement patterns and the mid-range movement often lead to a loss of range of motion and contractures of joints (Gordon, et al. 1996, Erhardt & Merrill, 1998, Bierman, J.).

Dyskinetic (also known as athetoid or dystonic) cerebral palsy is caused by a lesion in the basal ganglia. The frequency is 10% to 15% of the cases of cerebral palsy. The distribution is most frequently quadriplegic with occasional hemiplegia. Dyskinesia with tonic spasms may also be present in a monoplegic distribution. Children with dyskinetic cerebral palsy move from one end range to another (full flexion to full extension) and are unable to sustain movement in midranges. They have difficulty with co-contraction for balance of muscle function around a joint, and difficulty with postural control. They may use asymmetrical postures for stability (Gordon et al., 1996; Boehme, 1987b).

Ataxia occurs when the lesion is in the cerebellar region. Ataxia accounts for less than 5% of the cases of cerebral palsy. The distribution is quadriplegic. Ataxia is characterized by poor postural control and decreased tone of the trunk. Tremors are often observed distally (Boehme, 1987b).

Children with flaccid tone present with poor postural control and increased mobility around joints (Boehme, 1987a). The child has difficulty assuming and maintaining positions against gravity. Flaccidity often evolves into other forms of cerebral palsy or becomes part of a mixed form, such as athetosis with hypotonicity.

The following chart depicts some of the common characteristics of cerebral palsy by type. Children with milder forms may have less of the difficulties described below (Gordon et al., 1996; Erhardt & Merrill, 1998).

Table 6.2
Characteristics of Cerebral Palsy

	Spastic	Dyskinetic	Flaccid
Movement	Moves in mid ranges More involved increased risk of contractures/ deformities Synergistic movement patterns	Moves in end ranges Decreased midrange control	Hypermobility Subluxation of joints
Reflexes and Reactions	Reflexive movement patterns	Decreased equilibrium and righting reactions	Delays in protective, righting, and equilibrium reactions
Oral Motor and Respiration	Shallow respiration Decreased lip closure Tongue thrust Difficult verbal communication Feeding difficulties	Difficulties with volume of speech Feeding difficulties	Soft voice Decreased respiration Drooling Difficulties with facial expressions
Personality Characteristics	Passive Dependent	Emotionally labile May get frustrated	Visually attentive Decreased motivation

Associated conditions vary with the type of cerebral palsy. Cognitive limitations; visual deficits; hearing impairments; respiratory, digestive, and elimination difficulties; and seizures are associated with cerebral palsy. The following table describes the associated conditions frequently associated by the type of cerebral palsy (Gordon et al., 1996).

Table 6.3
Conditions Associated With Types of Cerebral Palsy

Spastic	Dyskinetic	Ataxia	Flaccid
Seizures	Hearing loss	Nystagmus	Obesity
Cortical blindness		Cognitive limitations	Sensory impairment
Deafness		Sensory impairment	Prone to upper respiratory infections
Prone to upper respiratory infections		Reliance on vision to assist with movement	
Cognitive limitations			
Imbalanced eye musculature			
Perceptual problems			
Learning disabilities			
Gastro-intestinal difficulties			

In addition to the associated medical conditions of cerebral palsy, there are conditions resulting from the motoric deficit. The child has a limitation and then develops compensations, which become habits, which may lead to contractures and eventually deformities (Alexander, Boehme, Cupps, & Kliebhan, 1987). The more severe the motoric deficit, the greater likelihood of abnormal motor development in the child with cerebral palsy.

Target Areas for Intervention

Occupational therapists who work with children with cerebral palsy need to have an awareness of medical interventions and other therapies that the child may be receiving. Children with cerebral palsy may receive oral medication or BOTOX™ injections to help with spasticity. An interthecal baclophen pump that releases spasticity medication in the body may be surgically implanted. A rhizotomy is a surgical procedure to reduce lower extremity spasticity that has implications for lower extremity dressing, transfer skills, and postural control. Surgical interventions include tendon releases, tendon transfers, and procedures to stabilize joints. Tendon releases and tendon transfers help to restore balance around a joint. Procedures to stabilize joints (arthrodesis) provide a fixed position for a joint. A child may have dynamic splints or serial casting to improve range of motion (Yasukawa, 1992). Equine facilitated therapy (horseback riding), hydrotherapy, and other specialty therapy programs may be available. Research is being conducted on the use of electrical stimulation to determine its effectiveness with children with cerebral palsy.

The occupational therapist has many opportunities to enhance the life of a person with cerebral palsy. Activities of daily living (ADL) skills are a main focus for intervention. ADLs need to be addressed in a developmental progression over the lifetime of a client with cerebral palsy, starting with basic dressing and mobility skills, progressing to more complex tasks such as toileting issues, and then on to more adult skills such as driving and meal preparation. Accessibility should be considered along with ADL training. The occupational therapist can play an important part in educating the child and family about universal design, and providing resources to help them plan for current and future needs. Technology for seating and positioning, environmental control, and communication are areas that often need to be addressed with this population. Although some children ambulate with braces, they may have difficulty with locomotion skills in the community. As these children get older and larger, ambulation may become less efficient as a primary means of mobility.

Children with cerebral palsy can exhibit delayed developmental skills. They often lack normal environmental opportunities that other children experience in addition to the possible neurological causes of developmental delay. Perceptual skills, fine motor coordination, play skills, body awareness, and social skills are possible areas of weakness for the child with cerebral palsy. They are also often at risk for low self-esteem and emotional problems.

Contextual Considerations

Clinical

The clinical evaluation should include information regarding the sensorimotor status, musculoskeletal, developmental status, and daily living skills of the child. The sensorimotor status provides information on the child's potential for independence by providing insight on the child's motor abilities and neurological status. A good understanding of the child's sensorimotor abilities may assist in determining the future potential of the child and the extent of adaptive equipment or modifications that he or she may require. Knowing the developmental level of any child receiving services is important to plan treatment activities. Because a large percentage of children with cerebral palsy will also demonstrate developmental, sensory, or other delays, it is important to consider these areas when performing the evaluation. One of the difficult challenges the therapist may face is finding an appropriate tool that can measure these skills without being heavily influenced by a child's motor impairment. Information on ADLs will provide insight on how the physiological and developmental skills are affecting the child's functioning and on how the family is coping.

The physiological evaluation includes information on the range of motion, muscle tone, strength and sensation of the upper extremities, trunk, and lower extremities. Since there are many different presentations of cerebral palsy, the therapist needs to identify the area or areas most affected. Then, the therapist needs to be able to identify the type of muscle tone involvement. It is sometimes difficult to differentiate between problems of spasticity, contracture, and dystonia, or distinguish hypotonia from weakness. It is also very important to look at reflex integration and determine its impact on functional performance. For example, a child who has not integrated the grasp reflex may have difficulty voluntarily releasing objects from the hand. Balance reactions and postural control are also key skills to evaluate.

Sensory impairment is often associated with cerebral palsy, especially in the hemiplegic population. The degree of sensory impairment is related to functional potential and spontaneity of use for the involved limb. It is especially important to evaluate sensation pre-operatively if upper extremity surgical intervention is being considered. Evaluation of two-point discrimination and stereognosis are frequently used to evaluate sensation.

The hemiplegic child poses a challenge for functional assessment because hemiplegia is a unilateral problem that typically affects the non-dominant extremity. Many upper extremity assessments either evaluate dominant unilateral function or the accomplishment of a specific skill. It is helpful to evaluate the involved extremity for its functional use as an assist to the dominant extremity. The best way to assess functional use is by informal observation during functional activities and assessment of the various degrees of thumb and palm deformity, a problem often associated with cerebral palsy due to muscular imbalance around the thumb (House et al, 1981).

There are many developmental assessments available. A general developmental assessment such as the *Peabody Developmental Motor Scales–2* (PDMS–2; Folio & Fewell, 2000); *Hawaii Early Learning Profile*™ (HELP; Furuno, O'Reilly, Hosake, Zeisloft, & Allman, 1984), or the *Learning Accomplishment Profile Revised Edition* (LAP-R; Glover, Preminger, & Sanford, 1988), will provide information for the infant or preschool aged child. Modifications may be necessary for children with significant motor involvement, and in some cases some tests will not be able to be used at all. The *Carolina Curriculum for Handicapped Infants and Infants at Risk* (Johnson-Martin, Jens, Attermeier, & Hacker, 1991); the *INFANIB* (Ellison, 1994); *Erhardt Developmental Prehension Assessment-Revised* (Erhardt, 1982b); *Erhardt Developmental Vision Assessment* (Erhardt, 1982a); or the *Pediatric Evaluation of Disability Inventory* (PEDI; Haley, Coster, Ludlow, Haltiwanger, & Andrellos, 1992) may be more appropriate for children with more significant motor impairment.

Children of school age can be evaluated using an assessment of visual motor skills, perceptual skills, and fine and gross motor coordination. Common assessments include the *Beery-Buktenica Developmental Test of Visual Motor Integration* (Beery, 1997); the *Motor-Free Visual Perception Test–Revised* (MVPT; Collarusso & Hammill, 1995); the *Test of Visual Perceptual Skills* (TVPS; Gardner, 1997); the *Jebsen Hand Function Test* (Jebsen, Taylor, Trieschmann, Trotter, & Howard, 1969); the *Melbourne Assessment of Unilateral Upper Limb Function—Revised* (Randall & Johnson, 1995); *Quality of Upper Extremity Skills Test* (QUESTl; DeMatteo, Law, Russell, Pollack, Rosenbaum, &Walter, 1992); the *Bruininks-Osteretsky Test of Motor Proficiency* (Bruininks, 1978); the *Gross Motor Functional Measure* (GMFM) (Russell, et al., 1989) and the *Pediatric Evaluation of Disability Inventory* (PEDI; Haley et al., 1992). It may be necessary to modify or eliminate use of some of the evaluations of motor coordination for children with more significant motor impairment.

A developmental ADL checklist can be helpful for children under the age of three, but these assessments often do not accommodate the child with a physical limitation. A rehabilitation-based checklist may incorporate the use of adaptive equipment. The *Functional Independence Measure*™ (FIM; State University of New York, 1993) and the *Functional Independence Measure for Children*™ (Wee-FIM; Hamilton & Granger, 1991) provides information on many areas and is often used in research. This type of assessment groups many skills together, which can affect its sensitivity to discreet functional changes and its usefulness in short-term treatment. The *School Function Assessment* (SFA; Coster, Deeney, Haltiwanger, & Haley, 1998) is an interview-based instrument that is useful in the examination of ADL and school-related functional skills.

Since children with cerebral palsy often display oral-motor impairment, any ADL assessment should address oral motor skills, such as lip closure, jaw and tongue control, as well as hand to mouth coordination. When evaluating ADL skills by taking a caregiver report, the interviewer can also use the opportunity to establish rapport with the caregiver, and gather data regarding other aspects of the family context as discussed below.

Family

The family values, priorities, and cultural preferences must always be considered. Information can be gathered using an informal interview. Open-ended questions may be more helpful than a yes/no checklist. This approach helps to establish a rapport and may gain information that might otherwise be overlooked. For example, "Tell me about a typical day," with supporting questions such as "Does anybody help you get dressed?" or "What kinds of food do you like to eat?" can provide information on family routines in addition to ADLs.

Families of children with cerebral palsy often express challenges coping with their own extended family, and with community reactions to their disability. It is especially difficult for children and adolescents to deal with problems associated with oral motor dysfunction. Drooling, unclear speech, and difficulty chewing and swallowing can be difficult to accept in a public or community environment. Children with cerebral palsy may have very obvious gait deviations, or may rely on adaptive devices such as crutches, walkers, or wheelchairs to get around in the community. This poses problems with accessibility and may limit their opportunities for interaction with non-disabled peers.

Children with cerebral palsy may have different needs for assistive devices during the transition from young childhood, to school-aged childhood, to adolescence, and to adulthood. The therapist needs to help the family and child determine what works best in each situation. The occupational therapist also needs to demonstrate sensitivity while gathering information about family resources, including medical coverage, formal and informal support groups, and information/educational resources. The occupational therapist can be a primary or secondary provider of information about coverage for medical expenses, support groups, special education, and rehabilitation laws. The information gathered may indicate that the family would like and benefit from referral to other professionals, agencies, or community programs for supportive help or additional resources.

The occupational therapist must be aware of future needs in order to provide the guidance necessary for addressing current needs. The family of the child who requires medical equipment such as wheelchairs, positioning equipment, orthotics, and splints must be made aware of reimbursement issues for medical equipment. Many third party payers (insurance, medical assistance) will provide services on a limited basis, provide one-per-lifetime coverage, or not cover durable medical equipment. The occupational therapist providing services individually or as part of a team can help select the appropriate equipment. The family may need information on alternate funding sources to help with expenses not covered by the family's insurance plan.

Practice Setting

Individuals with cerebral palsy often require occupational therapy in an acute care hospital, rehabilitation hospital, rehabilitation outpatient facility, early intervention, and school-based settings. In all of these settings, the occupational therapist functions as a member of multidisciplinary teams comprised of professionals from disciplines such as developmental neurology, orthopedic medicine, nursing, physical therapy, social work, psychology, therapeutic recreation, speech language pathology, and special education. Family members and other primary caregivers are also involved. Parents may be confused about the roles of the various professionals involved in their child's care and that confusion may be compounded if the child is receiving services from different settings simultaneously. It is important to establish and maintain communication between therapists, family, and other members of the team to ensure consistency of care and facilitate transitions between service settings as the child matures.

The acute care therapist may first encounter the individual with cerebral palsy in the neonatal nursery or through the high-risk follow-up programs. The parents should be provided with education and information about arranging therapy needs in the community. The occupational therapist must work with other professionals to assist the family with coping and preparing for a child with special needs. Positioning and handling techniques are important for caregivers to know in order to reduce spasticity and facilitate functional ability. The best source of information is *Handling the Young Child with Cerebral Palsy at Home* (Finnie, 1997). These children may also be prone to oral-motor difficulties that impair feeding abilities. The therapist should have special training or knowledge to provide intervention related to oral-motor skills. In some settings the speech therapist may be responsible for oral motor intervention.

The rehabilitation hospital-based occupational therapist often provides therapy services for a specific period of time following a surgical procedure, or for specific rehabilitation goals. For example, a child may have a rehabilitation admission for post-operative rehabilitation, ADL training, or adaptive equipment training. Occupational therapists and other members of the rehabilitation team would provide coordinated intervention for the identified needs. A clinical follow-up program may be based at the rehabilitation hospital. Periodic follow-up is important for children with cerebral palsy. As they grow and develop, there is potential for problems associated with joint contractures and deformity from muscle imbalances. The clinic-based therapist in the rehabilitation hospital should also be able to assist the child and family with transitioning to an adult setting for needed services.

The outpatient-based occupational therapist often provides ongoing services to help the child develop gross motor, fine motor, perceptual, visual motor, social, play, sensory processing, ADL, and oral-motor skills. The therapist may also make recommendations and facilitate the acquisition of special equipment. Since the child is often seen only once a week, the development of home programs that are designed to be implemented by parents and caregivers is essential for the child's ongoing developmental progress.

Occupational therapists working in an early intervention program may provide home-based and/or community-based services. The focus of intervention would be working in partnership with the family, fostering skills that enable the child to participate within the family and their community. The therapist works with the family to enhance gross and fine motor skills, visual motor and perceptual skills, play skills, sensory processing, oral motor, and ADL skills which impact the child's daily routines and school readiness. Therapists in this setting may also be involved with seating and positioning issues, and using assistive technology to facilitate communication and environmental access.

The school-based therapist provides therapy with an emphasis on skills needed in the school environment. The school therapist can work collaboratively with the rehabilitation or outpatient-based therapist as well as the classroom teacher in order to establish educationally relevant intervention plans. The focus of the school therapist in accordance with the Individuals with Disabilities Education Act (IDEA, 1997) is to be a supportive service to enable full participation in the school program and successful transition to adulthood. The child with cerebral palsy may experience perceptual and visual motor delays, as well as sensory processing problems. These may interfere with mobility, social skills, self-care, and the ability to manage school-related tools and supplies. In order for the child to participate in all aspects of the educational process with non-disabled peers, a variety of assistive technologies may be required. Therapists need to collaborate with technological support personnel and other members of the team in the development of high-tech and low-tech strategies for proper seating and positioning, environmental access, mobility, and communication.

Sociopolitical

There are three primary laws that relate to children with cerebral palsy. The laws relate to education, rehabilitation, and accessibility. The Individuals with Disabilities Education Act (IDEA, 1997) mandates that all children are entitled to a free and appropriate education in the least restrictive environment. The Rehabilitation Act ensures the equal rights of individuals with disabilities in all institutions, agencies, or organizations that receive federal funding or financial assistance. The Americans with Disabilities Act (ADA, 1997) guarantees equal opportunities for employment, accessibility, transportation, and government services. Additional legislation includes the Technology Act and Vocational Rehabilitation Service Act (Technology Related Assistance for Individuals with Disabilities Act, 1988; Vocational Rehabilitation Service Act, 1973).

The child with cerebral palsy has a legal right to be educated with his non-disabled peers. He has the right to appropriate technology to help him benefit from his education, with the goal of participating in the mainstream of society following completion of his educational program. When the child is 14 years old, the IDEA mandates the development of a plan that facilitates the transition from school to work. The school-based transition plan encompasses community living, employment, and socialization, and is informed by the abilities, interests, needs, and goals of the student. Vocational rehabilitation services mandated by the Vocational Rehabilitation Service Act assist the child with cerebral palsy to enter the world of work after completing school.

Lifestyle/Lifespan

It is important to help the individual and the family to be aware of issues that will be faced throughout the lifetime of an individual with cerebral palsy. These issues may relate to the financial, medical, family, and social aspects of life. The following table highlights the issues discussed below. Although the issues are discussed separately, there is often overlap.

Table 6.4
Accessibility Issues in Various Environments

Accessibility	Financial	Medical	Family	Social
Home	Daily supplies and medicine	Surgery to enhance function, prevent or correct deformity	Increased time for daily care	Interaction with peers
School	Home modifications	Require periodic follow-up for issues of growth and new equipment	Coping	Adaptive Sports
Community	Durable medical equipment	Medications to manage muscle tone	Sibling relationships	Leisure activities
Driving/ Transportation	Special driving/ transportation equipment or needs		Care of caregivers	

Accessibility issues for home modifications for a child with a cerebral palsy often include assistive devices to maximize function. For example, a buttonhook, tub transfer bench, positioning equipment, or a wheelchair may facilitate independence. Extensive home modifications may be necessary for a child with significant motor involvement. Specialized evaluation, training, and adaptations may be needed for driving. Some adolescents or young adults may not have the potential for driving but may require special equipment such as a van with a wheelchair lift for transport.

Financial issues will vary depending on the family's economic resources. Insurance may not cover the cost of some supplies, and this will affect household budgets. It is important to remember that families generally meet needs based on priorities for survival, with food and shelter being first on the list. Clothing and daily medical equipment may come next. Insurance reimbursement often has limitations, and money for medical equipment, adaptive equipment, and orthosis may have to be found. The occupational therapist needs to be aware of resources for the family, and about equipment that can "grow" with the child to promote maximum use during the child's growing years. Children with cerebral palsy may also change the focus of their needs as they grow. It is important to recognize that the use of equipment may vary over the lifetime of the child.

The child with mild cerebral palsy is often able to participate in typical community programs with minimal adaptations. Encouragement to participate in sports will be beneficial to the child for physical fitness and peer relationships. Children with more severe involvement may require specialized programs or accommodations to participate in sports or other community activities.

Clinical Decision Making Process

Defining Focus for Intervention

The practice setting helps to determine the focus of intervention. For example, the child in a school setting may require intervention for the development of visual perceptual skills, handwriting, fine motor and bilateral hand coordination, and self-care skills related to the school environment. Home-based activity programs based on an assessment of ADL status, range of motion (ROM), strength, motor coordination, cognitive abilities, perceptual status, social skills, and adaptive equipment requirements may be needed in a hospital setting. Children with cerebral palsy may benefit from short rehabilitation admissions or outpatient services to work on ADL skills. These admissions may be required periodically as the child is developmentally able to take on more responsibility for self-care. Transfers, wheelchair mobility, dressing, and bathing are some of the skills that are typical targets for intervention.

The age and developmental level of the child indicates the nature of intervention services. Family education and support, with a focus on the developmental and physical needs of the child, is paramount for the newly diagnosed infant with cerebral palsy. In the preschool years, environmental exploration and mobility issues often need to be addressed. Independent mobility, with or without assistive devices, has a positive impact on a disabled child's cognitive and emotional well being. As noted above, the school-aged child may need intervention related to learning difficulties or visual perceptual impairment. Self-care skills usually need ongoing attention across the life span.

The advent of adolescence presents physical, social, and emotional challenges for the child with cerebral palsy. Weight gain and growth can exacerbate mobility problems. Individuals who have ambulated with lower extremity braces as young children may find that they are unable to continue as functional community ambulators and may need to use a wheelchair. Unless appropriate adaptations are made, children with cerebral palsy may have fewer opportunities for interaction with the community. The adolescent with cerebral palsy is at risk of becoming isolated and demoralized at the stage where the development of peer networks and feelings of personal competence are crucial. Successful transition to adulthood may depend on the development of competence in home management skills, community mobility, and peer interactions. Strategies such as adapting a van for transportation, pet assisted living, involvement in church, and community and/or special interest groups may facilitate the transition to adulthood.

Establishing Goals for Intervention

The setting in which services are being delivered often dictates the amount of time available for service provision and defines the scope of intervention. The chronological and developmental age of the child also influences the goals that are established. It is important to consider the normal developmental progression, the functional level of the child when establishing goals and the needs and interests of the child and the family. The neuromuscular and physical data from the evaluation, combined with information on cognitive and perceptual skills, will help to define treatment goals. For example, a child with moderate cerebral palsy and minimal cognitive deficits may learn to use a power wheelchair for independent mobility; however, a child with moderate cerebral palsy and severe cognitive limitations may be dependent on a caregiver for transport in a manual wheelchair. Family attitudes, cultural practices, and values need to be considered. The physical environment is also an important consideration. Accessibility issues may influence the priority of a goal or dictate the level of independence that is realistic to expect. For example, if the child uses a wheelchair for mobility and is unable to access the bathroom, independent hygiene for tooth brushing may not be possible. Sociopolitical factors and lifestyle implications may also influence treatment goals. Reimbursement issues and relevant legislation may dictate the length or frequency of treatment and the consequent prioritization of treatment goals.

Goals are also based on medical intervention that the child receives. The child may have surgical intervention to improve range of motion and balance the function of a joint. An example would be lengthening or release of a muscle such as the adductor pollicus brevis and transfer of the flexor carpi ulnaris to the extensor carpi radialus brevis to facilitate thumb and wrist extension to enhance the grasp of objects. Post-operative management would include scar management, splinting, range of motion, muscle strengthening, muscle re-education, and functional skill training.

Designing Theory-Based Intervention

There are many theoretical frameworks in occupational therapy that can be used to provide services for children with cerebral palsy. Intervention and treatment is usually based on clinical decisions that integrate parts of many different theories. The following descriptions and examples of how different theories might be applied should not be considered an all-inclusive list.

Many treatment approaches are informed by the model of human occupation (Kielhofner, 2002), which focuses on the development and maintenance of the roles and behaviors associated with daily routines and consistent with the values of the individual. This approach assists the therapist in developing intervention strategies that are relevant to, and facilitative of, the child's myriad role requirements as sibling, student, son, daughter, worker, and/or community member.

Developmental theories and/or frames of reference focus on the patterns of skill acquisition as progressive and predictable. Children with cerebral palsy face many obstacles and interruptions in the development of skills related to the primary motor problems and secondary associated conditions. The therapist employs an understanding of normal development to assist the child in the design of treatment programs that provide for the progressive acquisition of the skills that are the substrate for functional activity. Other useful approaches include neurodevelopmental therapy and sensory integration. Neurodevelopmental treatment is a sensorimotor approach that is often the approach of choice for the child with cerebral palsy, although studies have not firmly established its effectiveness (Sharkey, 2002). Handling techniques and positioning principles are used to influence the sensorimotor system and foster the development of postural control, equilibrium and righting reactions, and a larger repertoire of movement patterns. In this approach, sensory input is used to prepare the body for the movement, facilitate the use of weak muscles, inhibit muscles with increased tone, and increase the variety of movement patterns. Examples of sensory input include tapping for facilitation of a muscle, weight bearing for co-contraction, and neutral warmth for inhibition of a muscle. Neurodevelopmental techniques are used to facilitate the development of motor skills in the child and to help a caregiver position the child to complete daily care needs.

Sensory integration is another theoretical approach that may be helpful when working with this population. There may be associated sensory processing problems with sensory registration and modulation as well as sensory defensiveness displayed with these children. Sensory integration treatment principles are often helpful when combined with neurodevelopmental therapy techniques.

Children with cerebral palsy also may benefit from treatment based on the rehabilitation or biomechanical frame of reference perspectives as a part of their therapy program. The rehabilitation frame of reference focuses on the performance of activities of daily living using compensatory methods, technology, and environmental adaptations (Dutton, 1995). Occupational therapy intervention may include the use of splints and serial casting to improve range of motion to mitigate limitations of motor function. It may also include adaptive techniques and assistive devices, such as pencil grips, soap holders, and adapted eating utensils to compensate for these limitations. The biomechanical frame of reference considers how range of motion, muscle strength, and endurance are related to the completion of purposeful activities (Dutton, 1995). These approaches are helpful in addressing the physical limitations presented by the child with cerebral palsy, and should be used in combination with other approaches that consider the other sensory and motor impairments that often co-exist in children with cerebral palsy.

Motor learning theories are also used in treatment approaches for children with cerebral palsy. Treatment is based on structured practice and feedback, fostering the development and refinement of specific motoric patterns such as grasp patterns. It may also develop motor behaviors, such as writing, which incorporate clusters of motor patterns.

Learning theory and rehabilitation theory are often combined to teach the child with cerebral palsy activities of daily living. For example, it may be necessary to break a task such as buttoning into small steps that are taught sequentially, and use an assistive device to achieve independence with buttoning.

In conclusion, treatment would be based on several theories that foster the development of roles and occupations, motor skills, and functional skills, plus developmental and learning principles. A treatment session may begin with handling techniques from neurodevelopmental therapy to prepare for movement that increases range of motion. Then, the biomechanical frame of reference may be employed through the use of strengthening strategies to support postural control and increase the variety of movement patterns. Once postural control is established, reaching into a shirtsleeve (for the development of activities of daily living from the rehabilitation frame of reference) may be the first step to donning a pullover shirt. The activity may be approached using learning perspectives to introduce the task in small parts. Learning to don a shirt and complete activities of daily living are roles/occupations of a growing child and part of the occupational behavioral theoretical models.

Evaluating Progress

Meeting established goals (usually annual long-term and short-term objectives) is the most tangible method of evaluating progress. Measurable goals typically focus on improving motor abilities and enhancing developmental skills, including self-care and the integration and use of appropriate equipment or technology in the child's daily life. In the clinic setting, repeated measures such as the *Functional Independence Measure for Children* (Hamilton & Granger, 1991) or the *Pediatric Evaluation of Disability Inventory* (PEDI); Haley et al., 1992) will help to monitor the changes that occur over time. Videotaping can be a powerful tool to evaluate subtle progress that is not measurable on standardized tests. Family and caregivers can also provide insight into significant or less significant improvements by reporting changes in the child's behavior or accomplishments at home. For example, positive changes in the child's mood or temperament, increases in the incidents of successful coping behaviors, or the increased ease with which a parent can dress a child may be indicative of improvement.

Determining Change in or Termination of Treatment

Change in or termination of treatment is warranted when the child does not appear to be capable of meeting an established goal, or when the child has met an established goal. In either event, the therapist needs to re-evaluate the situation to determine whether the goals should be modified or replaced. The new goal could reflect a change of focus or an adjustment in the expected outcome. Sometimes a particular treatment technique doesn't work for a child. For example, using a therapy ball to develop balance and righting reactions and to help inhibit or facilitate muscle tone and movement patterns is a very commonly used practice. If a child happens to be gravitationally and posturally insecure, he or she may be terrified of being on the ball, and another method of treatment may need to be found. Or, the treatment of sensory processing issues may need to proceed before work can be done with balance and righting reactions. Discharge from therapy may occur when the child has reached a maximum level of independence for his or her age and the child has acquired a sufficient level of foundational skills to promote independent problem solving and future skills acquisition.

Occupational therapy may be episodic during the child's lifetime. Occupational therapy may be reinstated when the child is old enough to learn a new skill, or learn the use of new or different technology. Times of transition or change in a child's life may also require therapy services to be modified or techniques to be changed.

Case Study

Description

Mark is a five-year-old with cerebral palsy, presenting with moderate left spastic hemiplegia. He ambulates independently with a molded ankle foot orthosis (MAFO) and an abnormal gait. Mark has a history of febrile seizures. He was the product of a full term pregnancy with a complicated delivery. He has a night splint for wrist, thumb, and finger extension and a day splint for wrist extension. The left upper extremity is used as a gross active assist for task specific activities. Protective reactions on the left are delayed, and righting and equilibrium reactions are impaired. Passive range of motion is limited in the end ranges of thumb abduction, supination, and elbow extension. Active range of motion is limited for shoulder external rotation, shoulder abduction and flexion, elbow extension, wrist extension, supination, and thumb extension. He can grossly extend his fingers to grasp and release an object with a weak grasp and demonstrates poor active assistance. Sensation is difficult to assess due to his age, however, it appears to be diminished. A flexor synergy posture is observed, and intensifies with energy and emotion.

Mark is in a preschool program and will transition into a school-based kindergarten program next fall. He is doing well, with visual motor and visual perceptual skill development scores in the 25th percentile on the *Beery-Buktenica Developmental Test of Visual-Motor Integration* (Beery, 1997). Fine motor skills are limited for bilateral tasks. He has difficulty with the use of scissors, buttoning, and zippers.

Mark lives with his mother, father, and younger sister in a two-story house. Mark is able to ascend and descend the stairs using a nonreciprocal gait pattern. Mark has friends in the neighborhood and tries to participate in typical preschool activities, but he has difficulty with bicycle riding and ball activities.

Mark requires assistance for dressing. He has difficulty manipulating fasteners and putting on and removing a pullover shirt, socks, and his MAFO. He is able to put on and remove his pants and shoes. Mark receives outpatient occupational therapy services once a week.

Long- and Short-Term Goals

The long-term goal of intervention for Mark is to enable him to increase independence with ADL tasks, for more normal participation with other children in preschool. This will be accomplished by focusing on the following:

1. Increase independence with self-care, in keeping with his peers.
2. Improve passive and active range of motion of the left upper extremity to enhance participation in school, play, and home activities.

3. Foster the development of bilateral hand skills with or without assistive devices in preparation for the tasks of kindergarten.
4. Facilitate socializing and play with neighborhood friends.

The short-term goals of intervention for Mark are:

1. Independently put on and take off pullover shirt, socks, and MAFO splints.
2. Put on and take off a light jacket using an over-the-head method, including zipping and unzipping using a large zipper pull.

Therapist Goals and Strategies

The therapist's goals include:

1. Improve range of motion in the left upper extremity.
2. Improve grasp and release in the left upper extremity.
3. Explore and expand opportunities to play with neighborhood children.

The therapist's strategies include:

1. Improve alignment of shoulder girdle and trunk with positioning and handling techniques to reduce muscle tone.
2. Engage in activities that facilitate righting reactions, equilibrium reactions, and weight shift in upper and lower extremities.
3. Work and discuss with caregivers strategies to increase socializing with peers other than ball and bike settings.
4. On an ongoing basis, evaluate the effects of splint usage.
5. Provide opportunities for carryover to the home and community environment.
6. Break down new tasks into small parts for learning, and teach this approach to caretakers.
7. Incorporate assistive devices as needed for environmental mastery, communication, and socialization.

Activity

Theraplast Ice Cream Cones

Theraputty will be rolled into large balls using both hands. The balls will be placed on top of a therapy cone held like an ice cream cone in the left hand. The right hand will add the "sprinkles" pegs while the left hand holds the cone. The theraplast ice cream cones will be made by Mark and offered to the therapist, to Mark's sister, and to his mother. Plans for carryover include Mark helping to organize and work at the ice cream table at the block party being planned in the neighborhood.

Treatment Objective

Mark will sustain grasp on an object with his left hand while manipulating the object with his dominant right hand.

Resources

The following resources can be helpful for gathering clinical data:

Physiological Data:

- Manual muscle test
- Active and passive range of motion
- Sensation
- Reflex testing
- Assessment of muscle tone
- Motor coordination

Developmental Assessments for 0–5 years:

- *Peabody Developmental Motor Scales–2*
- *Hawaii Early Learning Profile*
- *Pediatric Developmental Inventory*
- *Learning Accomplishment Profile–revised*
- *Carolina Curriculum for Handicapped Infants and Infants at Risk*
- *Movement Assessment of Infants*
- *Erhardt Developmental Assessment of Prehension*
- *Erhardt Developmental Assessment of Vision*

School-aged assessments:

- *Berry Test of Visual Motor* Skills
- *Gardner Test of Visual Perceptual Skills*
- *Motor-Free Visual Perception Test*
- *Bruininks-Osteretsky Test of Motor Proficiency*
- *Jebsen Test of Upper Limb Function*
- *Melbourne Assessment of Unilateral Upper Limb Function–revised*
- *School Function Assessment*
- *Gross Motor Functional Measure* (GMFM)

Activities of Daily Living:

- *Functional Independence Measure*
- *Functional Independence Measure for Children*

The following resources can be helpful for gathering family data:

Informal interview with open ended questions

Financial resources

Awareness of culture, value, priorities

Daily routines

The following are common practice settings:

Acute hospitalization

Neonatal intensive care unit (NICU)

Rehabilitation hospital (inpatient or outpatient)
Outpatient rehabilitation services
Community-based (early intervention, preschool, and school)

The following resources can be helpful for gathering sociopolitical data:

Individuals with Disabilities Education Act (IDEA) Amendments of 1997
Americans with Disabilities Act (ADA)
Rehabilitation Act
Vocational Rehabilitation Service Act
Technology-Related Assistance for Individuals with Disabilities Act
Medical Assistance
Disability (SSI)

The following can be helpful in understanding and managing lifestyle/lifespan issues:

Accessibility evaluation

- Home
- School
- Community

Evaluation of financial need for:

- Daily supplies and medicine
- Durable medical equipment
- Home modifications
- Transitioning to adulthood

Medical needs

- Regulation of tone via medication or surgery
- Nutrition and growth
- Orthopedic care
- Surgical correction or prevention of deformity
- Neurological care

Family needs

- Coping skills
- Increased time for daily care
- Sibling relationships
- Caregiver

Social requirements

- Interaction with peers
- Adaptive sports
- Leisure skills
- Self-esteem/confidence

Internet Resources

United Cerebral Palsy Association (UCPA):
www.ucpa.org

American Academy for Cerebral Palsy & Developmental Medicine (AACPDM):
http://aacpdm.org/

National Institute of Neurological Disorders and Stroke (NINDS):
www.ninds.nih.gov

National Information Center for Children and Youth with Disabilities (NICHCY):
www.nichcy.org

Council for Exceptional Children:
www.cec.sped.org

IDEA Partnerships/IDEA Law:
www.ideapractices.org

American Occupational Therapy Association:
www.aota.org

Neuro-Developmental Treatment Association (NDTA):
www.ndta.org

Alliance for Technology Access:
www.ataccess.org

National Disability Sports Alliance:
www.ndsaonline.org

References

Alexander, R., Boehme, R., Cupps, B., & Kliebhan, L. (1987). Motor development in cerebral palsy. In R. Boehm (Ed.), *Approach to treatment of the baby* (pp. 5–14). Milwaukee, WI: Boehm Workshops.

Beery, K. (1997). *Beery-Buktenica developmental test of visual-motor integration* (4th ed.). Parsippany, NJ: Modern Curriculum Press.

Bierman, J., (1991). *Lecture notes from 8-week pediatric NDT certification course.* Augusta, GA.

Boehme, R., (1987a). *The hypotonic child: Treatment for postural control, endurance, strength, and sensory organization.* Milwaukee, WI: Boehm Workshops.

Boehme, R., (1987b). *Developing mid range control and function in children with fluctuating muscle tone.* Milwaukee, WI: Boehm Workshops.

Bruininks, R. (1978). *Bruininks-Oseretsky test of motor proficiency.* Circle Pines, MN: American Guidance Service.

Callarusso, R. P., & Hammill, D. D. (1995). *Motor-free visual perception test—revised.* Novato, CA: Academic Therapy Publications.

Coster, W., Deeney, T., Haltiwanger, J., & Haley, S. (1998). *School function assessment.* San Antonio, TX: The Psychological Corporation.

DeMatteo, C., Law, M., Russell, D., Pollock, N., Rosenbaum, P., & Walter, S. (1992). *QUEST: Quality of upper extremity skills test.* Hamilton, ON: McMaster University, Neurodevelopmental Clinical Research Unit.

Dutton, R. (1995). *Clinical reasoning in physical disabilities.* Philadelphia: Williams & Wilkins.

Ellison, P. H. (1994). *The INFANIB.* Tucson, AZ: Therapy Skill Builders.

Erhardt, R.P., & Merrill, S. C. (1998). Chapter 29: Neurological Dysfunction in Children. In M. E. Neistadt, & E. B. Crepeau (Eds.), *Occupational therapy* (9th ed.). (pp. 582–608). Philadelphia: Lippincott, Williams & Wilkins.

Erhardt, R. P. (1982a). *Erhardt developmental vision assessment.* Laurel, MD: Ramsco Publishing.

Erhardt, R. P. (1982b). *Erhardt developmental prehension assessment.* Laurel, MD: Ramsco Publishing.

Finnie, N. (1997). *Handling the young child with cerebral palsy at home.* Berwick Upon Tweed, UK: Butterworth-Heinemann.

Folio, R., & Fewell, R. (2000). *Peabody developmental motor scales* (2nd ed.). Austin, TX: Pro-Ed.

Furuno, S., O'Reilly, K.A., Hosake, C.M., Allman, T.L., & Zeisloft, B. (1984). *Hawaii Early Learning Profile* (HELP). Palo Alto, CA: VORT.

Gardner, M. F. (1997). *Test of visual perceptual skills (non-motor).* Hydesville, CA: Psychological and Educational Publications, Inc.

Glover, M. E., Preminger, J. L., & Sanford, A. R. (1988). *The early learning accomplishments profile* (Rev. ed.). Winston-Salem, NC: Kaplan Press.

Gordon, C. Y., Schanzenbacher, K. E., Case-Smith, J., & Carrasco, R. C. (1996). Diagnostic Problems in Pediatrics. In J. Case-Smith, A. S. Allen, & P. N. Pratt (Eds.), *Occupational therapy for children* (3rd ed.). (pp.113–162). St. Louis, MO: Mosby.

Haley, S., Coster, W., Ludlow, L., Haltiwanger, J., & Andrellos, P. (1992). *Pediatric evaluation of disability inventory.* San Antonio, TX: The Psychological Corporation.

Hamilton, B. B., & Granger, C. U. (1991). *Functional independence measure for children (Wee-FIM).* Buffalo, NY: Research Foundation of the State University of New York.

House, J. H, Gwathmey, F. W, & Fidler, M. O. (1981). A dynamic approach to the thumb-in-palm deformity in cerebral palsy. *Journal of Bone and Joint Surgery, 63A,* 216–225.

Individuals with Disabilities Education Act (IDEA) Amendments of 1997 (P.L. No. 105–17). U. S. C., 1400.

Jebsen, R.H., Taylor, N., Trieschmann, R.B., Trotter, M.J., & Howard, L.A. (1969). An objective and standardized test of hand function. *Archives of Physical Medicine and Rehabilitation. 50,* 311–319.

Johnson-Martin, N., Jens, K. G., Attermeier, S. M., & Hacker, B. (1991). *The Carolina Curriculum for Handicapped Infants and Infants at Risk.* Baltimore: Brooks.

Keilhofner, G., (2002). *Model of human occupation, third edition.* Baltimore: Lippincott.

Randall, M., & Johnson, L. (1995). *The Melbourne assessment of unilateral upper limb function—revised.* Victoria, Australia: Royal Children's Hospital.

Ratanawongsa, B. (2001). *Cerebral palsy.* Retrieved January 24, 2003, from http://www.emedicine.com/neuro/topic533.htm

Russell, D.J., Rosenbaum, P.L., Cadman, D.T., Gowland, C., Hardy, S., Jarvis, S. (1989). The Gross motor function measure: A means to evaluate the efforts of physical therapy. *Developmental Medicine and Child Neurology,* 31, 341–352.

Scherzer, A. L., & Tscharnuter, I. (1982). *Early diagnosis and therapy in cerebral palsy.* New York: Marcel Dekker, Inc.

Sharkey, M. A. (2002). The debate: NDTA & AACPDM, Neuro-developmental treatment for cerebral palsy: Is it effective? *NDTA Network Newsletter, 9(5),* 1–9.

State University of New York. (1993). *Functional independence measure (FIM).* Buffalo, NY: Author.

Technology Related Assistance for Individuals with Disabilities Act (1988). Public Law 100–407.

Thorogood, C. (2001). *Cerebral palsy.* Retrieved January 24, 2003, from http://www.emedicine.com/pmr/topic24.htm

Vocational Rehabilitation Service Act (1973). Public Law 93–112.

Yasukawa, A. (1992). Upper extremity casting: Adjunct treatment of the child with cerebral palsy. In P. Case-Smith, & C. Pehoski (Eds.), *Development of hand skills in the child* (pp. 111–123). Bethesda, MD: AOTA.

Spina Bifida

7

Meryl S. Cooperman, MS, OTR/L
Roberta T. Ciocco, OTR/L

Synopsis of Clinical Condition

Prevalence

Spina bifida literally means "cleft spine" and is a neural tube defect that occurs in utero as a result of an incomplete closure of the spinal column. According to the Association of Spina Bifida and Hydrocephalus (2002), there are three types of spina bifida:

1. Spina bifida occulta, in which there is bony abnormality of the vertebrae with no damage to the spinal cord. This type is usually undetected and poses no clinical problems.
2. Meningocele, in which the meninges (the protective covering of the spinal cord) have been pushed through the vertebral defect in a sac called the meningocele. In this condition the spinal cord remains intact. Repair can result in little or no damage to the nerve pathways. Functional results for this group are very favorable.
3. Myelomeningocele is the most severe form of spina bifida. In this form, the spinal cord itself protrudes through the vertebral defect. In some cases the resulting sac is covered with skin, but sometimes the tissues and nerves are exposed. Surgery to close a newborn's back is usually performed within 24 hours of birth to minimize the risk of infection. In this population there is certain paralysis but the degree of functional impairment varies according to the level and severity of the defect.

The latter two conditions are considered spina bifida manifesta, and are the focus of this discussion.

Spina bifida occurs in approximately one in every one thousand live births. Within this group there is a 96% incidence of myelomeningocele and only a 4% incidence of meningocele, (National Information Center for Children and Youth with Disabilities, Spina Bifida, 2002).

Common Characteristics and Symptoms

The functional effects of spina bifida include weakness and or paralysis of muscles, loss of sensation, loss of bowel and bladder control, and possible associated neurological conditions. Some of the information in this chapter may also be applied to the pediatric spinal cord population. Although they don't share the associated neurological problems, they do have many commonalities with regard to physical, self-care, and environmental needs.

Frequently, a condition known as hydrocephalus is associated with spina bifida. Hydrocephalus is a buildup of fluid in the brain that if untreated can cause brain damage, seizures, or blindness. This condition is treated by a procedure called VP shunting in which a drain is implanted to divert the excess ventricular fluid to the abdominal cavity. It is not uncommon for children with a shunt to undergo multiple surgical revisions to keep the shunt functioning properly as they grow and develop. Some children with spina bifida also have seizure disorders that require treatment with medication.

Arnold Chiari malformation type II (ACM II) is also a common neurological deformity that is associated with spina bifida. ACM II is characterized by a downward herniation of the cerebellar tonsils and the fourth ventricle at the formen magnum. Approximately half of these children may also have a kink in the medulla, which can cause brainstem or cervical cord compression. ACM II requires surgical intervention, which usually consists of decompression by removing part of the cervical vertebra and the lower part of the skull; shunt placement, and reconstruction of the posterior fossa. Symptoms of ACM II may be serious. The following is a list of some of the symptoms that may occur (Struss, 2001):

Table 7.1
Symptoms of Spina Bifida

Systemic/Autonomic	Sensory	Cognitive	Motor
Apnea	Deafness	Learning disorders	Vocal cord paralysis
Dysphagia	Visual blurring	Language comprehension problems	Articulation problems
Gastroesophogeal reflux	Sensory impairment		Ataxia
Cyanotic episodes			Upper extremity muscle weakness
Slow heart rate			
Vomiting			
Seizures			
Arythmias			

Children with spina bifida and hydrocephalus often experience learning difficulties, low levels of motivation, and visual perception impairment. Nonverbal learning disorders (NLDs) are frequently seen with these children. A child with NLD presents with a specific cluster of neuropsychological, academic, and social emotional characteristics. The primary deficit is in nonverbal reasoning. These children often present with weak visual-spatial and visual discrimination abilities, poor organizational skills, difficulty with abstract and mathematical reasoning, and decreased social competence (Spina Bifida Association of America, 2002). Many children with spina bifida can also exhibit behaviors associated with attention deficit hyperactivity disorder (ADHD). Communication disorders may be present. For instance, the child may use "cocktail speech" or the mimicry of sophisticated language patterns without comprehension.

Recently, it has been discovered that children with spina bifida are prone to latex allergies. This may be due to their increased exposure to latex products from use of catheters and other medical products. Medical suppliers are now producing latex-free products for people who are susceptible to latex allergies. Care should be taken when treating someone with spina bifida to avoid using anything with latex, such as balloons, elastic bandages, and pacifiers.

Children with spina bifida can exhibit various orthopedic problems. Sometimes this is due to their vertebral instability and muscle paralysis. Kyphosis or scoliosis, which is a rounding or curving of the spine, is often a secondary complication of spina bifida. Hip dysplasia and other lower extremity deformities can also occur from muscle imbalances due to partial paralysis. As the child gets older, upper extremity tendonitis is sometimes an associated problem due to the stress and strain put on the arms for mobility and transfers. These children can also be more prone to injury and fracture of their lower extremities due to their lack of sensation and poor body awareness. Sensory loss can also pose other problems for children with spina bifida. They can develop decubitus ulcers, especially as they reach adolescence when weight gain and hormonal changes cause increased pressure over their bony prominences. It is important that these children are aware of safety precautions to avoid burns and abrasions of insensate areas.

Obesity is another frequent problem that children with spina bifida face due to their sedentary lifestyle. Children with spina bifida need to be encouraged to participate in physical activity whenever possible because they lack the benefit of burning calories in the kind of physical play activities that their able-bodied peers enjoy. Urinary tract infections are another common problem for those children who have to rely on self-catheterization. Children and adolescents with spina bifida are at risk for low self-esteem and emotional problems. They also tend to have poor social skills and motivational problems.

Target Areas for Intervention

The occupational therapist has many opportunities to enhance the life of a child, adolescent, or adult with spina bifida. Activities of daily living (ADL) skills are a main focus for intervention. ADLs need to be addressed in a developmental progression over the lifetime of a client with spina bifida, starting with basic dressing and mobility skills, and progressing to more complex tasks such as bowel and bladder management, and then on to more adult skills such as driving and meal preparation. Accessibility should be considered along with ADL training. The occupational therapist can play an important part in educating the child and family about universal design and providing resource information to help them plan for current and future needs. Seating and positioning are also areas that often need to be addressed. Although some children do ambulate with braces, they are often unable to be functional as community ambulators. As these children get older and larger, ambulation usually becomes less efficient as a primary means of mobility.

Children with spina bifida can exhibit delayed developmental skills due to neurological causes and diminished opportunities for environmental exploration. They are at risk for difficulties with visual motor coordination, body awareness, self-esteem, and social emotional adjustment.

Contextual Considerations

Clinical

The clinical evaluation must incorporate information regarding the integrity of the musculoskeletal system and developmental skills acquisition, including activities of daily living. The musculoskeletal integrity, in concert with developmental ability, determines whether the child may be capable of performing life tasks independently, either with adaptive techniques or equipment, or with varying degrees of caregiver assistance. Since children with spina bifida often have accompanying developmental difficulties associated with hydrocephaly in addition to physical limitations, it is important to combine the knowledge of the musculoskeletal status with developmental skills.

The physiological evaluation includes information on the range of motion, muscle strength, and sensation of the upper and lower extremities. The physical therapist on the intervention team can provide detailed information regarding lower extremity status. Lower extremity status is relevant for dressing the lower extremities, bowel and bladder care, skin management, bath and bathing, and transfer techniques.

There are many developmental assessments available. A general developmental assessment such as the *Peabody Developmental Motor Scales–2* (PDMS–2; Folio & Fewell, 2000), *Hawaii Early Learning Profile*™ (HELP; Furuno, O'Reilly, Hosaka, Zeisloft, & Allman, 1984), or *Pediatric Evaluation of Disability Inventory* (PEDI; Haley, Coster, Ludlow, Haltiwanger, & Andrellos, 1992) will provide information for the preschool-aged child.

Children of school age can be evaluated using an assessment of visual motor skills, perceptual skills, and fine motor coordination. Common assessments include the *Beery-Buktenica Developmental Test of Visual-Motor Integration* (Beery, 1997), *Test of Visual Motor Skills–Revised* (Gardner, 1997a), *Test of Visual Perceptual Skill–Non-motor* (Gardner, 1997b), the *Jebsen Hand Function Test* (Jebsen, Trieschmann, Trotter, & Howard, 1969), the *Bruininks-Oseretsky Test of Motor Proficiency* (Bruininks, 1978), the *Pediatric Examination of Educational Readiness-Revised* (PEER; Levine & Schneider, 1983) and *Pediatric Examination of Educational Readiness at Middle Childhood–Revised* (Levine, 1985). It may be necessary to modify some of the evaluations of motor coordination due to the child's physical limitations.

A thorough evaluation of ADL skills needs to incorporate skin checks and self-management of the bowel and bladder, in addition to the areas of dressing, feeding, hygiene, and grooming. A developmental ADL checklist can be helpful for young children (under 3). However, these assessments often do not accommodate a child with physical limitations. An adult rehabilitation- based checklist may incorporate transfer skills, skin checks, and the use of adaptive equipment. The *Functional Independence Measure*™ *(FIM;)* Hamilton & Granger, 1991b) and *Functional Independence Measure for Children*™ (Wee-FIM; Hamilton & Granger, 1991a) provide information on many areas and are often used in research. These assessments group many skills together, which make them insensitive to smaller changes when used for short durations and for goal setting. When evaluating ADL skills by caregiver or self-report, the interview should be structured to help establish a rapport and learn more about the family, as discussed in the following section.

Family

The family values, priorities, and cultural preferences must be considered. It is often possible to gather information using an informal interview with a few key questions. Open-ended questions may be more helpful than a yes/no checklist and help to establish rapport. For example, "Tell me about a typical day," with supporting questions such as, "What time do you wake up?" or "Does anybody help you get dressed?" or "What do you usually eat for breakfast/lunch/dinner?" can provide information on family routines in addition to ADLs.

The occupational therapist needs to demonstrate sensitivity while gathering information about family resources, including medical coverage, formal and informal support groups, and information or educational resources. The occupational therapist can be a primary or secondary provider of information about coverage for medical expenses, special education and rehabilitation laws, and care of the caregivers. The information gathered may indicate the need for a social service referral to assist in accessing counseling services and other forms of support in the community.

The occupational therapist must be aware of future needs in order to provide the guidance necessary for addressing current needs. The occupational therapist can help select a wheelchair that can grow with the child, to minimize costs for the family. The family of the child who requires medical equipment such as wheelchairs, shower/bath chairs, etc., must be made aware of the criteria for reimbursement. Many third-party payers will reimburse services on a limited basis but will not cover durable medical equipment. Medical assistance often covers this type of equipment. The family may need information on medical assistance to help with expenses not covered by the family's insurance plan.

It is important for the occupational therapist to support the concept of back care and proper positioning or lifting techniques for the caregiver. Families with young children may need to prepare themselves as their child grows and requires more assistance with transfers and ADL skills. Families with school-aged and older children with spina bifida may need guidance on using equipment and incorporating improved body mechanics into their care routines.

Practice Setting

Individuals with spina bifida require OT services throughout their lifetimes, in various settings. Occupational therapists may provide services in an acute hospital, rehabilitation hospital, rehabilitation outpatient facility, early intervention, and school-based settings. The occupational therapist functions as a member of a multidisciplinary team that is often comprised of professionals from disciplines such as neurology, orthopedic medicine, nursing, physical therapy, social work, psychology, therapeutic recreation, speech language pathology, and special education. The team also includes family members and other primary caregivers. Parents may be confused about the roles of the various professionals involved in their child's care, and that confusion may be compounded if the child is receiving services in different settings simultaneously. It is important to establish and maintain communication among therapists and other members of the team to ensure consistency of care and facilitate transitions between service settings as the child matures.

The acute care therapist may first encounter the individual with spina bifida in the neonatal intensive care unit (NICU). The child usually requires surgical intervention for the cele (deformity) and hydrocephaly (if present). Initial care may be limited to assisting with positioning and feeding issues. The parents should be provided with education and information about arranging therapy. The occupational therapist must work with other professionals to assist the family with coping and preparing for having a child with special needs.

The rehabilitation hospital-based occupational therapist often provides therapy services for a specific period following a surgical procedure, or for specific rehabilitation goals. For example, a child may have a rehabilitation admission for ambulation issues, activities of daily living, bowel and bladder management, and treatment of skin breakdown. Occupational therapy intervention would focus on environmental adaptation to accommodate for compromised ambulation skills, adaptive seating, personal hygiene aids, and training regarding the prevention and care of skin breakdowns.

The occupational therapist who works in outpatient settings often provides services to facilitate the ongoing development of fine motor, perceptual, visual motor, social, play, and ADL skills. Parent education is an important aspect of the intervention plan since the therapist often sees the child on a weekly or monthly basis.

Occupational therapists working in an early intervention program may provide home-based and/or community-based services focused on the development of gross and fine motor skills, hand skills, perceptual skills, visual motor skills, play skills, and ADL skills. The occupational therapist, in concert with other members of the intervention team, including the family, addresses environmental modifications, ergonomic seating, handling and positioning strategies, and planning for future needs.

The school-based therapist provides therapy with a focus on skills needed to be successful in the classroom. The school therapist can work collaboratively with the rehabilitation or outpatient-based therapist. The focus of the school-based therapist, in accordance with the Individuals with Disabilities Education Act (IDEA), is to be a supportive service to enable full participation in the school program. The child with spina bifida may experience accessibility issues with stairs in the school that affect class participation, perceptual issues that affect handwriting, difficulty with social skills, and dressing issues associated with managing outer garments and clothing for toileting and hygiene associated with toileting.

Sociopolitical

Three primary laws relate to children with spina bifida. The Individuals with Disabilities Education Act (1997) entitled all children to a free and appropriate education in the least restrictive environment and whenever possible with non-disabled peers (IDEA, 1997). The Rehabilitation Act (1972) ensures the civil rights of individuals with disabilities in all institutions, agencies, or organizations that receive federal funding or financial assistance. The Americans with Disabilities Act (ADA; 1991) guarantees equal opportunities for employment, accessibility, transportation, and government services. Additional legislation includes the Technology-Related Assistance for Individuals with Disabilities Act (1988) and Vocational Rehabilitation Service Act (VRSA).

As a consequence of legislation, a child with disabilities may receive occupational therapy and other related services—including supporting technology—in order to be educated with non-disabled peers, with a goal of preparation for life in the mainstream of society. When the child is fourteen years old, the IDEA mandates the development of a plan that facilitates the transition from school to life after school. The school-based transition plan includes community living, employment, and socialization. It is informed by the abilities, interests, needs, and goals of the student. Vocational rehabilitation services mandated by the VRSA assist the child with spina bifida to enter the world of work after completing school.

Federal, state, and local government programs—plus private agencies—may provide financial resources for individuals with spina bifida. Children with spina bifida may qualify for medical assistance based on their disability, not the financial resources of the family. Social Security Income (SSI) may also be available for the child and the family. Home modifications may be supported through programs ranging from Habitat for Humanity to local agencies. Some automobile manufacturers will pay a limited amount for modifications if a new vehicle is purchased. The VRSA will help fund home and vehicle modifications if they are necessary for the individual's employment.

Lifestyle/Lifespan

It is important to help the individual and the family to become aware of the issues that an individual with spina bifida will face throughout life. These include accessibility, financial, medical, family, and social issues. The following chart highlights the issues discussed below.

Table 7.2
Lifestyle/Lifespan Factors

Accessibility	Financial	Medical	Family	Social
Home School Community	Daily supplies for medicine and bowel and bladder Durable medical equipment Home modification Living arrangements for the future	Latex allergy Shunt care Skin management	Increased time for daily care Coping with ongoing medical needs Sibling relationships Care of the caregivers	Interaction with peers Adaptive sports

Many families will learn about accessibility issues in the home and community by encountering obstacles with their child. Individuals with spina bifida often locomote with crutches or a wheelchair. Speed, endurance, management of stairs and curbs, and climbing into and out of family vehicles will be some of the obstacles with which families will need to cope. The needs of the child may change as he or she grows and becomes heavier and needs larger equipment. Families often cope with accessibility issues for young children easily because managing a stroller is a common occurrence. However, as the child with spina bifida grows, the family will have to continue to cope with accessibility beyond the preschool years. The family with a young child with spina bifida may be able to carry the child up and down stairs to a second story bathroom or to enter or exit the family home. As the child grows, if the child is dependent on mobility devices, the family may need to consider home modifications or relocating to an accessible home.

Financial concerns will vary depending on the family's economic resources and the availability of private insurance and government assistance programs. Insurance may not cover the cost of some supplies, and this will affect household budgets. Diapers may be a routine expense that families anticipate with young children, but the child with spina bifida may require diapers for extended years. Diapers and other bowel and bladder supplies are often not covered by insurance. Daycare services, finding a babysitter, and other elements of family life may be more costly. Insurance reimbursement often has limitations, so that the cost of walkers, crutches, wheelchairs, lifts, adapted vans, and home modifications may not be covered. It is important to recognize that the use of equipment may vary over time, depending on the needs and interests of the child and family. The occupational therapist needs to be aware of resources for the family, the cost effectiveness of equipment, and environmental modifications that can "grow" with the child.

Medical issues will need to be addressed beyond the cost factors often associated with medical needs. Coping with the need for hospitalizations related to a shunt or orthopedic deformities will impact the life of the child and the family. Work schedules and family routines will need to be readjusted. If siblings are present, planning requirements will increase.

Latex allergies often result in lifestyle changes for the entire family. The most common latex object is probably the balloon. Parents will need to be advocates for their young children, and learn what toys and objects contain latex. It can be challenging to limit or restrict the exposure to latex in the community since it is often present. The older child with spina bifida and a latex allergy will need to be educated on avoiding and dealing with exposure.

Skin integrity is a very important issue. Young children with spina bifida generally are able to tolerate many positions and often do not experience skin breakdown. As the child grows, several factors increase the risk for skin breakdown. The child may need to learn to perform skin checks, practice pressure relief, and make other lifestyle changes. The onset of puberty results in increased sweat glands and weight changes that translate into an increased risk of skin breakdown. The child and family of the child with spina bifida must cope with these changes in addition to the emotions associated with puberty. Occupational therapists could provide resources for community programs or counseling to help with the adjustment to adolescents.

As caregivers age, it may become challenging to perform some of the daily care tasks of children who do not independently perform ADLs. Caregivers may require training to alleviate or prevent back strain and pain. Parents also may need to engage in long-term planning in the event that they are no longer able to provide care. Siblings may assume some or the entire primary caregiver role as adults or teenagers. When designing home programs for parents, the occupational therapist should consider the need to balance the daily needs of the child with spina bifida with those of siblings. Play activities that engage siblings can help to promote positive family relationships.

Social experience with peer groups in the community is often disrupted due to physical limitations and learning or social differences. Encouragement to participate in adaptive sports will be beneficial to the child for physical fitness and peer relationships.

Clinical Decision Making Process

Defining Focus for Intervention

Visual-perceptual skills, cognitive abilities, handwriting, fine motor and bilateral hand coordination, self-care, and social skills related to the academic environment are often the focus of school-based occupational therapy intervention.

ADL status, range of motion, strength, motor coordination, environmental accessibility, skin integrity, and adaptive equipment may be the focus of hospital-based intervention. Transfers, wheelchair mobility, dressing, bathing, and self-catheterization are typically addressed in short-term rehabilitation admissions or outpatient services.

The other major consideration is the age or timing of intervention. Early in the child's life, parent education, assessment, and facilitation of developmental skills are paramount. Assisting the child in achieving independent mobility takes precedence in the preschool years and impacts the child's feelings of self-efficacy and emotional well being. Most children are capable of independent wheelchair mobility by two years of age. The school-aged child may need intervention related to learning difficulties or visual perceptual impairment. Self-care skills are usually in need of ongoing attention. Putting on lower extremity braces, shoe tying, and self-catheterization can be quite challenging for the spina bifida child with perceptual problems and/or fine motor coordination deficits.

Adolescence brings some additional challenges for the child with spina bifida. Even though ambulation may be effective in the confines of elementary school or home setting, efficient participation in the middle and high school experience often requires the child to adapt to the use of a wheelchair in order to interact with peers in a variety of educational and social activities and reduce the risk of social isolation. Although increased mobility may afford many opportunities, prolonged sitting can foster weight gain and skin lesions. Driver education with adapted vehicles, self-care, and home management skills are target areas for intervention that will foster self-efficacy and independence, and prepare the child for the transition to adulthood. Certainly the occupational therapist also must consider the family and child's interests and needs, in addition to environmental problems and limitations or opportunities that may be guided by regulatory, legislative, or reimbursement situations.

Establishing Goals for Intervention

Depending on the chronological age, developmental age, and functional abilities of the child, the practice setting, and the needs and interests of the primary caregivers, the therapist may consider goals that compensate, remediate, or prevent disability. Although most children learn to tie their shoes around the age of five, a child with significant visual perception impairment may require the use of Velcro® closures to achieve independence in this skill at the expected age. The biomechanical and physical data from your evaluation may help guide goal development. Some of the children will present with a higher thoracic level cele. These children would usually have no sensory or motor preservation in the lower extremities and trunk and tend to have greater orthopedic deformity (i.e., kyphosis, scoliosis, and hip dislocation). Goals for independent mobility are geared towards wheelchair use with a complex seating system to address orthopedic deformities and diminished trunk control. Lower lumbar level celes will indicate little functional impairment of the lower extremities and goals would relate to independent management of orthotics.

Accessibility issues may influence the priority of a goal or dictate the level of achievable independence. For example, if the child's wheelchair does not fit through the cafeteria line, then a goal for the child to be independent in buying his or her lunch and negotiating the cafeteria line may not be appropriate. But engaging the child in preparing his or her own lunch and bringing it to school might be an appropriate and viable solution—one that will develop independence and prevent social isolation. Environmental limitations can provide great opportunities for engaging parents, children, and other involved parties such as teachers and classroom aides to develop relevant and viable treatment goals. The prioritization of goals may be dictated by legislative and reimbursement criteria that establish the focus and frequency of treatment.

Designing Theory-Based Intervention

This population presents with a variety of problems, therefore several theoretical models are applicable. The rehabilitation frame of reference focuses on acquiring ADL skills using compensatory methods, technology, and environmental adaptations (Dutton, 1995). This framework might be used in combination with principles of learning theory when teaching a child who has significant lower extremity paralysis to put on pants. The activity would be broken down into several steps such as putting the pants over the feet, pulling them up to the knees, laying down and rolling side to side to pull them up in the back, and finally buttoning and zippering. These steps might be introduced to the therapy session one or two at a time. Techniques may be modified and/or adaptive equipment may need to be introduced at various steps. Trial and error problem solving is often used to refine the process. Afterward, practice to reinforce the skill would be indicated.

The biomechanical frame of reference is used with individuals with neuromuscular or musculoskeletal problems. This frame of reference is based on principles of physics, physiology, neuroscience, and kinesiology, and is often used in combination with the rehabilitation frame of reference when adaptive equipment is necessary. For example, a complicated seating system may be indicated to provide a child with enough trunk stability and upper extremity use for functional activities. The final seating system design depends on an understanding and application of biomechanical and physiologic concepts inherent to joint position, movement, and fixed deformities.

The developmental frame of reference is certainly relevant to any pediatric population. Children with spina bifida face many obstacles and interruptions in the normal progression or acquisition of skills. The occupational therapist must have a good understanding of normal development in order to develop interventions that remediate or prevent disruption in the progression of developmental skill.

Neurodevelopmental treatment (NDT) is a sensorimotor approach that is used primarily with neurological and motor control problems. Although this approach is widely used with the child with cerebral palsy, handling techniques and positioning principals may be applicable to children with spina bifida. An example of an appropriate use of this frame of reference might be in the case of a child who has poor head control. Frequently, children with spina bifida have hydrocephalus and therefore have difficulty gaining stability because of lower limb and trunk paralysis. NDT handling techniques and positioning principals foster the development of efficient postural adjustments and distal limb movement, on a firm base of central trunk stability.

Sensory integration is another theoretical approach that may be very applicable to this population. Due to neurological involvement, these children often experience sensory processing problems. Problems with sensory registration and modulation, as well as sensory defensiveness, can be exhibited these children.

The model of human occupation (Keilhofner, 2002) focuses on the development and maintenance of roles and associated with daily routines. This approach assists in the development of intervention strategies that are relevant to and facilitative of the child's myriad role requirements and the child's ability to lead a productive and fulfilling life.

Evaluating Progress

Meeting established goals (usually annual long-term goals and short-term objectives) is the most tangible method of evaluating progress. Re-administration of testing may be necessary to evaluate progress in some areas, such as visual perception and visual motor integration. Interviews with the child and family can also provide a measure of progress. Parents usually take notice of new skills that their child is able to demonstrate in the home or community environment. Another measure of progress that is less objective is the adaptation and coping of the child and the family with the disability. Even if the child has not reached a goal of independence with bowel care, for instance, the family may have established a routine that is more comfortable for the child and the caregiver. Another example would be if a child with spina bifida, who is not yet independent with transfers, becomes able to request assistance and provide instruction to the person helping with the transfer.

Determining Change in or Termination of Treatment

Change in or termination of treatment is warranted when the child does not meet the goals established, or has met all the goals established. In either event, the therapist needs to re-evaluate the goals to see if new goals are appropriate. The new goals could represent a change of focus or expect higher levels of independence and function. Discharge from therapy may occur when the child has reached a maximum level of independence for his or her age, and the child has acquired a sufficient level of foundational skills to promote independent problem solving and future skill acquisition. Therapy may also be terminated when the child has reached a plateau of progress.

Occupational therapy may be episodic during the child's lifetime. Occupational therapy may be reinstated when the child is old enough to learn new skills. For example, therapy may be indicated when the child is old enough to learn bowel and bladder management, deal with skin integrity issues, or when he or she transitions from a school to a work environment. Occupational therapy in the elementary school may be discontinued and reinstated when the child transitions to a new school and has new expectations, such as using a locker and dressing and undressing for gym class.

Case Study

Description

Tia is an eight-year-old female with spina bifida. Her motor and sensory level is thoracic-10. She ambulates for exercise only with HKAFOs (Hip-knee-ankle-foot orthoses). She is currently not using her braces because she has a small open sore on her right lateral malleolus. Tia's main means of mobility is her lightweight wheelchair. Tia has a 30-degree thoracic scoliosis. She has worn a body jacket in the past, but she has recently been noncompliant with the brace because it restricts her mobility. Her orthopedic surgeon has agreed to let her try going without the brace for part of the day if her seating system can be redesigned to offer her more support. She currently has a planar seating system that consists of a solid seat and back with lateral trunk supports that are always loose and out of position.

Tia has a shunt for hydrocephalus. She has undergone six surgical revisions. Tia is in the second grade with part-time learning support in a resource room because she has trouble with math and reading. She is functioning at a beginning first-grade level in both areas. Tia also has visual motor and visual perceptual difficulties. She scored in the 16th percentile on the *Beery Developmental Test of Visual Motor Integration*. She has difficulty drawing diagonal lines and she frequently reverses her letters and numbers. On the *Gardner Test of Visual Perceptual Skills* she scored in the 25th percentile. Her lowest scores were on the subtests that involved visual memory, spatial relations, figure ground, and visual closure.

Tia lives with her mom, dad, and younger sister. They live in an older two-story house with wheelchair accessibility problems. The bathroom presents the biggest problem. Mom or dad has to carry Tia into the bathroom and lift her into the tub because the wheelchair doesn't fit into the bathroom. Mom has recently been experiencing back pain. The family has a car for transportation, but they are considering the purchase of a minivan because it is difficult to fit everyone and Tia's equipment into the car. Tia's mom is also having difficulty lifting the wheelchair in and out of the trunk. Tia has a few friends in the neighborhood and school with whom she occasionally plays. Most of her free time is spent playing with her younger sister. She is a very bubbly and engaging child.

Tia is independent in upper extremity dressing. She requires moderate assistance for lower extremity dressing and bathing. She is independent in level surface transfers and she is dependent with bowel and bladder care. Tia is being admitted to a pediatric rehabilitation center for an intense three-week rehab stay.

Long- and Short-Term Goals

The immediate goals of Tia's admission are:

1. Increase Tia's independence with self-care.
2. Complete a seating evaluation and make the appropriate modifications to Tia's seating system.
3. Address Tia's skin issues.
4. Evaluate the home and make recommendations to improve accessibility.

The long-term goal of intervention for Tia is to enable her to increase her independence with ADLs.

The short-term goals of intervention for Tia are:

1. Put on and take off pants and shorts.
2. Put on and take off socks and shoes.
3. Self-catheterize in bed, with setup and moderate assistance.
4. Transfer to a tub bench with a contact guard.
5. Bathe using equipment as necessary, with supervision.
6. Perform skin checks, with supervision.

Therapist Goals and Strategies

The therapist's goals include:

1. Provide recommendations and funding resource information for adaptive equipment.
2. Assist with evaluation and ordering of the new wheelchair seating system.
3. Assist with educating the child and family in independent skin checks.

The therapist's strategies include:

1. Provide opportunities to explore adaptive equipment to facilitate independence.
2. Try different adaptive techniques for positioning Tia's body for dressing activities.
3. Explore different teaching styles and task analyses (such as pictures, verbal cues, lists, and props) to compensate for perceptual deficits.
4. Provide opportunities for repetition and practice.
5. Evaluate the home (in person or through interviews).
6. Instruct the caregivers regarding the home program.

Activity

The Dressing Relay

Tia will navigate through an obstacle course. Skills such as rolling, picking up garments, getting into and out of her wheelchair, transferring to a tub bench, shoe tying, and putting on and taking off articles of clothing (from the dress-up bin) will be incorporated into the course. This activity can be graded over time. Initially, she would start with only a few simple tasks and then more stations with increased complexity would be added. Different skills, such as perceptual motor skills and upper extremity strengthening, could also be incorporated. Techniques will be taught to the mother for carryover into daily routines.

Treatment Objectives

Treatment session objectives may include Tia putting on her pants independently with the correct orientation.

Resources

The following resources can be helpful for gathering clinical data:

Physiological data:

- Manual muscle test
- Active and passive range of motion
- Sensation

Developmental assessments for 0–5 years:

- *Peabody Developmental Motor Scales–2*
- *Hawaii Early Learning Profile*
- *Pediatric Developmental Inventory*

School-aged assessments:

- *Berry Test of Visual Motor Skills*
- *Gardner Test of Visual Perceptual Skills*
- *Bruininks-Oseretsky Test of Motor Proficiency*

- *Jebsen Test of Upper Limb Function*
- *Pediatric Early Elementary Examination–Revised*
- *Pediatric Examination of Educational Readiness at Middle Childhood–Revised*
- *School Function Assessment*

Activities of daily living:

- Checklist
- FIM
- Wee-FIM

The following resources can be helpful for gathering family data:

Informal interview with open-ended questions regarding financial resources, culture, values, priorities, and daily routines.

The following are common practice settings:

Acute hospitalization

NICU

Rehabilitation hospital (inpatient or outpatient)

Outpatient rehabilitation services

Community-based (early intervention, preschool, and school)

The following resources can be helpful for gathering sociopolitical data:

Individuals with Disabilities Education Act (IDEA) Amendments of 1997

Americans with Disabilities Act

Vocational and Rehabilitation Services Act

Technology-Related Assistance for Individuals with Disabilities Act

Medical Assistance

Disability (SSI)

The following can be helpful in managing and understanding lifestyle/lifespan issues:

Accessibility evaluation:

- Home
- School
- Community

Financial needs:

- Daily supplies and medicine
- Durable medical equipment
- Home modifications
- Transitioning to adulthood

Medical needs:

- Latex allergies
- Shunt care
- Skin management
- Bowel and bladder care
- Orthopedic care

Family needs:

- Coping skills
- Increased time for daily care
- Sibling relationships
- Care of the caregiver

Social needs:

- Interaction with peers
- Adaptive sports

Internet Resources

Spina Bifida Association of America:
www.sbaa.org

World Arnold Chiari Malformation Association:
www.pressenter.com/~wacmal/

National Information Center for Children and Youth with Disabilities (NICHCY):
www.nichcy.org

Council for Exceptional Children:
www.cec.sped.org

IDEA Partnerships/IDEA Law:
www.ideapractices.org

American Occupational Therapy Association:
www.aota.org

Published Resources

Sandler, A. (1997). Living with spina bifida: A guide for families and professionals. The University of North Carolina Press.

Lutkenhoff, M, and Oppenheimer, S. G. (Eds). (1997). Spinabilities: A young person's guide to spina bifida. Bethesda, MD. Woodbine House.

References

Americans with Disabilities Act of 1990, Pub. L. No. 101–336, 104.

Association for Spina Bifida and Hydrocephalus. (2002). *What is spina bifida*? Retrieved Dec. 5, 2002, from http://www.asbah.org/whatissb.html

Beery, K. (1997). *Beery-Buktenica developmental test of visual-motor integration* (4th ed.). Parsippany, NJ: Modern Curriculum Press.

Bruininks, R. H. (1978). *Bruininks-Oseretsky test of motor proficiency*. Circle Pines, MN: AGS.

Dutton, R. (1995). *Clinical reasoning in physical disabilities*. Philadelphia: Williams & Wilkins.

Folio, R., & Fewell, R. (2000). *Peabody developmental motor scales* (2nd ed.). Austin, TX: Pro-Ed.

Furuno, S., O'Reilly, K., Hosaka, C. M., Zeisloft, B., & Allman, T. (1984). *The Hawaii Early Learning Profile™*. Palo Alto, CA: VORT.

Gardner, M. F. (1997a). *Test of visual motor skills–revised.* Hydesville, CA: Psychological and Educational Publications Inc.

Gardner, M. F. (1997b). *Test of visual perceptual skills–non-motor.* Hydesville, CA: Psychological and Educational Publications, Inc.

Haley, S. M., Coster, W. J., Ludlow, L. H., Haltiwanger, J. T., & Andrellos, P. J. (1992). *Pediatric evaluation of disability inventory.* San Antonio, TX: The Psychological Corporation.

Hamilton, B. B., & Granger, C. U. (1991a). *Functional independence measure for children (Wee-FIM™).* Buffalo, NY: Research Foundation of the State University of New York.

Hamilton, B. B., & Granger, C. U. (1991b). *Functional Independence Measure.* Buffalo, NY: Research Foundation of the State University of New York.

Guide for the Uniform Data Set for Medical Rehabilitation (FIM™). State University of New York at Buffalo. 1996.

Individuals with Disabilities Education Act (IDEA) Amendments of 1997, Pub. L. No. 105–17.

Jebsen, R. H., Taylor, N., Trieschmann, R. B., Trotter, M. J., & Howard, L. A. (1969). *Jebsen hand function test.* Bolingbrook, IL: Sammons Preston, Inc.

Keilhofner G. (2002). *Model of human occupation.* Baltimore: Lippencott.

Levine, M. D. (1985). *Pediatric examination of educational readiness in middle childhood (PEERAMID).* Cambridge, MA: Educators Publishing Services, Inc.

Levine, M. D., & Schneider, E. A. (1983*). Pediatric examination of educational readiness (PEER).* Cambridge, MA: Educators Publishing Services Inc.

The National Information Center for Children and Youth with Disabilities, Spina Bifida. (2002). Retrieved Dec. 5, 2002, from http://westworld.com/~barbara/index28spinabif.

Rehabilitation Act of 1973. PL 93-112.

Spina Bifida Association of America. (2002). *Helping students with NLDs achieve academic and social success.* Retrieved Dec. 5, 2002, from http://www.sba.org/doc/insights/helping_students_with_NLDs.pdf.

Struss, L. (2001). *Terms/definitions with an overview of Arnold Chiari malformation.* Retrieved Dec. 5, 2002 from_http://www.pressenter.com/~wacma/lisapaper.htm

Technology Related Assistance for Individuals with Disabilities Act (1988). Public Law 100-407.

Vocational Rehabilitation Service Act (1973). Public Law 93-112.

Genetic Conditions

8

Kristie P. Koenig, Ph.D., OTR/L

Synopsis of Clinical Condition

Prevalence and Etiology

The human genome is no longer a complex riddle. An international team of researchers has successfully sequenced and mapped the human genome, which is made up of 30,000 to 40,000 human genes. This information can be thought of as a basic set of inheritable "instructions" for the development and function of a human being (National Human Genome Research Institute, n.d.). Humans have 23 pairs of chromosomes, including 22 identical pairs of autosomes one pair of sex chromosomes. The sex chromosomes are identical (XX) if the human is female, and disparate (XY) if the human is male. Risks that lead to genetic conditions include abnormalities in the chromosomes, single gene mutations that produce genetic diseases and conditions, and more complex multi-factorial risks.

It is estimated that 2% to 3% of newborns have a major genetic defect (Blackman, 1997). These include, but are not limited to, Down syndrome, muscular dystrophies, cystic fibrosis, fragile X syndrome, sickle cell anemia, and Tay-Sachs disease. Incidence rates for genetic conditions vary according to the specific condition. The prevalence of genetic conditions in newborns is tracked as a vital statistic, as is infant mortality, birth weight, etc. For example, in the Bureau of Vital Statistics' National report (Martin, Hamilton, Ventura, Menacker, & Park, 2002) the incidence rate of Down syndrome is listed as 46.9 per 100,000 live births. This is compared to Hurler's syndrome with a rate of 1 per 100,000, a much more rare condition.

A thorough understanding of all genetic conditions is outside the scope of this chapter, due to the multitude of conditions that have their origins in the genetic map. An understanding of incidence, inheritance patterns, and common genetic conditions that the therapist may encounter in practice is necessary for best practice.

Genetic causes can be classified as (1) chromosomal abnormalities, with too little or too much genetic information present; (2) single-gene disorders, where there is adequate genetic material but there is alteration in the genetic material within the chromosomes; and (3) multi-factorial disorders caused by an interplay of genetic and environmental factors. The latter is the most prevalent.

An example of a chromosomal abnormality would be trisomy 21 or Down syndrome, where there is an extra chromosome 21. Chromosomal abnormalities can be identified through karotyping. A single-gene disorder can be an alteration in a single or pair of genes on either the autosomes or the sex chromosomes. The inheritance pattern can be recessive or dominant in nature and causes such conditions as cystic fibrosis, fragile X syndrome, tuberous sclerosis, and Duchenne and Becker muscular dystrophies. The defective condition can be an autosomal dominant or recessive condition or an X-linked dominant or recessive condition.

Autosomal recessive inheritance indicates that an abnormal gene must be in a paired condition (i.e., both parents have the gene) in order for the child to inherit the disease. For each pregnancy, there is a 25% chance the child will have the paired genes and the condition will be expressed. In autosomal recessive inheritance patterns there is also a 50% chance the child will become a carrier for the condition. Males and females are at equal risk. The risk of an unaffected offspring being a carrier is 66%, with a 33% chance of being an unaffected non-carrier. Typically, both parents are carriers but have no symptoms of the condition. For many conditions, these carrier states can be identified through early diagnostic testing. There are several common genetic conditions that are an autosomal recessive inheritance, including cystic fibrosis in the Caucasian population, Tay-Sachs disease in the Ashkenazi Jewish population, and sickle cell disease in the African American population.

Autosomal dominant conditions indicate that the abnormal gene is present on one of the non-sex chromosomes. There is no carrier state for autosomal dominant conditions. If the gene is present, the child will have the condition. For each pregnancy, there is a 50% chance that the child will have the condition. Huntington's chorea is an example of an autosomal dominant condition. Genetic counseling accompanies the prenatal screening that identifies carrier and affected states.

X-linked inheritance disorders may be recessive or dominant. X-linked dominant diseases are considered very rare and usually lethal if a male inherits the gene, since he only has one X. This is why fathers cannot pass the trait to their sons, since fathers provide the Y that determines that the sex of the child will be male. A mother can be a carrier with differential risks for male as compared to female offspring. For each pregnancy that is a male, the child has a 50% chance of being affected. Since the female is XX, for each pregnancy that is female with a carrier mother the child has a 50% risk of being a carrier (Schopmeyer & Lowe, 1992).

Multi-factorial or polygenic disorders have a more complex causal pattern, and can include cardiac malformations, cleft lip and palate, and myelomeningocele (Blackman, 1997). Multi-factorial conditions suggest a more complex interplay between the genetic material and environmental factors. In these cases, genes do not have a yes-no impact on whether an individual has a genetic condition. Instead, there may have more subtle influences in combination with other genetic and environmental influences.

Common Characteristics and Symptoms

Two well-known genetic conditions, Down syndrome and fragile X syndrome, are the most common causes of developmental disabilities and mental retardation in the general population (Schopmeyer & Lowe, 1992). Down syndrome has a higher incidence rate (4 to 5 per 1,000 births) and is seen more commonly than fragile X syndrome. However, fragile X syndrome, with its X-linked recessive pattern, is the most common inherited cause of mental retardation in males, with an estimated incidence of 1 per 4,000 (Bailey, Hatton, Tassone, Skinner, & Taylor, 2001). Down syndrome is not an inherited genetic condition, but rather a chromosomal abnormality. These two conditions have similarities and differences, but are frequently seen in pediatric occupational therapy practice.

Fragile X syndrome is a single-gene disorder carried on the X chromosome. The disorder can be passed through several generations in the carrier state, with each generation having a higher risk of having the gene that causes the syndrome (Bailey, Skinner, Hatton, & Roberts, 2000). Typically, this gene is transmitted stably from parent to child. However, in individuals with fragile X syndrome there is a mutation and expansion in one end of the gene which does not allow the FMR1 gene to be expressed, so no FMR1 protein is made. The production of this protein is believed to be essential for normal brain functioning (Bailey et al., 2001). Both males and females can have this syndrome, however, males are usually more severely affected than females. Individuals with fragile X syndrome may experience delays in all areas of development, especially in the areas of cognition and communication. In contrast to children born with Down syndrome, children with fragile X may look and behave normally at birth. Males may develop distinguishing physical features that include an elongated face, large ears, hypotonia, and hyperextensibility at the finger joints (Schopmeyer & Lowe, 1992). Behaviorally, children with fragile X syndrome may demonstrate hyperactivity, tactile defensiveness and other sensitivities to sensory stimulation. They may also demonstrate autistic-like behaviors such as hand flapping and avoidance of eye contact. Miller et al. (1999) found that children with fragile X syndrome manifested the most severe sensory processing disorders of all the clinical groups studied (i.e., autism and attention deficit hyperactivity disorder). The sensory processing deficits can have an impact on occupational performance. Baranek et al. (2002) found that children with fragile X syndrome who avoided sensory experiences had lower levels of school participation, self-care, and play skills than children with fragile X who did not avoid sensory experiences. Often it is the behaviors that result in a child being referred to occupational therapy, even prior to a diagnosis of fragile X syndrome.

Down syndrome (also called trisomy 21) is the most common chromosomal abnormality, with an overall incidence rate from 1 per 600 to 1 per 800 (National Down Syndrome Society [NDSS], n.d.). As the name trisomy 21 indicates, the condition involves a triplication of genetic material. Although Down syndrome has an unknown etiology, the age of the mother is a documented risk factor. If a mother is under the age of 25, she has a 1 per 1,600 chance of having a child with Down syndrome. At 35 years of age, the risk increases to 1 per 340. If the mother is over the age of 43 the risk increases dramatically to 1 per 40. (National Information Center for Children with Youth and Disabilities, n.d.). The primary genetic cause of Down syndrome is an error in genetic cell division called non-disjunction, resulting in a triplication at chromosome 21. Translocation and mosaicism are also two additional chromosomal abnormalities which result in Down syndrome, but at a significantly lower rate than nondisjunction (NDSS, n.d.).

At birth, the characteristic physical features are usually identifiable, including a flattened nasal bridge, minimal space in the oral cavity with resulting tongue protrusion, short hands with short fingers, a palmar simian crease, hypotonia, hyperextensibility at the joints, and decreased or inefficient sucking patterns (Case-Smith, 2001). In addition, there are specific medical concerns associated with a diagnosis of Down syndrome, including possible cardiac abnormalities that require surgical repair, an increased risk for leukemia, increased risk of respiratory infections, and atlantoaxial dislocation of the vertebra (Case-Smith, 2001).

Target Areas for Intervention

The child with Down syndrome typically experiences delays in the attainment of most developmental milestones, including motor, language, learning, and adaptive skills. Postural and fine motor skills are typically decreased, affecting independence in activities of daily living including functional mobility, self-feeding, dressing, and tool use. There may be sensory processing and integration issues as well, with defensive behavior or a failure to register sensory input. Children with Down syndrome have a higher than normal incidence of visual acuity deficits requiring correction. The occupational therapist plays a vital role on the treatment team, addressing the myriad issues associated with a diagnosis of Down syndrome. Common to both fragile X syndrome and Down syndrome are developmental delays that typically cross several areas of development, including motor, language, social, adaptive behavior, functional independence, play skills, sensory processing, and cognitive skills.

Contextual Considerations

Clinical

The clinical evaluation of the child with genetic conditions can be varied due to the differential nature of genetic conditions, but there are some common elements that should be addressed. The clinical evaluation is dependent upon the service delivery setting, age of the child, and reason for referral. In general, the purpose of the occupational therapy assessment with a child with a genetic condition is to assess strengths and weaknesses in broad areas of development, including gross and fine motor skills, cognitive skills, sensory processing, and adaptive functioning in the areas of activities of daily living, play, education, and work.

Since children with genetic conditions often present with delays in many areas of development, evaluation data that provides a broad perspective of developmental functioning is beneficial. Standardized and criterion-based assessments such as the *Bayley Scales of Infant Development–II*™ (Bayley, 1993), the *Battelle Developmental Inventory* (Newborg, Stock, Wnek, Guidubaldi, & Svinicki, 1988), the *Miller Assessment for Preschoolers*™ (Miller, 1988), and the *Hawaii Early Learning Profile*™ (Furono, O'Reilly, Hosaka, Zeisloft, & Allman, 1984) provide data in a broad number of developmental areas. These can include motor, cognitive, language, social, and adaptive skills related to dressing, bathing, play skills, and feeding.

Feeding can be an issue, especially in children with Down syndrome. Many non-standardized procedures are used to assess a child's oral-motor and feeding skills, including oral motor structures, control and praxis; oral sensitivity; a comprehensive feeding history; and (for the older child) an observation of self-feeding skills.

Children with genetic conditions are frequently delayed in their attainment of motor milestones. Data from criterion-referenced and standardized tests, including the *Peabody Developmental Motor Scales–2* (Folio & Fewell, 2000), the *Bruininks-Oseretsky Test of Motor Proficiency* (Bruininks, 1978), and the *Erhardt Developmental Prehension Assessment* (Erhardt, 1994), will provide the therapist with information on how the child's gross motor and fine motor skills compare to a developmental norm. But test results should be supplemented by clinical observations related to functional gross motor and fine motor skills (e.g., climbing stairs, getting on or off a bus, and tool use in the classroom).

Children with genetic conditions may have sensory defensiveness that may impact their engagement and participation in life activities. The *Sensory Profile* (Dunn, 1999) is a standardized assessment, based on caregiver interviews, which provides information on the child's ability to process and respond to a variety of sensory information.

Functional assessments that look at developmental skills within context include the *School Function Assessment* (SFA) which evaluates a child's (K through 6th grade) performance, level of participation, and need for assistance in school activities, including physical, and cognitive and behavioral tasks (Coster, Deeney, Haltiwanger, & Haley, 1998). The *Vineland Adaptive Behavior Scales* (VABS) measures communication, daily living skills, socialization, and motor skills with a behavioral rating scale (Sparrow, Balla, & Cicchetti, 1984). An important component to these functional assessments is to consider the child's cognitive abilities and level of mental retardation, which for children with genetic conditions, can range from mild to severe.

According to the *Diagnostic and Statistical Manual of Mental Disorders* (*DSM–IV–TR*; American Psychiatric Association, 2000), mental retardation (MR) can be classified into mild, moderate, severe, or profound range. Individuals with mild MR can acquire basic math and reading skills and work in semiskilled jobs with vocational training. Individuals with moderate MR may be able to learn "survival skills" that will help them with community integration, such as writing a legal signature, reading for safety, using public transportation, basic money management, and working with the help of a "job coach" and supervision. Individuals with severe MR typically need programs that focus on basic self-care skills and structured prevocational skills. Children classified with profound MR have delays in many functional areas and are usually dependent for all areas of basic self-care skills including feeding, dressing, and toileting. Children with profound MR typically have severe CNS impairment and often require family support and respite programs due to dependence on the caregiver. Within each classification of MR there can be a wide range of adaptive functioning and cognitive skills.

Cognitive abilities, as they relate to functional occupational performance, include the ability to attend and follow directions, plus memory skills, general knowledge of basic concepts, judgment and self-awareness, and problem solving. In addition to looking at the classification system and standardized intelligence testing as a guide, these abilities should be informally evaluated within the context of functional occupational performance. For example, when out in the community, does the adolescent with Down syndrome have the cognitive ability to independently purchase an item from a retail store? These types of naturalistic observations will provide data on areas which may require direct intervention in order for the individual to be successful, or determine levels of assistance that may be required.

Family

Families that have a child with a genetic condition often are very aware of the nature of the condition either before the child is born or immediately at birth. Prenatally, there are screening tests that assess the risk of having a child with a genetic condition, and diagnostic testing that tells whether or not the fetus has the condition. To detect Down syndrome, two screening blood tests are available, the triple screen and alpha-fetoprotein plus, which are used in conjunction with a sonogram and age of the mother to assess risk (NDSS, n.d.). These screenings accurately detect 60% of fetuses with Down syndrome, but many women get false positive results and others get false negative results. A prenatal diagnosis of Down syndrome can be made with chorionic villus sampling (CVS) at 8 to 12 weeks gestation, amniocentesis at 12 to 20 weeks, and precutaneous umbilical blood sampling (PUBS) after 20 weeks gestation (NDSS, n.d.). All of these procedures carry a small risk of miscarriage but are 98% to 99% accurate in confirming a diagnosis of Down syndrome. Genetic counseling is given in conjunction with prenatal genetic testing.

If the pregnancy continues, the early diagnosis often puts the family in touch with support groups, early intervention services, and a wealth of internet resources related to the specific conditions. This is a different dynamic than a parent who suspects something is wrong with their child's development, but may not get a diagnosis for several years. The early diagnosis does not negate the need to focus on family-centered care, which takes into account the priorities, values, goals and culture of the family. The child with Down syndrome or fragile X syndrome is not going to "grow out of it," or be cured. A genetic condition is life-long and, if inherited, has implications for subsequent pregnancies.

The family's routines, habits, and priorities will be altered with the birth of a child with Down syndrome or fragile X syndrome. For example, feeding a child with Down syndrome may be prolonged and more difficult for the caregiver versus an expected bonding experience. It is vital to keep in communication with the family on an informal basis as well as structured interviews to get a sense of what a typical day is like, what areas of family functioning are being impacted, and parental stress levels around routines and daily habits. The therapist can offer suggestions and adaptive equipment that may make feeding and self-care skills easier. Many times, close communication with the family is a focus of early intervention services, but decreases dramatically when the child enters school. By scheduling time to maintain communication with the family via logs or phone calls, in addition to face-to-face contact at Individualized Educational Plan (IEP) meetings, the therapist can also educate the family about the role of intervention and how service delivery models may change as the child goes through formal schooling. The occupational therapist has an important role in stressing advocacy for the family and providing resources for the family of a child with a genetic condition. This may include "futuring" or finding out what the family's vision is for their child, to determine when occupational therapy services are most appropriate and what the focus of intervention should be, based on the relevant occupations of the child within the context of the family.

Practice Setting

Children with genetic conditions interface with medical, educational, and community-based practice settings. Most children with Down syndrome or fragile X syndrome would be seen primarily in early intervention, school-based, and private practice. The determination of practice setting is largely based on the child's age. From birth to age five services can be delivered in the Neonatal Intensive Care Unit (NICU), the acute or rehabilitation hospital, community-based services including early intervention that is home and/or center-based, and private practice. Infants with Down syndrome often have medical complications, including feeding, respiratory difficulties, and congenital heart defects that require the services of the NICU. The therapist will focus on positioning, strategies to improve feeding, and facilitation of developmental milestones. If a child with Down syndrome requires cardiac surgery to correct a heart defect, a therapist may deliver services in the acute and rehabilitation stages of the child's recovery, including positioning to decrease swelling and promote postural drainage immediately post surgery, and intervention to improve endurance to activity. During the rehabilitation phase of intervention, goals would be associated with returning the child to post-surgery levels of functioning and communicating with family and community-based therapists.

Early intervention services are provided within the "natural environment" from birth to age three, which often means home-based services or services that are delivered in a primary day care setting. The therapist typically works as part of a treatment team with children with Down syndrome and fragile X syndrome in early intervention, due to multiple areas of developmental delay. From the ages of three to five, children with Down syndrome and fragile X syndrome may continue to be seen in the home, but are often transitioned to center-based programs, such as regular daycare programs or pre-schools, where they are integrated with children without disabilities. The transition to school-based services is then made, with the majority of therapy services received during the course of the school day. The therapist works with the child to ensure that he or she can benefit from special education programming, with a focus on developing fine motor skills, social skills, activities of daily living, prevocational, and vocational readiness skills. During the transition from school to adulthood, the therapist may deliver services in a variety of community-based programs that service individuals with developmental disabilities such as Down syndrome and fragile X syndrome. These settings include (but are not limited to) institutional programs, group homes, supported employment, and sheltered workshops. Practice settings may also include adult day care programs and long-term care facilities that provide services for adults with developmental disabilities.

Sociopolitical

The laws concern services and education for children with disabilities also apply to children with genetic conditions. Specifically, the Individuals with Disabilities Education Act (IDEA, 101-476, 1997), reauthorized in 2002 entitles all children with disabilities to a free and appropriate education and related services. In addition, many children with genetic defects are diagnosed at birth and qualify for early intervention services. Under Part C of the IDEA, which outlines services for children from birth to age 3, Down syndrome and fragile X syndrome are classified as an established risk factor, which include conditions that have a high probability of resulting in developmental delay (IDEA, 1997). Occupational therapy is a direct service provider for children from birth to 3 years of age, offering services in natural environments, following a philosophy of family centered practice.

IDEA (1997) mandates special education services for children from 3 to 21 years of age who are identified and coded with a disability. Most children with a genetic condition that affects development would be classified to receive special education services. Occupational therapy is a related or supportive service that is utilized when a child needs occupational therapy to benefit from his or her education program. School-based occupational therapy services may also be provided through civil rights legislation under the Rehabilitation Act of 1973, (PC 93–112) with a "504 plan" which ensures that students with disabilities are given equal access to school activities, and reasonable accommodations are made to allow students to access these activities. Children with Down syndrome and fragile X for example, would be classified and coded with a condition that would entitle them to education services under the IDEA, and provide for occupational therapy services as a related service if necessary for the child to benefit from his or her program.

The reauthorization of the IDEA 2002 (IDEA Amendments of 2002) also strengthened the legislative mandate for transition planning, education, and vocational services for individuals with disabilities. Transition planning and programming must be in place by the time the child is 14 years of age, to focus on success and participation in society after 21 years of age. Often, students with Down syndrome and fragile X will begin to explore vocational options, engage in prevocational tasks to build foundational skills, practice instrumental activities of daily living, and engage in community-based activities.

Lifestyle/Lifespan

Depending upon the specific genetic condition, there will be a variety of lifestyle and lifespan issues to consider. For example, individuals with Down syndrome can lead productive lives, live independently or with minimal supervision, have a diverse and rich social life, and become gainfully employed. The level of success in the community is dependent upon the severity of the disability, community resources and supports, and a focus on independent functioning and quality of life from the outset. The key to success in the community is often related to the level of the individual's adaptive skills, and this should be the focus throughout the lifespan and during times of transition (i.e. elementary to middle school, school to work, etc.).

Individuals with genetic conditions may have a reduced life expectancy or a higher incidence of medical complications. Individuals with Down syndrome have a life expectancy of approximately 50 years, with a higher incidence of dementia and Alzheimer's disease, and increased risk of mortality from specific causes like leukemia, and an elevated risk of other cancers (Hill et al., 2003).

Clinical Decision Making Process

Defining Focus for Intervention

There are several elements of the context that assist in determining the focus of the occupational therapy intervention. The key elements include the practice setting; the age of the client; the priorities of the family, client, and treatment team; and, finally, the presenting problems gathered from formal and informal evaluation procedures. The age of the client, for example will determine if the focus of occupational therapy intervention should be on developing foundational skills, compensating for a lack of skill that may not develop, modifying the environment, adapting the task, or a combination of several these methods. With children with Down syndrome and fragile X syndrome, all of these methods will most likely be utilized to (1) develop foundational motor skills that support gross and fine motor function; (2) compensate for decreased cognitive skills with adapted instructions or use of assistive technology for expressive language impairments; and (3) adapt work related tasks to modified work environments to ensure a successful transition after school-based interventions.

Establishing Goals for Intervention

Just as there are key elements that determine the focus of intervention, these same elements assist in the establishment of goals for intervention. Goals are going to be directly related to the age of the child, client factors that influence the potential for independence, and the setting where services are delivered. It should also be grounded in the priorities of the family and/or caregivers. Services that are delivered in the schools must have goals directly related to the child's ability to benefit from their educational program, while considering the curriculum context. The ultimate goal of occupational therapy is to promote and support people's ability to engage in meaningful occupations (American Occupational Therapy Association, 2002). For a child with Down syndrome or fragile X, this may mean engagement in play, school, prevocational or work-related activities, or basic and instrumental activities of daily living. The timing of long-term goals is dependent on the practice setting. In schools, a long-term goal is typically for the duration of a school year. In rehabilitation hospital settings the duration is shorter, typically one to two months. Short-term goals (also referred to as behavioral objectives) are steps to meet the long-term goal. Short-term goals should have measurable criteria in order to evaluate progress. Goals for children with Down syndrome and fragile X syndrome should be grounded in adaptive skills, since those are instrumental to successful participation in the community.

Designing Theory-Based Intervention

As discussed, children with genetic conditions typically have developmental delays in several areas, including motor, cognitive, language, sensory, play, and activities of daily living. Several frames of reference that are used in pediatric practice are applicable to this population.

Developmental theories (Llorens, Erickson, Piaget, Freud, Havinghurst, etc.) shape the therapist's conceptualization and knowledge of normal development, which is essential to pediatric practice. Developmental theories guide the intervention initially, to build necessary foundational skills in an expected developmental sequence. For example, the therapist would try to develop postural stability and mobility skills with a child with Down syndrome in prone and supine positions before working in a quadruped or sitting position. Also, by having a solid understanding of normal development and the theories that explain expected progressions, the therapist can recognize deviations in development that may need compensation.

The model of human of occupation (Kielhofner, 1995) is essential to frame intervention with this population. Different occupations that provide meaning and purpose to the individual are engaged in throughout the lifecycle. The child with Down syndrome will not be in a student role forever, and therapy must focus on this shift in roles and expectations. By using an occupation-based perspective, the therapist can frame interventions that will facilitate successful engagement, with the abilities the individual possesses. For example, it may not be necessary to continue to work on handwriting legibility and spacing if the child or adolescent can write and sign his name. This may be the highest level of functioning in this area that the individual can obtain. Time may be better spent looking at other performance skills he or she may need to be successful in the student role, as a family member, and in a future worker role. Inherent in the model of human occupation is an examination of the roles, routines, habits, and volitions of the child and family members; as well as the environmental context. This framework is essential to practice with any population.

Sensory integration is a theoretical framework that can be utilized to improve sensory integration and processing. Children with fragile X syndrome are often hypersensitive to sensory stimulation, which can lead to behavioral responses that include avoidance and withdrawal, non-adaptability, and a need to control the amount of stimulation that is received. A therapist can utilize the principles of sensory integration theory to influence how a child responds to sensory stimuli and reduce extremes in behavioral response patterns (i.e., increase accepted foods, eliminate hitting during grooming activities, impact sleep patterns, etc.).

Evaluating Progress

Progress is assessed based on the goals that were established. Goal attainment warrants a revision of the goals to continue with progress, or a determination of whether services are no longer indicated. Outcomes should be functional and based on the child or adolescent's occupational role performance. Is he or she succeeding in participating and engaging in occupations that are relevant to the age, the diagnosis, and the practice setting? A review of established goals, formal re-evaluation, and interviews with parents and teachers are the best way to evaluate progress.

Determining Change in or Termination of Treatment

Occupational therapy services should be utilized intensively upon the diagnosis of a genetic condition, to work with the child and family to maximize functioning in delayed areas, and impact the ability to participate in occupational roles. The focus of intervention should change as the child develops, as should expectations for participation in different activities. As these expectations shift, the occupational therapist can provide intervention to enhance specific skills, habits, or behaviors; adapt or change the context; or work as a consultant with the child's caregivers or other adults who are frequently with the child to enable participation in activities. Termination of services is appropriate when the goals have been met and the child or adolescent is functioning at his or her maximal level and/or has reached a plateau. Occupational therapy in context implies that services may be terminated in one context, but as the context changes, services may be required in order to achieve maximum functioning in the individual's occupational roles.

Case Study

Description

Adam is a 14-year-old boy with Down syndrome. Adam has received early intervention services and special education services throughout his schooling. He is in the first year of high school, in a full inclusion class with a one-to-one aide, and participates in special education programming for half of his school day. Adam has mild to moderate mental retardation and has good receptive language skills, but limited expressive language skills. He uses a Picture Exchange Communication System (PECS) and simple sign language to supplement his limited vocabulary. He becomes easily frustrated and angry when he is not understood. Socially, Adam doesn't initiate interaction with his peers, but enjoys social interaction if initiated by his classmates. Because Adam is 14 years of age, transition planning services are being developed and implemented. His curriculum currently consists of exploring potential areas of employment and focuses on a life skills approach.

A multidisciplinary team, which includes Adam, his parents, his aide, both his special education and regular education teacher, an occupational therapist, speech and language pathologist, and the school psychologist have met to formulate a transition plan. The plan utilizes Adam's strengths and interests to begin to explore vocational activities in which he might be the most successful. Adam has identified an interest in working with papers and "having an office." He has always liked having his own task that he can try to see through to completion, versus working collaboratively with a group of individuals. Adam can be easily distracted when there are increased auditory stimuli in the environment. A review of his IEP and his most recent three-year evaluation results made the team members aware of his strengths and weaknesses, and of teaching strategies that have worked with Adam in the past. He appears to have some relative strengths with visual perceptual motor skills.

In transition planning, critical considerations include the client's priorities, goals, and interests. These must intersect with the abilities and potential skills that the team has identified. Adam has identified an interest in "working with papers," and has documented strengths in the areas of visual perceptual skills. He likes working as independently as possible and prefers to "do it on his own," with task completion being highly valued. He has a tendency to get easily distracted in the classroom. The team chose a "real world" sorting activity that lets him work independently, utilizes his strengths, and could potentially lead to vocational work if he is successful. The task was broken down into key elements in order to have Adam achieve a sense of mastery and task completion.

Long- and Short-Term Goals

The long-term goal of intervention for Adam is to enable him to independently sort incoming mail for 30 minutes on three consecutive days with 100% accuracy.

The short-term goals of intervention for Adam are:

1. Match 10 names to the correct letter box with 80% accuracy.
2. Complete a sorting and matching task with no more than two verbal reminders to remain on task.

Therapist Goals and Strategies

The therapist's goals include:

1. Improve Adam's on-task behavior.
2. Enhance Adam's visual discrimination and matching abilities.
3. Improve Adam's motor speed.

The therapist's strategies include:

1. Use visual cueing with colors to improve task orientation and focusing.
2. Provide opportunities for repetition, practice, verbal cueing, and reward.
3. Conduct task analysis to gain understanding of potential strengths and weaknesses.
4. Upgrade the activity to include the time, speed, and accuracy necessary to perform the job in a real context.

Activity

Last Name First

Adam will be given a green highlighter and an initial template of envelopes that show several ways a last name can appear. For example, "Mr. Smith," "Mr. James Smith," "The Smith's," "The Smith Family," and "To the parents of Thomas Smith." Adam will be required to initially scan each envelope and locate the last name on the envelope. If correct he will be required to highlight the last name and put in the "done" box. If incorrect, Adam will be verbally cued to put the envelope aside and continue. After the activity is completed, Adam will count the number of correct pieces of mail and give himself a score. Each incorrect piece of mail will be reviewed with Adam in a teach-and-learn process.

Treatment Objective

Adam will correctly highlight the last name on 15 random pieces of mail without verbal cueing.

Resources

The following resources can be helpful for gathering clinical data:

Developmental evaluations:

- *Bayley Scales of Infant Development* (BSID–II)
- *Battelle Developmental Inventory* (BDI)
- *Miller Assessment of Preschoolers* (MAP)
- *Hawaii Early Learning Profile* (HELP)

Motor Evaluations:

- *Peabody Developmental Motor Scales–2* (PDMS–2)
- *Bruininks-Oseretsky Test of Motor Proficiency*
- *Erhardt Developmental Prehension Assessment*

Sensory Processing:

- *Sensory Profile*

Functional Behavior Assessments:

- *School Function Assessment* (SFA)
- *Vineland Adaptive Behavior Scales* (VABS)
- Naturalistic Observations of functioning and participation in relevant occupations

The following resources can be helpful for gathering family data:

Early diagnostic testing and genetic counseling

Family priorities, values, and culture

Daily routines associated with basic and instrumental activities of daily living

Informal interviews to elicit relevant occupations

The following are common practice settings:

0 to 5 years:

- NICU
- Early intervention
- Acute/rehab hospital due to medical complications (i.e., cardiac surgery with Down syndrome)
- Private practice

5 to 21 years:

- Schools
- Private practice

Adulthood:

- Supported employment
- Sheltered workshops
- Group homes
- Nursing homes
- Institutional settings

The following resources can be helpful for gathering sociopolitical data:

IDEA

Section 504 of Rehab Act

Vocational Rehab Services

The following can be helpful in understanding and managing lifestyle and lifespan issues:

Key transitions include:

- Early intervention to school-based services
- Transition services documented starting at age 14
- Transition from school-based services to adult MR services providing housing, job opportunities, and social services
- With Down syndrome, a higher incidence of dementia and Alzheimer's disease may require additional services

Internet Resources

National Down Syndrome Society:
www.ndss.org

National Fragile X Foundation:
www.fragilex.org

National Institute of Health-Genetic Conditions Section:
www.rarediseases.info.nih.gov

National Human Genome Research Institute:
www.genome.gov

National Information Center for Children and Youth with Disabilities:
www.nichcy.org

Council for Exceptional Children:
www.cec.sped.org

References

American Occupational Therapy Association. (2002). Occupational therapy practice framework: Domain and process. *American Journal of Occupational Therapy, 56,* 609–639.

American Psychiatric Association. (2000). *Diagnostic and statistical manual of mental disorders* (4th ed., text revision). Washington, DC: Author.

Bailey, D. B., Hatton, D. D., Tassone, F., Skinner, M., & Taylor, A. K. (2001). FMRP and early development in fragile x syndrome. *American Journal of Mental Retardation, 106,* 16–27.

Bailey, D. B., Skinner, D., Hatton, D., & Roberts, J. (2000). Family experiences and factors associated with diagnosis of fragile x syndrome. *Journal of Developmental and Behavioral Pediatrics, 21(5)*, 315–321.

Baranek, G. T., Chin, Y. K., Greiss Hess, L. M., Yankee, J. G., Hatton, D. D., & Hooper, S. R. (2002). Sensory processing correlates of occupational performance in children with fragile x syndrome: Preliminary findings. *American Journal of Occupational Therapy, 56*, 538–546.

Bayley, N. (1993). *Bayley scales of infant development–II™* (2nd ed.). San Antonio, TX: The Psychological Corporation.

Blackman, J. A. (1997). *Medical aspects of developmental disabilities in children birth to three* (3rd ed.). Gaithersburg, MD: Aspen Publishing, Inc.

Bruininks, R. H. (1978). *Bruininks-Oseretsky test of motor proficiency.* Circle Pines, MN: AGS.

Case-Smith, J. (2001). *Occupational therapy for children* (4th ed.). St. Louis, MO: Mosby.

Coster, W., Deeney, T. Haltiwanger, J., & Haley, S. (1998). *School function assessment (SFA).* San Antonio, TX: The Psychological Corporation.

Dunn, W. (1999). *Sensory profile user's manual.* San Antonio, TX: The Psychological Corporation.

Erhardt, R. P. (1994). *Developmental prehension assessment-revised.* San Antonio, TX: The Psychological Corporation.

Folio, R., & Fewell, R. (2000). *Peabody Developmental Motor Scales* (2nd ed.). Austin, TX: Pro-Ed.

Furuno, S., O'Reilly, K., Hosaka, C. M., Zeisloft, B., & Allman, T. (1984). *The Hawaii Early Learning Profile.* Palo Alto, CA: VORT.

Hill, D. A., Gridley, G., Cnattingius, S., Mellemkjaer, L., Linet, M., Adami, H., et al. (2003). Mortality and cancer incidence among individuals with Down syndrome. *Archives of Internal Medicine, 163*, 705–711.

Individuals with Disabilities Education Act (IDEA) Amendments of 1997 (P. L. No. 105-17). U.S.C., 1400.

Kielhofner, G. (1995). *A model of human occupation theory and application* (2nd ed.). Baltimore: Williams & Wilkins.

Martin, J. A., Hamilton, B. E., Ventura, S. J., Menacker, F., & Park, M. M. (2002). Maternal demographic characteristics. *National Vital Statistics Reports, 50 (5)*, 1–102.

Miller, L. J. (1988). *Miller assessment for preschoolers.* San Antonio, TX: The Psychological Corporation.

Miller, L.J., McIntosh, D.N., McGrath, J. Shyu, V. Lampe, M., Taylor, A.K., Tassone, F., Neitzel, K., Stackhouse, T., & Hagerman, R. (1999). Electrodermal responses to sensory stimuli in individuals with fragile X syndrome: A preliminary report. *American Journal of Medical Genetics*, 83, 268–279.

National Down Syndrome Society (n.d.). *What causes Down syndrome?.* Retrieved August 1, 2003, from http://www.ndss.org.

National Human Genome Research Institute. (n.d.) *International consortium completes human genome project.* Retrieved May 2, 2003, from http://www.genome.gov.

National Information Center for Children with Youth and Disabilities (n.d.). *Down syndrome fact sheet.* Retrieved May 2, 2003, from http://www.nichcy.org.

Newborg, J., Stock, J. R., Wnek, L., Guidubaldi, J., and Svinicki, J. (1988). *Battelle developmental inventory.* Itasca, IL: Riverside Publishing Company.

Rehabilitation Act of 1973, 29 U.S.C. §504.

Schopmeyer, B. B., & Lowe, F. (1992). *The fragile X child.* San Diego: Singular Publishing Group, Inc.

Sparrow, S., Balla, D., & Cicchetti, D. (1984). *The Vineland adaptive behavior scales, interview edition: Survey form manual.* Circle Pines, MN: AGS.

Pediatric Upper Limb Conditions 9

Roberta T. Ciocco, OTR/L
Meryl S. Cooperman, MS OTR/L

Synopsis of Clinical Condition

Prevalence and Etiology

Pediatric upper limb conditions comprise a very broad diagnostic group. This chapter will refer to two different groups within this category: those with anatomical or structural anomalies, and those without structural deformity. The following is a listing of the primary patient populations that will be touched upon in this chapter.

Upper limb conditions with structural anomalies include:

- Congenital and acquired transverse upper limb deficiency
- Phocomelia
- Arthrogryposis
- Radial and ulnar deficienies (longitudinal deficiency)
- Congenital hand deformities (i.e. syndactyly, cleft hand)

Upper limb conditions without structural anomalies include:

- Brachial plexus injuries

It is helpful to understand the timing and general principles of embryological limb development when discussing congenital conditions with structural deformity. The development of the limbs takes place between the third to eighth weeks of gestation. The type of limb deformity that occurs will be dictated by the time of insult. Three causes or sequences are generally attributed to problems with limb development. The first is a malformation sequence. This means that there is a malformation in the embryo that already exists at the time of limb development. A resulting problem of this scenario would be radial deficiency. The second possibility is a deformation sequence. In this case, an abnormal external mechanical or structural force causes the deformity. An example of this type of problem would be congenital constriction bands. The third possibility is a disruption sequence. In this situation, the healthy embryological tissue is subjected to injury or breakdown. An example of this would be a deformity caused by an infection such as rubella or a drug-induced deformity.

The incidence of congenital limb deformities is difficult to estimate because there is such a diversity of problems with varying occurrence frequencies. Some of the less severe problems, such as syndactyly, are reported to occur at a rate of 1 in 600 births.

Other more severe deformities are reported to occur at a rate of 1 in 100,000 births (Glynn, 2002; McDonnell, Scott, & McKay, 1988).

The following classification system that was developed by Swanson (1976) is used today by hand surgeons and physicians to label the various types of deformity.

Type I–Failure of formation:

- Transverse arrest (amputations)
- Longitudinal arrest
  - Preaxial (radial deficiency)
  - Central (cleft hand)
  - Postaxial (ulnar deficiency)
  - Intercalated longitudinal arrest (phocomelia)

Type II–Failure of differentiation

- Soft tissue (arthrogryposis)
- Skeletal (delta phalanx)
- Tumorous conditions

Type III–Duplication (polydactyly)

Type IV–Overgrowth (macrodactyly)

Type V–Undergrowth (hypoplasia)

Type VI–Constriction band syndromes

Type VII–Generalized anomalies and syndromes

Common Characteristics and Symptoms

Most children with congenital hand deformities are otherwise normal, healthy children. Occasionally there are associated medical issues, such as cardiac problems, blood disorders, or other visceral problems. With some of the syndromes, other parts of the body can be affected, such as in the case of arthrogryposis, where the lower extremities can also be affected. Often there is a significant difference in the size of the involved hand as well as other deformities. Atypical appearance is often the cause of self-consciousness and social-emotional distress. Frequently, multiple surgical procedures are performed for cosmetic as well as functional reasons. When surgery is not a viable alternative, orthotic or prosthetic devices are often employed. Surgical and mechanical interventions are usually focused on the achievement of hand-to-mouth and grasp-and-release movements. Regardless of the treatment course, there is usually a need to have regular long-term contact with a medical facility that specializes in upper-limb orthopedic treatment. Table 9.1 lists the most typical surgical interventions for some of these diagnoses (Glynn, 2002).

Congenital or obstetrical brachial plexus injuries are not associated with structural deformity and are typically caused by a traction injury to all or part of the brachial plexus at the time of delivery. The incidence of obstetrical palsies is reported to be between .04 and 2.5 cases per 1,000 live births (Hunter, et. al., 2002). This problem is almost always unilateral. There are two main types of injury. The first is an upper plexus injury which is referred to as Erb's Palsy. In this case, the C-5 and C-6 musculature and sensation is most affected.

Table 9.1
Typical Surgical Intervention

Diagnosis	Functional/Structural Problem	Surgical Procedure
Radial Deficiency	Significant wrist radial deviation	Centralization procedure. Use of an external fixator to gradually realign hand on wrist
	Absence of thumb	Pollicization (surgical rotation of index finger into position of thumb)
	Elbow flexion contracture	Soft tissue release
Transverse Deficiency at metacarpal or phalangeal level	Shortened digits making grasp of large objects difficult	Web space deepening
		Bone distraction
	Poor or absent thumb	Toe to thumb transfer
Syndactyly	Two or more fingers joined together. Can be just soft tissue or involve bony fusion	Digit separation—method of skin coverage may vary (flaps, z-plasty, or skin graft)
		Correction of bony deformity
Arthrogryposis	Reoccurring wrist flexor contractures with no available motors for transfer, requires full-time use of orthotic to keep wrist at neutral position	Arthrodesis of wrist when skeletally mature (may also require proximal row carpectomy)
	Lack of active elbow flexion with good passive range	Flexorplasty using either the triceps, latissimus or pectoralis muscle
	Decreased passive elbow or wrist motion	Joint release or tendon lengthening

There is very poor shoulder control and often some weakness at the elbow. The second and less common type of injury is the lower plexus or Klumpke's Palsy. In this case, the C-7 and C-8 muscles and distal sensation are usually affected. A child with this condition would present with good proximal strength but very weak wrist and hand musculature. Although it is rare, both the upper and lower plexus can be injured with resultant total arm paralysis and sensory impairment. There are few associated medical problems with these children. They can sometimes have shoulder dystocia or fractures of the clavicle. Horner's Sign (eye ptosis and myosis) is sometimes seen with severe brachial plexus injury (Mackinnon, 2002).

Children with obstetrical brachial plexus palsy usually have some degree of spontaneous recovery within three to five months. Children who do not demonstrate biceps function within that time period are often considered for a nerve graft or nerve transfer. The results of nerve grating vary, but usually some improvement is seen within six months of surgery. However, there may be residual deficits. Over time, muscle imbalances due to partial paralysis can cause deformity. The most common problems are elbow flexion and internal rotation deformities. Surgery may be indicated to prevent future deformity, improve function, or release contractures prior to tendon transfers. Tendon transfers are often used to improve the function and appearance of the arm. An evaluation conducted by the entire intervention team (including the occupational therapist, the physical therapist, the pediatric physiatrist, and the hand surgeon) must ascertain muscle strength, sensation, and functional skills before surgical intervention. The following table summarizes possible surgical options for the shoulder and elbow (Hunter et al., 2002).

Table 9.2
Surgical Options for Shoulder and Elbow

Involved Joint	Functional Problem	Surgical Procedure
Shoulder	Lack of external rotation	Latissimus to infraspinatus transfer
		Derotational osteotomy of the humerous
	Lack of shoulder abduction	Transfer of the trapezius to the lateral aspect of the humerus
		Bipolar latissimus dorsi transfer
	Severe shoulder dysfunction without possible motor donors	Shoulder arthrodesis
Elbow	Lack of elbow flexion	Flexorplasty using either the latissimus, pectoralis major, triceps, flexor-pronator muscles
		Free muscle (gracilis) transfer
	Lack of extension	Latissimus to triceps
		Biceps to triceps

Tendon transfers are less common in lower plexus injuries because there are usually less options for donor muscles to transfer in the wrist and hand. An evaluation conducted by the entire intervention team including the occupational therapist, the physical therapist, and the surgeon must ascertain muscle strength, sensation, and functional skills before surgical intervention.

Target Areas for Intervention

The occupational therapist can provide the family and child with education, guidance, and support throughout the various stages of development. Children with upper limb conditions often require direct intervention in infancy and periodic intervention throughout childhood and adolescence for splinting, range of motion, adaptive equipment, functional skills training, and prosthetic training, if necessary. Those who require surgical intervention will often require occupational therapy services for post-operative rehabilitation.

Contextual Considerations

Clinical

The clinical evaluation must incorporate information about sensorimotor and developmental status, and activities of daily living (ADL). An ADL evaluation provides information regarding the skills that the child may be capable of completing independently or with the assistance of adaptive equipment, and provides insight into the coping strategies of the child and family. The sensorimotor evaluation includes information on the range of motion, muscle strength, and sensation of the upper extremities. Upper limb conditions with structural anomalies pose a challenge for testing because landmarks may be absent or in an alternative position. This is because the bone structure may be incomplete or absent. If prosthetics options, specially designed orthosi, or other technologies are being considered, it is important to be knowledgeable of the skills needed to support and operate the device. For example, a conventional body-powered prosthetic is operated by scapular protraction and retraction.

Manual muscle testing is also challenging for young children, who may not understand the directions or be fully cooperative with specific muscle testing. To obtain accurate information, the occupational therapist needs to be competent in manual muscle testing, including knowledge of substitute patterns of movement. Children with brachial plexus injury or other forms of paralysis often use patterns of substitution for weak or paralyzed muscles. A few common substitutions include using lateral trunk flexion to assist with shoulder abduction, and shoulder abduction to assist with elbow flexion.

Many upper limb conditions are unilateral, and the involved extremity is typically the non-dominant extremity. This poses a challenge for assessment because most assessments evaluate either unilateral function or the accomplishment of a specific skill. It is helpful to evaluate the involved extremity for its functional use as an assist to the dominant extremity. The *University of New Brunswick Test of Prosthetic Function* (UNB; Sanderson & Scott, 1985) is a standardized test for the use of a below-the-elbow prosthesis as an assist to an intact extremity. A clinical assessment using the format of the UNB is helpful to determine the effectiveness of intervention for many unilateral limb conditions.

Children with upper limb deficiencies also pose a challenge for evaluation because fine motor assessments are based on an intact structure. A child with an absent thumb will not be able to perform a pincer grasp without surgical intervention. A child with paralysis of the wrist extensors will not be able to demonstrate a mature grasp pattern with wrist extension. Therefore, the therapist must be able to extrapolate information and focus on the accomplishment of functional skills.

There are many developmental assessments available. A general developmental assessment, such as the *Peabody Developmental Motor Scales–2* (PDMS–2; Folio & Fewell, 2000), the *Hawaii Early Learning Profile*™ (HELP; Furano, O'Reilly, Hosaka, Zeisloft, & Allman, 1984), or the *Pediatric Developmental Inventory* (PEDI; Haley, Coster, Ludlow, Haltiwanger, & Andrellos, 1992) will provide information for the preschool-aged child.

Children of school age can be evaluated using an assessment of visual motor skills, perceptual skills, and fine motor coordination. Common assessments include the *Test of Visual Motor Integration* (Beery, 1997), the *Gardner Test of Visual Perceptual Skills-Revised* (Gardner, 1997), the *Jebsen Hand Function Test* (Jebsen, Taylor, Trieschmann, Trotter, & Howard, 1969), the *Bruininks-Osteretsky Test of Motor Proficiency* (Bruininks, 1978), the *Pediatric Examination of Educational Readiness* (PEER; Levine & Schneider, 1983), and the *Pediatric Examination of Educational Readiness at Middle School* (PEERamid; Levine, 1985). It may be necessary to modify some of the evaluations of motor coordination due to physical limitations.

A developmental ADL checklist can be helpful for young children (under age three), however, these assessments often do not accommodate the child with a physical limitation. An adult rehabilitation-based checklist may incorporate the use of adaptive equipment. The *Functional Independence Measure* and *Functional Independence Measure for Children*™ (Hamilton & Granger, 1991) provide information on many areas and are often used in research. These assessments group many skills together, which make them less sensitive to incremental changes if used for short-term goal setting. When evaluating ADL skills through parent report, the interview should be structured to help establish rapport and learn more about the family.

Family

The family values, priorities, and cultural preferences must be considered. It is often possible to gather information using an informal interview with a few key questions. Open-ended questions may be more helpful than a yes/no checklist and help to establish rapport. For example, "Tell me about a typical day" with supportive questions, "What time do you wake-up?" "Does anybody help you get dressed?" and "What do you usually eat for breakfast/lunch/dinner?" can provide information on family routines in addition to ADLs.

Families of children with a limb condition often express challenges coping with their own, extended family, and community reactions to the presence of the limb condition. In our society, the hands and arms are used for communication and are part of our social being. The family often views the loss of the upper limb's communication potential as very detrimental. As the child grows, he or she may become more aware of the loss of the social communication of the extremity. The occupational therapist needs to be aware of the social communication function of the upper extremity and be sensitive to interventions that influence this role. There may be times when function is a priority over cosmesis, and other times in the child's life during which cosmesis is the primary concern.

Children with limb deficiencies vary in their choice of assistive devices during the transition from young child, to school-aged child, to adolescent, and to adult. It may be difficult for the family to accept the desires of the child if the child chooses to use devices that are different from the family's expectations. It is the responsibility of the therapist to ensure the child has the most successful experience possible with an assistive device in order that the child can make an informed decision. The therapist may need to help the family understand why a child may prefer different options.

The occupational therapist needs to demonstrate sensitivity while gathering information about family resources including medical coverage, formal and informal support groups, and information and educational resources. The occupational therapist can be a primary or secondary provider of information about coverage for medical expenses, support groups, special education, and rehabilitation laws. The information gathered may indicate the need to refer to a social worker to help with contacting agencies and receiving supportive counseling.

The occupational therapist must be aware of the potential equipment needs over time of an individual in order to guide the selection of devices. The family of the child who requires medical equipment such as prosthetics and splints must be made aware of reimbursement issues for medical equipment. Many third party payers (insurance, medical assistance) will provide services on a limited basis, provide one-per-lifetime coverage, or not cover durable medical equipment. Some insurance carriers cover one prosthetic device per lifetime. The occupational therapist providing services individually or as part of a team, which includes prosthetists, can help with selecting prosthetic components and aspects of a functional splint. The family may need information on medical assistance to help with expenses not covered by the family's insurance plan.

Practice Setting

Individuals with limb deformities often receive occupational therapy in acute care hospitals, early intervention programs, rehabilitation hospitals or outpatient facilities, and school-based settings. A child with an upper limb condition may receive occupational therapy service at a variety of settings simultaneously and/or over time. Parents may be confused about the role of occupational therapy as the child transitions from community-based early intervention settings to school-based settings. It is important to establish communication between settings to ensure program consistency.

The acute care therapist may first encounter the individual with an upper limb condition in the nursery. The occupational therapist must work with other professionals to assist the family by providing education regarding the child's special needs and information about community resources.

The rehabilitation hospital-based occupational therapist often provides therapy services for a specific period of time following a surgical procedure, or for specific rehabilitation goals. Occupational therapy and other members of the rehabilitation team would provide intervention in the form of prosthetic, adaptive equipment, or splint training and clinical follow-up programs

Occupational therapists based in early intervention and outpatient programs provide ongoing home and community-based services to help the child develop fine motor, perceptual, visual motor, social, play, and ADL skills, plus refine the use of assistive devices.

The focus of school-based therapy is the development of educationally relevant skills which will facilitate maximum levels of participation in the school program. The management of school related tools and supplies, peer socialization, and dressing and hygiene related to toileting, are frequently identified areas for intervention.

Sociopolitical

Three primary laws relate to children with limb conditions. The laws relate to education, rehabilitation, and accessibility. The Individuals with Disabilities Education Act (IDEA, 1997) was reauthorized in 2002 and entitles all children with disabilities to a free and appropriate education with related services in the least restrictive environment. A child may also be eligible for early intervention services starting at birth. Occupational therapy services are provided in school settings under IDEA. The Americans with Disabilities Act (ADA) extends civil rights protections to individuals with disabilities, supporting equal opportunities for employment, accessibility, transportation, and government services. The Technology Act (Technology Related Assistance for Individuals with Disabilities Act, 1988) supports the acquisition of adaptive equipment and assistive technology for people who require it.

Lifestyle/Lifespan

It is important to help the individual and the family become aware of issues that will be faced throughout the lifetime of the individual with upper extremity limb conditions. Table 9.3 highlights major areas of concern.

Accessibility issues for home modifications for a child with an upper limb conditions often include assistive devices to maximize one-handed completion of tasks. For example, a rocker knife, cutting board, hair dryer holder, etc. may facilitate independence. Extensive home modifications may be necessary for the child with multiple limb deformities. Adaptations are typically needed for driving, such as a knob on the steering wheel.

Financial issues will vary depending on the family's economic resources and insurance coverage. Insurance reimbursement often has limitations and medical equipment expenses for prosthetics, adaptive equipment, and orthoses may be encountered. It is important to recognize that the use of equipment may vary over time, depending on the needs and interests of the child and family. The occupational therapist needs to be aware

Table 9.3
Life Span Considerations

Accessibility	Financial	Medical	Family	Social
May need adaptations for specialized sports equipment May need adaptation for driving a car Minor home modifications	Reimbursement for prosthetics and splints may be limited	Surgery to enhance function may be offered Require periodic follow-up for issues of growth and new equipment, and equipment repair	Increased time for daily care Coping Sibling relationships	Interaction with peers Loss of upper extremity for body language/social communicator Cosmesis versus function

of resources for the family and about equipment that can "grow" with the child to promote maximum length of use during the child's growing years.

The child with an upper extremity limb condition is often able to participate in typical community recreation programs with minimal adaptations. Encouragement to participate in sports will be beneficial to the child for physical fitness and peer relationships.

Clinical Decision Making Process

Defining Focus for Intervention

In school, the foci for intervention are skills that will enable the child to benefit from the educational setting, such as handwriting, fine motor, bilateral hand coordination necessary for schoolwork, and self-care skills. Hospital clinic outcomes are concerned with changes in range of motion, muscle function and functional movement. Pre-surgical evaluation, splinting, prostheses, and adaptive equipment are often provided in this setting. Outpatient prosthetic training, splinting, scar management, muscle re-education, and functional skills training may be necessary in the post-operative phase.

Passive prosthesis, along with parent education and home programming, is usually prescribed at four to six months of age. At about 18 months of age, the child should begin occupational therapy in the form of prosthetic training with a functional prosthesis. As the child matures, more technologically sophisticated equipment, such as a myoelectric prosthesis, may be employed. Also, personal goals related to school performance, prevocational skills, social acceptability, and extracurricular activities such as sports or the arts will govern the thrust of treatment.

Establishing Goals for Intervention

The setting, developmental level of the child, family values, interests and expectations, as well as reimbursement issues often dictate the length or frequency of treatment, and influence the prioritization of goals for intervention. For example, the expected proficiency with a prosthetic device for a nine-month-old differs from that of a two-year-old or a six-year-old. If tendon transfer surgery is anticipated, then range of motion and muscle and joint strength become treatment priorities.

Designing Theory-Based Intervention

Although many frames of reference would be appropriately applied to this population, the biomechanical frame of reference is most frequently employed. The biomechanical frame of reference is used with individuals with neuromuscular or musculoskeletal problems. This frame of reference is based on principals of physics, physiology, neuroscience, and kinesiology (Case-Smith, Allen, & Nuse Pratt, 1996). This frame of reference is often used when adaptive equipment, orthotic, or prosthetic intervention is required. The therapist must understand the biomechanical and physiologic forces that are acting on the child, as well as understanding the mechanical advantages and disadvantages of the specific device. Joint position, fixed deformities, sensory function, functional needs, and dynamic movement patterns may be a few of the major factors that need to be considered in determining the final orthotic or prosthetic design.

The developmental frame of reference is certainly relevant to any pediatric population. Children with upper limb deficiencies are faced with many challenges to the normal progression or acquisition of skills. Understanding normal development will assist the therapist in designing treatment plans that mitigate or compensate for these challenges, and facilitate the child's ability to engage in age-appropriate life tasks that are associated with school, self-care, and play.

Many frames of reference consider the evaluation of ADLs. The principles inherent to motor learning theory are used to teach the child specific ADL tasks. This framework might be used when teaching a child who has significant upper extremity paralysis to don a shirt. The activity would be broken down into several steps and gradually introduced into the therapy sessions. Techniques may be modified and adaptive equipment may be introduced at various steps. Trial and error problem solving is then used to refine the process. Home programs might be used to provide the repeated practice that is required to reinforce the skill.

The model of human occupation is also very useful. This frame of reference focuses on the life roles that the individual needs to assume in order to develop and maintain a personally meaningful and productive lifestyle, and then establishes which behaviors facilitate the performance of the life tasks and daily routines associated with those roles. This approach is driven by the values, needs, and aspirations of the child and family (Case-Smith, Allen, & Nuse Pratt, 1996).

Evaluating Progress

Traditionally, progress is based on meeting established goals. Measurable goals typically focus on independence with ADLs, and the use and care of assistive technology. In the clinic setting, repeated measures such as the *Functional Independence Measure* (FIM; Uniform Data System for Medical Rehabilitation, 1993) and a specific checklist will help to monitor the changes that occur over time. Videotaping can be a powerful tool to evaluate subtle progress that is not measurable on standardized tests. Another measure of progress that is less objective is the adaptation and coping of the child and the family to the disability.

Determining Change in or Termination of Treatment

Change in or termination of treatment is warranted when the child does not meet the goals established, or has met all the goals established. In either event, the therapist needs to re-evaluate goals for relevance. New goals could indicate a change of focus or higher levels of independence. Discharge from therapy may occur when the child has reached a maximum level of independence for his or her age, and the child has acquired a sufficient level of foundational skills to promote independent problem-solving and future skill acquisition.

Case Study 1

Description

Joe is an 11-year-old male with a short left congenital below-elbow amputation. He has been wearing a prosthesis since he was six months old. He started with a conventional body-powered prosthesis and progressed to a myoelectric unit by the age of four years. He currently uses both a conventional voluntary closing and myoelectric prosthesis. He wears the myoelectric unit to school and uses the conventional unit (or no prosthesis at all) for sports activities and play at home. Joe is proficient with both prostheses but he still will often complete tasks one handed. His scores on the *University of New Brunswick Test of Prosthetic Function* (Sanderson & Scott, 1985) were as follows:

Prosthesis	Skill	Spontaneity
Conventional	30/40	25/40
Myoelectric	27/40	23/40

Joe is very well adjusted to his disability and he has no difficulty socially interacting with his peers. Joe is very athletic. He plays on a travel soccer team and is an avid swimmer. Recently he has taken an interest in ice hockey. He tried holding the stick with his conventional prosthesis but he did not feel that he had enough control to "get a good shot off." At his clinic visit he asked the team for help with this problem. The prosthetist suggested trying a special terminal device designed to hold a hockey stick. The device could be easily interchanged on his conventional prosthesis because it had a quick disconnect wrist unit. Joe was then set up for two sessions of occupational therapy to try out the device. The goals of his outpatient therapy are as follows:

Long- and Short-Term Goals

The long-term goal of intervention for Joe is to evaluate the success of the prosthetic device, teach him how to use and care for the device, and be able to play ice hockey using the new prosthetic terminal device.

These goals will be reached in part through successfully achieving the following short-term goals:

1. Independently interchange the terminal device.
2. Secure the stick using the sound extremity and the new prosthetic device.
3. Shoot a puck into a net from a distance of 10 feet with fair accuracy.

Therapist Goals and Strategies

The therapist's goals include:

1. Provide resource information for adaptive sports.
2. Assure that the fit of the prosthesis is appropriate and that everything is functioning properly.
3. Assist with education of the child and family in the care and use of the prosthesis.

The therapist's strategies include:

1. Provide opportunities to explore use of the adaptive equipment to facilitate skill in its use.
2. Try different techniques for positioning body or prosthesis to accomplish the task.
3. Provide opportunities for repetition and practice.

Activity

Indoor Hockey Game

Joe will attempt to shoot a street hockey puck into a portable net. The angle and approach on the net will be varied after five attempts from each position.

Treatment Objectives

Joe will get the puck in the net 50% of the time without dropping his hockey stick.

Case Study 2

Description

Mara is a 15-month-old female with a right obstetric brachial plexus palsy injury involving the upper nerve roots (i.e., Erb's palsy). She is six months post a nerve graft to the biceps. She receives occupational therapy services once per week as an outpatient at a rehabilitation facility, and is followed through a clinic program at the hospital that performed the surgical procedure. Mara has not had any other medical issues. She is a first child born to an intact family. Her development has been mildly delayed for bilateral upper extremity weight bearing activities such as reciprocal creeping and pulling to stand. She is currently cruising, has learned to pull to stand using only her left upper extremity, and is able to sit independently. Social, language, cognitive, and fine motor and play skills are within normal limits, using modified techniques to compensate for her right upper extremity weakness. Table 9.4 presents the results of the initial evaluation for outpatient therapy.

Table 9.4
Musculoskeletal Evaluation Results for Mara

	Right Upper Extremity		
Muscle/Movement	**Strength**	**Active Range**	**Passive Range**
Biceps	2+/5	0–100°	WNL
Shoulder flexion	2+/5	10°–80°	10°–170°
Shoulder abduction	2/5	0–80°	WFL
Shoulder external rotation	2–/5	0–45°	0–70°
Wrist extension	2/5	0–45°	0–70°
Supination	2/5	0–60°	0–80°

Sensation of the right upper extremity appears impaired as she inconsistently responds to touch.

Long- and Short-Term Goals

The long-term goal of intervention for Mara is to improve bilateral coordination to develop independence in activity of daily living skills.

This goal will be reached in part through successfully achieving the following short-term goals:

1. Mara will bring a 2-handled cup to her mouth using both hands.
2. Mara will put on and take off a hat with both hands.

Therapist Goals and Strategies

The therapist's goals include:

1. Increasing range of motion and strength of right elbow flexion.
2. Improving bilateral integration and spontaneous use of the right upper extremity.

The therapist's strategies include:

1. Improving strength by grading size and weight of objects to manipulate.
2. Engaging in sensory-based activities to the right upper extremity.
3. Positioning of activities to promote awareness of the right arm.

Activity

Dramatic Play with Hats

Various hats used for dress-up play will be used including an army helmet, a fireman's hat, a baseball cap, a construction hat, a space helmet, etc,. that will be placed on the head of the child, parent, and therapist.

Treatment Objective

Mara will use both upper extremities to put on a hat and bend her elbow 120° against gravity.

Resources

The following resources can be helpful for gathering clinical data:

Physiological data:

- Manual muscle test
- Active and passive range of motion
- Sensation

General Development for ages 0 to 5:

- *Peabody Developmental Motor Scales–2*

- *Hawaii Early Learning Profile™*
- *Pediatric Developmental Inventory*
- *University of New Brunswick Test of Prosthetic Function*

School-Aged Assessments:

- *Jebsen Test of Upper Limb Function*
- *Berry Test of Visual Motor Skills*
- *Gardner Test of Visual Perceptual Skills*
- *Bruininks-Osteretsky Test of Motor Proficiency*
- *Pediatric Early Elementary Examination–Revised*
- *Pediatric Examination of Educational Readiness at Middle Childhood–Revised*
- *School Function Assessment*

Activities of Daily Living:

- Checklist
- FIM™
- Wee-FIM™

The following resources can be helpful for gathering family data:

Informal interview with open ended questions

Awareness of financial resources, cultural concerns, values, priorities, and daily routines

The following are common practice settings:

Acute hospitalization

Rehabilitation hospital (inpatient, outpatient, and clinic setting)

Outpatient rehabilitation services

Community-based (early intervention and school)

The following resources can be helpful for gathering sociopolitical data:

IDEA

Disability Act

Rehabilitation Act

Vocational Rehabilitation

Technology-Related Assistance for Individuals with Disabilities Act

Medical Assistance

Disability (SSI)

The following can be helpful in managing and understanding lifestyle and lifespan issues:

Accessibility needs:

- Home
- School
- Community

Financial needs:

- Durable medical equipment

- Home modifications

Medical needs:

- Clinical follow-up
- Surgical intervention

Family needs:

- Coping skills
- Decreased social communication
- Sibling relationships

Internet Resources

United Brachial Plexus Network:
www.ubpn.org

Brachial Plexus Palsy Foundation email address:
brachial@aol.com

The Association of Children's Prosthetic-Orthotic Clinics:
www.ACPOC.org

Published Resources

Booklets from the Area Child Amputee Center (235 Wealthy S.E., Grand Rapids, Michigan 49503):
Children with Hand Differences: A Guide for Families
Children with Limb Loss: A Handbook for Families.
Children with Limb Loss: A Handbook for Teachers

Caseley, J. (1991). Harry, Willy, and Carrothead. (New York, Greenwillow Books)

References

Beery, K. (1997). *Beery-Buktenica developmental test of visual motor integration* (4th ed.). Parsippany, NJ: Modern Curriculum Press.

Bruininks, R. H. (1978). *Bruininks Oseretsky test of motor proficiency.* Circle Pines, MN: AGS.

Case-Smith, J., Allen, A., & Nuse Pratt, P. (1996). *Occupational therapy for children.* Saint Louis, MO: Mosby.

Folio, R., & Fewell, R. (2000). *Peabody developmental scales,* (2nd ed.). Austin, TX: Pro-Ed.

Furuno, S., O'Reilly, K., Hosaka, C. M., Zeisloft, B., & Allman, T. (1984). *The Hawaii early learning profile.* Palo Alto, CA: VORT.

Gardner, M. F. (1997). *Test of visual motor skills–revised.* Hydesville, CA: Psychological and Educational Publications Inc.

Glynn, B. D. (2002). *Congenital hand deformities.* Retrieved 12-5-2002, from www.eMedicine.com/plastic/topic298.htm

Haley, S., Coster, W., Ludlow, L., Haltiwanger, J., & Andrellos, P. (1992). *Pediatric evaluation of disability inventory.* San Antonio, TX: The Psychological Corporation.

Hamilton, B. B., & Granger, C. U. (1991). *Functional independence measure for children.* Buffalo, NY: Research Foundation of the State University of New York.

Hunter, Mackin, et. al. (2002). *Rehabilitation of the hand and upper extremity* (5th ed.). St. Louis, MO: Mosby.

Individuals with Disabilities Education Act (IDEA) Amendments of 1997 (P. L. No. 105-17). U. S. C., 1400.

Jebsen, R. H., Taylor, N., Trieschmann, R. B., Trotter, M. J., & Howard, L. A. (1969). *Jebsen hand function test.* Bolingbrook, IL: Sammons Preston, Inc.

Levine, M. D. (1985). *Pediatric examination of educational readiness in middle childhood.* Cambridge, MA: Educators Publishing Services, Inc.

Levine, M. D., & Schneider, E. A. (1983). *Pediatric examination of educational readiness.* Cambridge, MA: Educators Publishing Services.

Mackinnon, S. E. (2002). *Brachial plexus injuries, congenital.* Retrieved 12-5-2002 from www.emedicine.com/orthoped/topic466.htm

McDonnell, P., Scott R., & McKay, A. (1988). Incidence of congenital upper-limb deficiencies. *Journal of the Association of Child Prosthetic-Orthotic Clinics.* 23(1), 8.

Sanderson, E. R., & Scott, R. N. (1985). *University of New Brunswick test of prosthetic function.* New Brunswick, Canada: Bioengineering Institute, University of New Brunswick.

Swanson, A. B. (1976) A classification for congenital malformations. *Journal of Hand Surgery, 1976 Jul; 1*(1), 8–22.

Uniform Data System for Medical Rehabilitation. (1993). *Functional independence measure.* Buffalo, NY: The State University of New York at Buffalo.

Social Skill Deficits 10

Nancy Allen Kauffman, Ed.M. OTR/L

Synopsis of Clinical Condition

Social skills are learned behaviors and actions, either purposeful or automatic, which enable a person to develop and maintain relationships. These skills must occur appropriately within a societal system and in a variety of environments, and require a coping style that is both effective and adaptive. Social cognition is more than just knowledge of interpersonal skills. It is the act of having both awareness *and* judgment regarding them. Pro-social skill is a term applied to positive behaviors that anticipate social obstacles and take steps to meet them.

Social interactions can serve two purposes. One type of interaction allows a person to give or receive an object or instruction or help, as in, "Please pass the salt." The other serves to establish, sustain, or deepen a relationship, as in, "How was your weekend?" or a warm handshake, or, "Guess what my mother said!" The latter includes expressions of feelings, mutually shared humor, conversations about dreams and values.

Social ability requires a series of social initiative and response steps in each encounter to achieve fluidity. One must identify the social situation, select the skills needed, carry out those skills, perceive the other person's response, and then adjust additional social actions accordingly. Social problem solving involves predicting consequences for each potential social response and selecting the most appropriately adaptive one.

Prevalence and Etiology

Social skills deficits occur more often in people with special needs than in the average population, even if social difficulty is not a discriminating feature of the diagnosis as it is in the autism spectrum. Other diagnoses, including language impairments, spina bifida, Turner's syndrome, neurofibromatosis, trichotillomania, and early gestational age or low birth weight, have all been associated with a higher than average incidence of social difficulties as children grow and develop.

Research in the domain of social skills is relatively new, and prevalence figures are sparse. The national Interagency Committee on Learning Disabilities (1987) recommended that social skills deficits be included in the definition of learning disabilities. As recently as 2000, the text revision of the fourth edition of the American Psychiatric Association's (APA) *Diagnostic and Statistical Manual of Mental Disorders* had not yet included social skills deficits among potential "Learning Disorders" (APA, 2000). (Its category of learning disorders did, however, include reading, mathematics, and written expression). Instead, "relational problems" were a fairly undefined mental health postscript under "other conditions," and no prevalence figures were reported.

Several conditions with known prevalence figures and concomitant social skill deficits include expressive language disorders (3% to 7% of the school-age population), mixed expressive-receptive language disorders (3%), attention deficit disorder (ADD) with and without hyperactivity (3% to 7%), selective mutism (fewer than 1% of people seen in mental health settings), and autism (2 to 20 per 10,000 people, with some evidence of possibly increasing prevalence). Other disorders that sometimes include social deviations include reactive attachment disorder, obsessive-compulsive disorder, and social anxiety (APA, 2000).

Autism is four or five times more prevalent in males than females, and Asperger's disorder, a condition on the autism spectrum, is at least five times more frequent in males. The prevalence of attention deficit disorders in males over females ranges from 2:1 to 9:1 with the predominantly inattentive type in the lower range. Five percent of siblings of persons with autism also exhibit the condition, and first-degree biological relatives of individuals with ADD or attention deficit hyperactivity disorder have greater than average difficulty with hyperactivity, impulsivity, and inattention (APA, 2000).

The large preponderance of males with social skill deficits may be due to a genetic predisposition associated with the X chromosome, which preliminary research suggests may contain the social cognition gene sites.

Persons who have difficulty acquiring social skills may fail to grasp skills initially because of language-related impairments, incomplete or impaired social perception (as in persons with nonverbal learning disabilities or the diagnoses on the autism spectrum), attentional issues (such as ADD, with or without hyperactivity), or environmental conditions (including family modeling or cultural differences).

On the other hand, social skills may be learned adequately by people who can describe and define them, yet who also fail to perform them reliably because of attentional issues, expressive language deficits, processing delays, sensory overload, organizational difficulties, inconsiderateness, defiance, or lack of motivation.

Common Characteristics and Symptoms

People may exhibit either delays in and/or deviations from social development. An example of a delay occurs in people who monologue about their own interests during conversation without noticing that the listener needs a chance to respond. This behavior is typical of toddlers who have not yet learned to be interested in the responses of others. An example of a deviation is reciting lengthy dialogue memorized from movies or videos in place of conversation. This behavior is not representative of a typical developmental phase.

People with difficulty using appropriate social skills often have trouble making or keeping friends. Some may have familiar old friends, but wish they could fit in socially with others who reject or ignore them. Some avoid interacting with other people on purpose, preferring instead to read, use computers for prolonged periods, or engage in other engrossing solitary activities. People with social deficits rarely make or receive personal phone calls or invitations, and their friendly overtures fail to bring them the desired results. Birthday parties and group mall visits may be either nonexistent or painful experiences.

Many people with social skill deficits have difficulty seeing situations from another person's point of view, or even recognizing that other perspectives than their own exist at all. They fail to notice needs or feelings of others without prompting, and may act or speak disrespectfully and inconsiderately to peers or adults both outside and within the family.

Some people with social inadequacies are not creative social problem solvers or innovators. They may be rigid in handling interpersonal exchanges, uncreative in resolving differences, or unimaginative in planning play or other group pastimes. Comprehension of abstract nuances, and "reading between the lines" of verbal and nonverbal cues, may elude them. In fact, Thompson (1997) reports that 65% of all communication is nonverbal. Therefore, people with nonverbal learning disabilities fail to benefit from about 65% of interaction skills, and sometimes even more.

The dyssemic individual described by Nowicki and Duke (1992) stands out from peers motorically and in space awareness, as well as socially. The social skill needs of individuals with hyperactivity or acting-out behaviors are often more noticed in schools, work environments, and families than are the needs of people who just quietly fail to grasp abstract inferences and social implications. Clinicians must be particularly alert to the social needs of unobtrusive, even withdrawn people who have difficulty with eye contact, understanding instructions, telling news about their friendships, or generally "catching on" to social interactions.

Gresham and Elliott (1999) use the acronym CARES to identify domains they chose to measure in their *Social Skills Rating System:* cooperation, assertion, responsibility, empathy, and self-control. Snopkowski (2001) identified seven themes likely to be atypical in children with ADD who show social skill problems: verbal presentations, nonverbal presentations, emotional responses, play/work skills, awareness of others, initiating and maintaining relations, and feelings about themselves.

Social skill deficits, if left untreated, are often persistent, and may result in general social adjustment problems and negative relationships in adulthood. These inadequacies affect workplace relations (with superiors, coworkers, and customers), family interaction (with spouses, offspring, and extended relatives), and friendship building. This may lead to depression and other psychopathology in later years if left unchecked. They may complicate or exacerbate treatment of other mental disorders or general medical conditions.

Target Areas for Intervention

The occupational therapist works as part of a team, which always includes the individual client, and may include the referring family, personnel from the school or work environment, psychologists, counselors, social workers, psychiatrists, speech therapists, neurologists, and other professionals. The occupational therapist helps gather information about primary and secondary social skill deficits that interfere with adjustment in the school, home, community, or workplace. For example, social skills are a primary deficit in the autism spectrum—part of the defining characteristics of the disorder. On the other hand, social skills may be secondary to other conditions that must be addressed instead of (or in addition to) the social competency itself. The primary issues may need to be addressed before or concurrently with social skill issues.

Table 10.1
Examples of Secondary Social Skill Deficits

Primary Deficit	Secondary Social Skill Deficits	Treatment Options to Precede or Run Concurrently with Social Skills Treatment
Sensory defensiveness	Person may withdraw from personal contact or avoid slightly crowded or mildly noisy social environments that could have been the site of friend-making opportunities.	Ameliorate interfering sensory defensiveness issues.*
Inadequate body scheme with resulting faulty spatial perception	Person may invade others' personal space or keep too much distance for comfortable interactions.	Sensory integration and other techniques to improve body awareness, motor planning, and overall space perception.*
Coordination disorders	Young child's embarrassment about handwriting, drawing, playground, or athletic competence may result in unrealistic oversensitivity and defensiveness in the presence of more competent children or actual rejection or ignoring by them.	Treat the coordination disorder.*
Attentional and impulsiveness issues; difficulty with self-regulation	Lack of focus during social interactions or interfering hyperactivity may spoil social opportunities.	Alert Program techniques from How Does Your Engine Run? program (Williams & Shellenberger 1996) Possibly refer for neurological or other medical evaluation.*
Learned family interaction styles that put off others	Argumentativeness, disrespectful speaking, put downs, whining, and griping may be verbal exchanges learned at home that interfere with friend-making elsewhere.	Possibly address this in an OT-run activity group focusing on attitude and manner of communicating, or refer to a family therapist.*
Language processing disorders	Failure to comprehend stated or implied social or game rules, or delays in processing information (thereby delaying social response time) may result in impatience or ignoring by others.	Refer to speech/language clinician, particularly one with thorough understanding of pragmatics.
Defiance	Defiant individuals may acquire the friendship of other defiant people, but attempts to socialize them with more compliant individuals may sabotage therapeutic efforts for the whole group.	Refer deep-seated defiance to other mental health professionals if the defiance repeatedly interferes with the group process.

Note: Asterisk (*) indicates a sampling of potential primary deficits suitable for occupational therapy intervention.
Adapted and reprinted with permission by Occupational Therapy Programs (© 2002).

The occupational therapist helps the team prioritize social goals. Next the therapist may, as appropriate, focus on resolving primary deficits using the treatments marked in the chart above with an asterisk (*). In addition, the occupational therapist may establish social competence groups using activity to address the following identified primary social goals:

- Awareness of and empathy towards others' needs and feelings
- Communication styles and content
- Social problem solving
- Ability to balance leader and follower roles, and handle responsibility

Contextual Considerations

Clinical

The occupational therapist interviews the potential client and possibly other family members to begin to identify inadequate social competencies. In addition, the therapist gathers written or oral reports from other sources (when confidentiality will not be compromised) such as the school or work setting, and therapeutic personnel working with the person elsewhere, paying particular note to both structured and unstructured situations. A full psychological or neuropsychological report is particularly helpful for giving an overview of the person's cognitive strengths and weaknesses, often a revealing adjunct to the social information. Information about medications is important so side effects can be taken into account.

The occupational therapist uses formal and informal measures to identify primary and secondary social skill goals in need of intervention. The *Canadian Occupational Performance Measure* (Law et al., 1994) is a structured interview intended as an outcome measure to detect change in a client's self-perception of occupational performance in any realm. Administered at the beginning of occupational therapy service and at appropriate intervals thereafter, it yields standardized results, and comes with a training video and accompanying self-instructional workbook. The *Social Skills Rating Scale* (Gresham & Elliott, 1990) yields standardized results for children in grades K to 12 in the five social skill areas mentioned previously. The accompanying manual and forms also include considerable information about planning and carrying out intervention based on the results of the assessment.

Measures of social adaptability in the birth-to-three population can serve as an informal gauge of the *sequence* in which early social and adaptive skills are acquired even when assessing somewhat older children. Examples are the *Early Coping Inventory,* (Zeitlin, Williamson, & Szczepanski, 1988), which rates reactive behavior, self-initiated behavior, and sensorimotor organization; and the social-emotional development sections of the *HELP Strands* (Parks, 1995).

One method of identifying social skill issues is through an informal structured meeting with the client. In the *COLLAGE Program,* this method has been used to identify social goals for well over 1,000 socially impaired people ages 4 to 40. A demonstration video is available (Kauffman, 2002).

Table 10.2 shows examples of important clinical considerations to keep in mind when establishing or leading group therapy programs (Kauffman, 2002).

Table 10.2
Sampling of Treatment Ideas for Developing Social Skills

Categories/ Constructs to be Modified	Relevant Treatment Concepts	Potential Strategies	Precautions
Verbal presentations (content)	Via modeling and coaching, group member observes and experiences successful verbal interactions.	Whole-group conversation in a circle every session. More complex small group chat later while concurrently sharing snack, including tastes, passing items, spills, etc.	Many members will try to direct comments to adult leaders only, not peers. Must redirect.
Nonverbal presentations (psychomotor)	Motivation to use self-regulation may be enhanced by improved skill at reading others' nonverbal and verbal cues depicting annoyance or frustration at the irritating behaviors.	Carpet samples to delineate space in conversation circle. "How Does Your Engine Run" techniques. Empower to recognize their own limits & take action: (e.g. request wheelbarrow walk if feeling over-aroused, or sit out game if unable to handle losing that day, etc.).	Those with ADD often hear criticism of psychomotor behaviors. Avoid repeated censoring. Instead encourage self-awareness, reading others' reactions, self initiating change.
Emotional responses	An emotion is usually not the social problem. Person's response/behavior is the problem.	Photograph or videotape group members acting out emotions. Label times they recall experiencing those emotions. Group members act out suitable response choices.	Do not necessarily avoid creating unpleasant emotions in activities; instead, help group members deal with them as they arise.
Play and work with others	The gifted, creative, or egocentric often strongly envision end products and play methods to their liking, and push hard for independence or leadership. Slower or passive members may have rarely experienced having others accept their ideas.	Constructions or murals, with requirements for jointly created end products. (Provide support and understanding for the frustration of the former group, encouragement and patience for latter group. Point out: Goal = "everyone has contributed and accepted each others' ideas," not "the end product is a prize winner").	May require restarting project several times until all members are contributing.
Awareness of self/others & valuing others	Use of two therapists allows one to remove a member into hallway for individual review of current social interaction and immediate feedback. Recognizing and predicting others' viewpoints is a major treatment goal.	Out in hallway for confidentiality, prompt member to identify what just happened socially and problem-solve for himself/herself how to carry out the interaction more effectively and adaptively next time.	Avoid telling or even suggesting. Encourage persons to figure out the problem and the solution for themselves, and the advantage to themselves of the new solution.

(*Continued*)

Table 10.2 (*Continued*)

Categories/ Constructs To Be Modified	Relevant Treatment Concepts	Potential Strategies	Precautions
Initiating/ maintaining interpersonal relations	Speaking respectfully to others is a major treatment goal. Expect it of (1) group members to each other and (2) members' manner of speaking to their families. Use "natural" opportunities during group sessions: interview newcomers, greet and handshake visitors, send group cards to ill members.	Encourage families to tape record their dinner or car conversations, and "score" themselves on respectful language and voice. Have member make phone call for group's pizza order, bowling alley schedule, or call to therapist's cell phone for practice. Indicate with colorful labels on group's big calendar, all calls/visits initiated or received that week.	Beware adding new member to "delicately bonded" group that is just starting to value each other. Let the valuing swell first.
Feelings about self	Research implications suggest: begin treatment early, thus preventing the negative feelings of self more likely in older children.	Empower group to carry out their ideas for activities, often generated during conversation time (rather than always having leaders impose activities on them). Seeing their ideas in action often builds esteem.	Be cautious about scheduling low-esteem person as one of oldest in group. Rather than building esteem as leader, person may feel further intimidated by social antics of less competent children. His or her fragile ego may be scared away. Compliments may sound hollow to the self-critic. Instead, encourage self-evaluation, but require both negative & positive aspects of performance.

Family

Children with social skill difficulties may be found in well-adjusted families. The child may stand out as different from other members of the family because of basic neurological makeup, or the child may be reflecting learned social behaviors that result in social deficits. In either case, the family may benefit from specific child management suggestions from the therapist or referral to parenting classes to help expand behavioral strategies to promote social development. Parents may need reassurance to help alleviate guilt they feel, often unjustified, about their contribution to their child's social inadequacies.

Siblings of socially impaired children may bear the brunt of their brother's or sister's social ineptness if unsatisfying social interactions characterize much of their playtime together. Also, the need to appease the inflexible or non-insightful member of the family may result in constant accommodation to that family member's needs, to the exclusion of siblings' and parents' needs. The therapist may help the family identify potential frustrations and create family accommodations, such as arranging to prevent the socially impaired child from repeatedly spoiling play dates at home for the sibling and friends. Some families successfully hold "family meetings" with all members encouraged to suggest issues they think need resolving and recommend solutions that family members could jointly carry out.

Practice Setting

The occupational therapist in any setting should be alert and address social competence delays that may currently or potentially interfere with their clients' interpersonal development. In the school environment, social skill difficulties emerge most often in the unstructured periods of the day rather than during teacher-directed activities. Particularly difficult situations arise during recess, in the lunchroom, at the bus stop, in the hallways, and on the school bus. These social hot spots require reciprocal interactions and correct interpretations of other people's feelings and intended meanings. In addition, many schools now require academic project or study groups that, while academic in their primary goal, also require collaborative planning and cooperative decision making. Schools are learning that such groups are excellent preparation for the realities of the adult workplace, where collaboration and cooperation will often be required with co-workers, customers, and bosses.

School interventions can take the form of (1) consultation with teachers or playground and lunchroom aides, (2) classroom intervention (for example, during project-group meetings), or (3) pull-out activity groups of children from several classes at once. Or, therapists may arrange a buddy system or "lunch pal" for a socially inept child to be paired with a socially competent model who brings the student along for inclusion in his or her social group of lunch friends.

Occupational therapists may run activity-oriented groups with names such as "Lunch Bunch," "Friday Friend," or "Kare Kids" to address social goals in school at the moment activities are taking place and the need for interaction arises. Each group may be limited to children with similar social difficulties, or may include typical students as models. The therapist's activity groups benefit greatly from being co-facilitated by a speech therapist, counselor, other occupational therapist, or member of another helping profession. This adds therapeutic viewpoints as well as the option of brief individual therapeutic input for one group member while others continue the activity led by another adult.

Social goals may also be addressed in therapy groups that were previously established to work on functional goals such as motor development, sensory integration, or graphomotor skills, or issues of a particular diagnosis, such as spina bifida or cerebral palsy. This can occur in schools, hospitals, clinics, or therapy centers. Less often, socially impaired children are referred directly into occupational therapy groups for the purpose of social skill building. Some social competence groups are freestanding, community based programs. New potential locations for such programming are after-school care programs for children of working parents, and camp settings—especially camps for handicapped children who are more likely to have social skill delays.

Social skills programming is also useful for adults with social delays. The adult program may be either freestanding or affiliated with a clinic, hospital, or religious organization. It can focus on interactions with family members, employers, or coworkers. It can also emphasize social cognition skills needed for establishing independent living arrangements, including building friendships, developing relationships with neighbors, or getting along with a roommate.

Sociopolitical

The reauthorization of the Individuals with Disabilities Education Act (IDEA, 1997) recognized that behavioral issues can interfere with a child's education and goals. These issues are to be addressed in the child's individual educational plan (IEP). Also, in recent years, the United States has experienced a new appreciation of the importance of the social environment of schools as TV screens and newspapers have documented the shooting of classmates and teachers by students who were loners or misfits, or the target of taunts. Workshops and publications offering help for bullies and the bullied have emerged, and school districts are beginning to adopt whole social competence curricula for their students, faculty, and parents.

A trend toward home schooling has expanded considerably, in part because parents have chosen to allow their children to avoid school social environments they deem unsuitable. Sometimes parents regard school social environments as unsuitable for any child; more often they consider them unsuitable for the out-of-the-ordinary social adjustment of their particular child.

American culture allows and encourages many choices in material purchases, vocations, lifestyles, and other alternatives. Providing therapeutic input to expand an individual's social options is in keeping with this environment of choices. The goal is not to require ultra-responsible social behavior uniformly or cooperative endeavors without exception, or to disallow time spent alone or projects completed independently. The goal is to allow a person wider choices of social responses in keeping with the context of each situation.

Lifestyle/Lifespan

Social cognition difficulties are likely to emerge at certain times in the life cycle. Often they are first identified as children enter kindergarten or preschool, where interactions with peers are for the first time a major part of the child's daily experiences. Other times when ineffective social cognition may emerge again are during periods of change in the social requirements of a contextual setting:

1. Entry into middle school and high school.

   For children with Asperger's disorder, it has been noted that susceptibility to anxiety, depression, victimization, and feelings of isolation increases in adolescence as self-awareness increases. This may be true of other neurological conditions as well.

   During the school years, academic difficulties occur more often in students with social disorders than in other students. This correlation does not imply that one necessarily causes the other. Difficulty with comprehension, abstract or inferential thinking, and organization may impact both the academic areas and the social domain. During these years, occupational therapists should be aware of and involved in the work of local school district transition councils, or other systems established to help smooth the conversion of the student from the role of student to the role of adult citizen.

2. Entry into college, including living with a roommate.
3. Early adulthood, including adapting to the working world.

   History of social skill difficulties in childhood and adolescence has been shown to be related to difficulty in adulthood with life friendships, workplace competence, and adult health.
4. Marriage, as two familys' customs combine, and as one partner may expect more or different social interaction within the marriage and among friends.
5. Carrying out the role of parenting.
6. Moving to a new community at any age.
7. Moving to a different country or culture at any age.
8. Retirement, and its concomitant change in daily companionship.
9. Coping in the elder years with the death of lifelong relatives and well-established friends, thereby creating a need for establishing new social relationships at a time when social initiative-taking is likely to be reduced.

Clinical Decision Making Process

Defining Focus for Intervention

The therapist first prioritizes the social skill difficulties, selecting out those that may result from (or be exacerbated by) underlying causes like those marked with an asterisk in Table 10.1. The therapist provides consultative or direct treatment (such as for sensory integration deficits), or makes a referral to another professional (for example, a speech and language clinician for a language processing evaluation).

The therapist forms activity groups based on these goals. The focus is on creating a social interaction environment that allows situations and scenarios that have been ineffectively resolved elsewhere to unfold naturally. For example, the activities may be selected to create frustration or provide a gentle opportunity to lose. The therapist guides group members to develop more effective methods of coping with such challenges to achieve a higher level of personal satisfaction.

The social skills focus of intervention may be similar to those of other professionals. However, the approach of the occupational therapist differs in that therapeutic activity is used as the actual facilitator of change.

Establishing Goals for Intervention

Goals are established by individual interview with the client, family, and other caregivers. Written reports identifying social skill needs may be available from schools, through evaluations by other professionals, and sometimes from work proficiency reports. Standardized questionnaires may be employed to identify further needs. From these sources, specific long- and short-term goals of occupational therapy intervention should be written. These goals should be reevaluated periodically and revised as needed.

Designing Theory-Based Intervention

The developmental frame of reference (Shortridge & Walker, 1993) assumes that individuals achieve mastery in all areas of development in a continuous process as they age. If physical, environmental, or psychological events interrupt the process, a gap in the developmental progression may result which undermines further development. Occupational therapists provide activities and experiences to promote development and prevent maladaption.

It is important for the therapist to know and understand the developmental frame of reference, particularly with regard to the sequences in which social interactions and play skills are acquired through the lifespan. It is unreasonable to introduce games with complex rules to a group of four-year-olds, as at that age they are mastering cooperative and role play. It is inappropriate to treat lightly a 15-year-old's inability to grasp the perspective of another, as this is essential for the development of healthy ongoing relationships at this age. The level of cognitive development should be considered in addressing social skills. For example, the gifted individual may relate better in a group of slightly older people, while the mildly retarded individual may be more comfortable in a either a mixed age group or one of slightly younger children.

The sensory integration frame of reference (Walker, 1993) assumes that the central nervous system receives, organizes, and uses sensory information from the environment to plan and execute appropriate and effective responses. Physical input of touch pressure has been found to be calming and organizing for some children. A therapist may use this and other sensory integration techniques to supplement social skills work. For example, a rambunctious 10-year-old group member may engage in wheelbarrow walking or Indian wrestling for a few minutes before rejoining the group. Also, the therapist may recommend to the teacher that the child carry books to the library, or help move the table and chairs into position before beginning a classroom group project with other students.

Behavior theory (positive reinforcement) and learning theory (modeling) inform the sequence and motivation of some group activities. For example, when a mildly defiant group member sabotages the parachute activity, the therapist may remind everyone that as soon as the group has cooperatively kept the ball from rolling off the surface of the parachute for 45 seconds, it will be snack time (the sabotaging member's favorite activity). If stickers or other artificial rewards are needed repeatedly for motivating a whole group to cooperate, the activities should be reevaluated and modified. Occupational therapy activities should be inherently motivating. As social skill develops, social rewards replace artificial rewards and intermittent behavioral reinforcement schedules can replace the need for continuous reinforcement. Verbal coaching (responding to the client's lead) will replace prompting (telling them what to do) as soon as possible. Modeling by pointing out another group member's excellent handling of a social situation will soon supplant demonstration by adult leaders.

The model of human occupation assumes that the focus of therapy should be on the person's roles, routines, habits, and motivation in his or her environment and stresses the importance of mastering a variety of roles (Miller, 1993). Many people with social skill delays have never mastered the role of being a friend. Although a child may want to make friends, the habits and routines that he or she has employed to do this may need to be altered or replaced to be effective. In addition, the occupational therapy group can establish an environment that allows group membership skills to be explored, practiced, and mastered. Group member skills include that of group leader, follower, initiator, collaborator, and mediator-negotiator. Pre-event rehearsal allows practice of an approaching social situation likely to be fraught with potential social hazards (such as birthday parties, or Thanksgiving with a crowd of relatives).

Evaluating Progress

Although every formal treatment session is an ongoing evaluation of social growth, the progress of the client *outside* the clinic is the more important measure. Progress there may not evenly parallel the changes seen within the safe environment of the accepting, professionally managed therapeutic setting. Is the client making or keeping friends? Being more considerate? Conversing reciprocally? Taking initiative? Noticing other people's needs?

Observations in informal social settings can either be done by the occupational therapist or can be reported by other team members (including the client himself or herself, family members, or other professionals). Periodic progress interviews with these team members to evaluate how social cognition is being manifested in the neighborhood, school, playground, workplace, or family are important. Written comparison of current social functioning in the clinical setting with the original goals and early progress notes helps document progress. Standardized reevaluation tools and questionnaire-type tests may be important for research purposes or for documentation to insurance companies or referring sources. However, being able to recite social rules or niceties does not necessarily mean they are being applied adaptively in the natural environment. Evaluation of social skills progress is documented not by what people *know* to do, or *talk* about doing, but by what they actually *do* in everyday social contacts.

Determining Change in or Termination of Treatment

The need for small modifications in the treatment approach is evaluated informally at every session. Keeping records of successful strategies or rewards helps the therapist know which strategies are working most effectively. Change in the total approach to providing treatment is warranted if the current methods for improving social skills are not yielding positive movement toward the established goals within six to eight weeks of the start of treatment. Change can take the form of:

- Referral elsewhere, for example if oppositional defiant behavior has not begun to mellow, and particularly if it is disrupting treatment for other members of a therapy group.
- Addition or substitution of other forms of occupational therapy treatment, for example sensory integration or motor coordination treatment, if lack of competence in either of these areas appears to be hampering progress in the social domain.
- A new approach within an existing group therapy setting, for example, adding brand new behavioral reinforcement strategies to increase motivation, such as prizes, points, or fascinating stickers.

If fairly long-term social skills work appears warranted (as in the case of Asperger's disorder), progress may at times seem minor, but often then spurts forward as repeated strategies for prompting particular skills finally "register."

Discharge is considered when social goals established by the client and family are met to a reasonable degree, and/or the client is experiencing satisfying social interactions. Discharge planning may include (1) joining or expanding involvement with relationship-building organizations in the community (Scouts or church groups), (2) joining programs related to the person's recreational or business interests (chess club, or horticultural group) or (3) participating in diagnosis related groups (wheelchair basketball, Special Olympics, or a discussion group for individuals with spina bifida).

Case Study

Description

Tyler is a 10-year-old fourth grader in a typical classroom. He is quick and accurate in math computation, and can read aloud well, even when new vocabulary is introduced. He is an excellent speller. Tyler has difficulty understanding the full meaning of what he reads, and receives resource room help for reading comprehension. Recently his math skills have faltered because he is struggling to understand the more difficult word problems that the fourth grade math curriculum brings. In addition, he does not complete the timed math calculation "Mad Minutes" because his handwriting is so labored, and it further lowers his math average. Some kids tease him about his poor handwriting and drawing, and he silently wishes the teacher wouldn't hang his papers on the bulletin board.

Timid and shy around other children, he often notices that they give him disapproving looks even when he tries to get their attention via his math accuracy. He feels disliked by many of his classmates. On the playground he watches longingly as the other kids play, and often swings by himself. He doesn't catch on to the rules of four-square, the current favorite recess activity, and he has in the past felt rebuffed when he has tried to join a group playing less complicated games.

He plays video games in his room after school. The many kids in his neighborhood don't invite him to join their activities, and when he sees them at the school bus stop he doesn't know what to say to them. He likes going to meetings of his Boy Scout troop, and the members are polite to him, but he overhears them speaking of visits to each other's houses which never include him.

Tyler has been referred to occupational therapy because his labored handwriting slows down his written schoolwork. The therapist notices that Tyler rarely looks at her, and does not return the greetings of children in the hall as he approaches her. She asks him who some of his friends are, and he looks blank and thinks a long time. Then he begins naming children, and the therapist soon realizes he has named over half the children in his fourth grade class (an indication that he has not yet experienced a true friend).

The therapist conducts an informal structured interview with him, learning that two of his classmates repeatedly bully him verbally during lunch and he wishes he could find someone pleasant to share both lunchtime and after-school free time. She observes him on the playground and notices that he watches the classmates engaged in group activities, but fails to look at the handful of other children also on the periphery of the play yard. She talks to the teacher, who assures her he is a cooperative, well-behaved student. She cannot think of anyone who seems like a particular friend of his, and has noticed that he sometimes takes offense at innocuous remarks of classmates who try to be nice to him. She reports that the last parent-teacher interview revealed that he doesn't say much to his parents about his school day, and is becoming increasingly withdrawn from them.

In addition to working with Tyler's fine motor delays, the occupational therapist talks with the school counselor about starting the social skills group they have often considered. They decide to include Tyler and two other students from the playground periphery as well as three students from younger classes who are antagonizing other children by their inconsideration and frequent "me first" behavior. The goals of the group program include:

1. Notice and read other people's needs and feelings with accuracy.
2. Increase conversation skills and verbal negotiating abilities.
3. Ask for and offer help to others with effective results.
4. Initiate playful and verbal interactions in a manner that results in a positive response.
5. Develop confidence based on a realistic appraisal of their skills and others' perception of them.

Long- and Short-Term Goals

The long-term intervention goal for Tyler is to increase his comprehension of verbal and nonverbal social cues.

The short-term goals for the social skills group include:

1. Accurately label and later verify facial expressions displayed, devoid of verbal cues.
2. Identify gestures and body movements that reveal social or emotional information.
3. Notice vocal inflection and tone of voice, correctly interpreting emotional content.

Therapist Goals and Strategies

The therapist's goals for the intervention include:

1. Use the school environment to Tyler's advantage for promoting social competence while also increasing confidence.
2. In addition to the whole-group social skill goals listed above, help Tyler to (a) expand comprehension of organizational structure (rules) of commonly used school games and play activities and (b) interpret innocuous verbal and non-verbal social cues of classmates and neighborhood peers without taking offense or interpreting them negatively.

The therapist's strategies for the intervention include:

1. Suggest to the counselor-collaborator that their weekly social skills group meet over lunch, thereby removing Tyler, and probably other group members, from a currently unsuccessful social environment.

2. Schedule his weekly fine motor therapy sessions to include one or two slightly less competent writers (to increase social opportunities under adult guidance without risking self-comparisons that would further erode self-esteem).
3. Consult with the teacher about possible confidence-building tactics, for example: (a) ask Tyler which of his papers to display on the bulletin board and (b) set up times for him to help a first- or second-grader with word recognition reading skills or math fact computations.
4. Consult with teacher about strategies to increase Tyler's comprehension of reading inferences and math word problems (for insight regarding possible carryover of such strategies to improve social comprehension).
5. Have the social skills group write, illustrate, and demonstrate four-square and perhaps other familiar school play activities as though to teach it to a younger group.

Activity

Photo Collage

Have group members each create one large collage of snapshots of themselves acting out various emotions. For further programming, use the same collage on another day and add captions under each picture describing one or more times when a group member experienced that emotion. Later a border could be added using cues that help identify the emotion being depicted: scowl, smile, eyes wide open, drooped shoulders, arms crossed, etc.

Treatment Objectives

Increase awareness of and accuracy for interpreting emotional responses and feelings of others.

Resources

The following resources can be helpful for gathering clinical data:

Canadian Occupational Therapy Measure (COPM)

Social Skills Rating System (SSRS)

HELP for Special Preschoolers

COLLAGE Occupational Therapy Programs (COLLAGE-OTP)

Personal interviews or review of professional reports

Observations in group settings

Physicians Desk Reference (PDR) or *The Internet Drug Index (www.rxlist.com)* concerning facts about medications

The following resources can be helpful for gathering family data:

Neighborhood support groups

Neighborhood parenting courses and behavior management service providers

Online Asperger's Syndrome Information and Support (O.A.S.I.S.;http://www.udel.edu/bkirby/asperger/)

Learning Disabilities Association of America (http://www.ldanatl.org)

Children and Adults with Attention Deficit/Hyperactivity Disorder (CH.A.D.D.) website (http://www.chadd.org/)

List of conference videos that families and professionals can use to develop social skills (http://collage-opt.org)

The following are common practice settings:

Schools

Hospitals or clinics

Community-based services

After-school care

Camps

The following resources can be helpful for gathering sociopolitical data:

Workshops and publications about school violence, bullies, and bullying

Home schooling laws

Curricula for creating a positive social climate throughout whole school district

IDEA (1997) behavior programs

Published Resources

Gresham, F., & Elliott, S. (1990). *Social skills rating system,* Circle Pines, MN: AGS.

Hutchins, S., Comins, J., & Offiler, J. (1991). *The social skills handbook: Practical activities for social communication.* Oxon, UK: Speechmark Publishing Ltd.

Inside Out: What Makes A Person with Social Cognitive Deficits Tick? M. Winner www.socialthinking.com

Sheridan, S. M., & Dee, C. C. (1993). *Helping parents help kids (...with social difficulties).* Department of Educational Psychology, Children's Medical Center, University of Utah. Salt Lake City: UT.

Williamson, G., & Dorman, W. (2003). *Promoting social competence.* San Antonio, TX: Therapy Skill Builders.

References

American Psychiatric Association. (2000). *Diagnostic and statistical manual of mental disorders:* (4th ed., text revision). Washington, DC: Author.

Gresham, F., & Elliott, S. (1990). *Social skills rating system,* Circle Pines, MN: AGS.

Individuals with Disabilities Education Act (IDEA) Amendments of 1997 (P. L. No. 105-17). U. S. C., 1400.

Interagency Committee on Learning Disabilities (1987). *Learning disabilities: A report to the U.S. Congress.*

Kauffman, N. A. (2002). *COLLAGE occupational therapy programs initial interview.* Request at http://www.collage-otp.org

Law, M., Baptiste, S., Carswell., H., McColl, M., Polatajko, H., & Pollack, N. (1994). *Canadian occupational performance measure* (*COPM;* 2nd ed.). Toronto, Canada: The Canadian Association of Occupational Therapy Publications.

Miller, R. J. (1993). Gary Kielhofner. In R. J. Miller & K. F. Walker (Eds.), *Perspectives on theory for the practice of occupational therapy* (pp. 179–208). Gaithersburg, MD: Aspen Publishers.

Nowicki, S. Jr., & Duke, M. P. (1992). *Helping the child who doesn't fit in.* Atlanta, GA: Peachtree Publishers, Ltd.

Parks, S. (1995). *HELP for Preschoolers.* Palo Alto, CA: VORT.

Shortridge, S. D., & Walker, K. F., (1993). Lela A. Llorens. In R. J. Miller & K. F. Walker (Eds.), *Perspectives on theory for the practice of occupational therapy* (pp. 65–90). Gaithersburg, MD: Aspen Publishers.

Snopkowski, A. (2001). *The social skill needs of children with attention deficit disorder or attention deficit hyperactivity* (Masters Thesis, Temple University, 2001).

Thompson, S. (1997). *The source for nonverbal learning disorders.* East Moline, IL: Linguisystems.

Walker, K. F. (1993). A. Jean Ayres. In R. J. Miller & K. F. Walker (Eds.), *Perspectives on theory for the practice of occupational therapy* (pp. 104–138). Gaithersburg, MD: Aspen Publishers.

Williams, M., & Shellenberger, S. (1996). *How does your engine run? A leader's guide to the Alert Program for self-regulation* (Rev. ed.). Albuquerque, NM: Therapy Works, Inc.

Zeitlin, S., Williamson, G., & Szczepanski, M. (1988). *Early coping inventory.* Bensenville, IL: Scholastic Testing Service.

Learning Disabilities

11

Nancy Allen Kauffman, Ed.M., OTR/L

Synopsis of Clinical Condition

Learning disabilities are "specific neurological disorders that affect the brain's ability to store, process, or communicate information" (National Center for Learning Disabilities, 2003). They are identified in individuals whose academic achievement levels are considerably below those expected for their age, schooling, and intelligence. Learning disabilities must be identified by *individually administered* standardized tests, and must interfere significantly with academics or with those activities of daily living that require specific academic competence (American Psychiatric Association, 2000).

Federal law uses the term specific learning disability (SLD) for any type of learning disability. The American Psychiatric Association (APA, 2000) uses the term learning disorders, and suggests criteria of 2 standard deviations (SD) between academic achievement and IQ to identify a significance level, with a standard of just 1 to 2 SD employed when a co-morbid (i.e., also occurring) condition compromises the IQ test results. School districts vary in their eligibility criteria for specialized educational services for learning problems.

Educational teams, psychologists, or medical professionals who make the diagnosis of any type of learning disability (LD) must consider the context of the person and must rule out cultural, ethnic, and economic factors, as well as poor teaching and lack of opportunity—all of which are not causes of true learning disabilities. Also, learning disabilities may occur in individuals with vision or hearing impairment, mental retardation, or pervasive developmental disorders, but only if difficulties with learning are beyond those commonly associated with these conditions (APA, 2000).

Prevalence and Etiology

The U. S. Department of Education (2001) has identified that learning disabilities affect approximately 5% of all children enrolled in public schools. The APA (2000) suggests 2% to 10% of the student population have one or more learning disorders, depending on the criteria used. Of these, 4 in 5 may have a reading disorder (4% of students), and at least 1 in 5 may have a mathematics disorder (1% of the school age population). Approximately 10% to 25% of people with attention deficit hyperactivity disorder, depression, disorders of conduct, or oppositional defiance also have learning disabilities.

According to functional magnetic resonance imaging (fMRI) studies (Gorman, 2003; "Focus on Brain Imaging Research," 2003) funded by the National Institute of Child Health and Human Development (NICHD), dyslexic children (who are poor readers by definition) exhibit unusual brain images when performing phonetic tasks while reading. Untreated, these unusual brain images remain into adulthood.

The automatic word-forming area for processing printed information is located in the brain near and behind the left ear. Unlike better readers, who activate the left occipito-temporal region of the brain, dyslexic readers without extra training use instead the left front, and portions of the right side of the brain as a backup system. Though they can compensate and eventually learn to read, they remain less fluent than good readers. Research has identified brain changes that occur when poor readers receive proper training, allowing them to become proficient readers. Although dyslexia is not curable, a firm foundation in phonological awareness appears to be a key to improvement.

Nonverbal learning disorder is believed to result from damage to the white matter connections (long myelinated fibers) in the right hemisphere (Thompson, 1997). Attention deficit disorder, a condition often co-morbid with learning disorders, has been studied by brain imaging research focusing on the limbic system, basal ganglia, cingulate system, and prefrontal cortex. As a person's attention shifts, research shows that the portion of the brain being activated also shifts. Research on etiology of LD has looked at other hereditary factors, birth trauma, and medical or neurological indicators that are often seen in those who experience a learning disorder, but one-to-one correlations have not yet been established.

Common Characteristics and Symptoms

Learning disorders may occur in the areas of reading, mathematics, written expression, or a combination of these. They may be associated with abnormalities in cognitive processing, for example visual processing, auditory processing, attention, or memory. They are often associated with social adjustment difficulties.

Dyslexia is a serious neurological impairment of reading skills, out of proportion to intellectual ability or teaching methods. It can be either inherited or congenital (Hart & Hopkins, 2002). Dyscalculia is characterized by difficulty in math computation, memory for math facts, and concepts of time and money (National Center for Learning Disabilities [NCLD], 2003). Language disorders may include receptive and/or expressive language impairment, and is likely to compromise the learning process. Nonverbal learning disorder is a neurological condition characterized by dysfunction in motor coordination, visual-spatial organizational skills, and social competence (Thompson, 1997). Some individuals with a learning disability in one or more areas may be sufficiently competent in other areas to qualify as gifted in their general intellectual development.

Motor coordination delays occur in the learning disabled population more often than in the typical population, although the delays may be subtle and not deviant enough to be formally diagnosed as dyspraxia (affecting general motor planning and manual dexterity) or dysgraphia (affecting written expression).

The APA reports that demoralization and low self-esteem may be associated with learning disabilities, particularly as individuals begin to recognize the discrepancy between their academic performance levels and that of their peers. Left untreated, a further loss of self-esteem and actual decrease in functional capacity may occur. The school dropout rate for this population is nearly 40%, or about 1.5 times the average, and difficulties with employment and social adjustment in adults with learning disabilities are more prevalent than in the non-LD population (APA, 2000). Therefore, educational and therapeutic interventions that help compensate for or overcome learning disabilities and associated difficulties early in a child's life serve a preventative role.

The identification of children eligible to receive special education and/or support services for a learning disability is a delicate task. The defining question is whether the potential for the person's educational achievement is being compromised by a factor that can be ameliorated by specialized programming. Test results must be applied carefully to this question, not to determine an arbitrary degree of discrepancy required for either an LD diagnosis or allowable therapeutic intervention. If a student's IQ measures lower than actual intellectual potential, the IQ results may cause educational and therapeutic personnel working with the individual to simply decrease their level of expectation and therefore fail to institute remedial and therapeutic techniques that could improve outcome. An example is the case of the potentially gifted student with obscure learning impediments.

Numerous factors can lower IQ scores other than the previously mentioned issues. For example, a particular cognitive processing disorder or language impairment can reduce IQ scores, as can mental illness (e.g., schizophrenia), emotional disorders (e.g., anxiety), and attentional issues—thereby resulting in a reduced discrepancy between measured potential and current level of educational functioning. Other conditions that can have a negative effect on IQ scores include medical conditions (e.g., anemia), sensory deficits (e.g., visual or hearing impairment, or a sensory integration deficit), ethnic and cultural factors (including English as a second language), and educational problems (e.g., poor teaching, lack of opportunity, or absenteeism). The important issue is whether the occupational therapist can take steps to significantly improve the student's learning success, not the degree of the discrepancy.

Target Areas for Intervention

The occupational therapist treating individuals with disabilities in a school setting works as a member of the intervention team to help solve problems that impact the learning process and, ultimately, preparation for adult living. The therapist brings a novel approach to concerns such as visual processing, motor coordination, sensory integration issues affecting attention and focus, organization, memory, the transition process, integration of information processing with sensory systems, and social skills. The therapist also considers architectural barriers and positioning concerns. The goal of intervention is not to improve deficit areas, but to positively affect the learning process.

See Table 11.1 for examples of therapeutic approaches in each of these focus areas that may positively affect academic learning and ultimate adjustment to life (B. Maxwell, personal communication, May 16, 2003). These are examples to encourage therapists to think broadly of services they are able to provide to the LD population. The transdisciplinary team approach that includes the practice of role release encourages the teachers to adapt and experiment with the therapist's concepts—and the therapists to use their knowledge to adapt the curriculum or presentation of the material to meet the student's specific learning needs. Providing insight to parents and teachers on why their strategies are working invites creative thinking and broader application of educational strategies. The overriding goal for working with the learning disabled (provided they have no other diagnoses) is for individuals to learn successfully without compromising their self-concept and social adjustment.

With all treatment strategies, therapists should carefully document results, consider the documentation made by others, and research the topic. This will help to establish certainty regarding treatment effectiveness.

Table 11.1
Examples of Therapeutic Treatment Approaches With Learning Disabled Students

Underlying Deficit Areas That May Negatively Impact Learning and Preparation for Adulthood	
Visual Processing	Introduce a moveable reading jig to expose one line at a time during reading. Eliminate the jig as soon as possible.
	Adapt math number lines or history timelines with raised touch points and color markers to enhance understanding.
	Advise teachers on the use of language, touch, and kinesthesia to augment visual demonstrations.
	Suggest types of lined paper and lines in copy books with perceptual, motor, and attention competence in mind.
Motor Coordination	Introduce dexterity tasks for classroom and home use that are interesting and self-motivating to the students. Score progress in accuracy and speed to further motivate independent use elsewhere.
	Introduce to teachers or administrators one or more suitable handwriting curricula for student, classroom, school, or district use, with ongoing consultation or individual treatment only for start-up or for particular problems that emerge. Report current research on effects of book bags on posture/motor development.
	Suggest that teachers clip heavy cardboard above and below the writing line to help new writers keep on lines and become accustomed to their own neat, tidy end result.
	Recommend assistive technology keyboarding early for impaired handwriters. Laptop computers, Alpha Smarts, and Co-Writers travel to classes and homes. Write-Out-Loud provides auditory feedback.
Sensory Integration Issues Affecting Attention and Focus	Suggest preferential seating, probably in the front center of classroom or near the teacher's desk to avoid visual distractions, classmates' sounds, and people brushing by accidentally.
	Encourage placement of special ed. classrooms away from the band room and views of the playground.
	To increase proprioceptive input at school or home, encourage students to deliver snack milk cartons from the school cafeteria, or mom's laptop to the bedroom, or the groceries from the car during study breaks.
	Schedule sensory integration treatment, if stipulated, shortly before the class that requires the most concentration.
	Store some of a child's books and materials across the room, to require walking around periodically to retrieve necessary materials.
	Propose heavy marching to classes, jumping or hopping during study breaks, or "pushing" walls out.

(Continued)

Table 11.1 (*Continued*)

Underlying Deficit Areas That May Negatively Impact Learning and Preparation for Adulthood	
Organization	Sort similar but not matching keys or buttons into groups defined by the student, requiring identification of common characteristics.
	Cut comic strips into individual squares, then sort by sequence.
	Make up headlines for paragraphs of information, thereby sorting out key topic from details.
	Experiment with a variety of assignment books and calendars to individualize more effective planning methods. Emphasize this as a lifetime work habit.
	Monitor book bags, desks, and notebooks for tidiness, sequencing, and completeness. Install a desk side pouch if needed for overflow. Use graphics organizer software or personal data assistant.
	In classroom, store a child's schoolbooks and folders in a sectioned magazine rack or file-folder filer, separated by subject. Promote the organizing characteristics of vestibular activities.
	In purchased textbooks, highlight information with different colors for section or paragraph headings, versus detail facts, to help perception of the relationship of chunks of information.

Contextual Considerations

Clinical

The occupational therapist collaborates with other team members in consensual decision making to identify (1) problem areas interfering with educational progress and (2) plans for carrying out needed supports and services to effect success in the learning process. To do this, the therapist uses formal evaluation measures, reports from the learning disabled individual, and any available written or oral reports available from relevant others (i.e., parents, teacher, spouse, boss, or job coach). When practical, the therapist observes the individuals in their natural environments, such as the classroom, playground, home, or workplace, to observe for contributing obstacles or strengths affecting learning. The therapist also reviews other professionals' relevant written reports. To better understand the latter, observe administration of the more commonly used tests such as the Wechsler Intelligence Scale for Children®–Fourth Edition (Weschler, 2002) to gather information about sensory, motor, organizational, or visual perceptual requirements of the items. This helps the therapist more accurately interpret written reports.

Under the Individuals with Disabilities Education Act (IDEA, 1997), therapists in schools are charged with the task of providing "recommendations of strategies and methods that can help the child learn and participate across the school environments" (Muhlenhaupt, 1998, p. 28). As a school "support service," occupational therapy is required to help children benefit from their educational placement. School therapists ask themselves, "If I were the classroom teacher, what might I do differently to get across to this individual the lessons I am trying to teach?" and, "How could the school program be different to help the individual absorb the information needed to prepare for adulthood?" The school therapist focuses on the context of a child's learning and activity, on high expectations that focus on positive results, and on the student as a capable learner.

The occupational therapist may be in a position to recommend unique sensory, perceptual, or motor enhancements to the learning process. If the occupational therapist's evaluations identify deficits in foundation skills that contribute to a breakdown in academic development, the goal of treatment is not to improve the foundation skill. The goal is to use the information to suggest strategies that will improve academic functioning. Although this may include improving one of the foundation skills, the goal is academic functioning. Some schools may identify the functional skill areas they expect a therapist to address, such as handwriting, adapting the environment, or assistive technology. In contrast, therapists working in a private or clinic setting may have more freedom to address underlying sensory integration issues and the neurological inefficiencies which contribute to the disability. They may be able to address sensory or gross motor inadequacies that may be impacting non-academic but important segments of life.

Visual perception and memory may be measured by the *Test of Visual Perceptual Skill–Revised* (TVPS–R) which consists of seven subtests for ages 4 to 13 (Gardner, 1997), or the *Motor-Free Visual Perception Test* (MVPT-R) for ages 4 to 12 (Colarusso & Hammill, 1995). *Raven's Progressive Matrices* (Raven & Raven, 1991) may be useful for ages 6 through adulthood to further define visual perception, particularly in LD individuals in whom spatial competencies may be a strength, but who have serious language processing handicaps. Sometimes they can grasp the concept of the more global task, though they don't understand the specific pieces of the perceptual task.

The *Wide Range Assessment of Visual Motor Abilities* (WRAVMA; Adams & Sheslow, 1995) manual points out that, though spatial and motor skills may be adequate in an individual, the person may have a deficit in the integration of the two skill areas, and it is necessary for the examiner to identify where the breakdown occurs. The WRAVMA for ages 3 years 0 months to 17 years 11 months separately measures fine motor skills (using a pegboard task) and visual-spatial skills (using only a crayon X or line to indicate answers). Additionally it measures the integration of visual and motor skills with fill-in and form-copying tasks.

Similarly, the revised fourth edition of the *Developmental Test of Visual-Motor Integration* (Beery, 1997) for ages 3 years 0 months to 17 years 11 months has been expanded. It not only includes the original series of forms to copy, but also two new supplemental standardized tests administered separately: visual perception ("Point to which answer is correct") and motor coordination ("Trace inside the wide 'road' of each shape"). All three portions of the test use the same stimulus forms.

If optical competencies appear to be contributing to learning difficulties, the therapist should screen for ocular control (for example, following a moving target) and for visual acuity, if it has not been done by nursing personnel. Dexterity as a contributor to eye-hand coordination may be evaluated along with other motor areas using the *Bruininks Oseretsky Test of Motor Proficiency* (Bruininks, 1978). This test will also identify balance problems that could contribute to difficulty sitting for long periods, or leaning heavily on the desk for trunk stability, which can interfere with graphomotor skills.

Organizational difficulties with functional life skills such as a disorganized book bag or forgetting appointments should be identified and addressed in treatment. The occupational therapist should observe the way clients approach a task and identify their learning and memory styles. He or she should also try informal organizing tasks such as sorting batches of unmatched keys or buttons according to attributes they notice as primary. Later, the therapist should have them pick another "important" attribute and sort again. The client's choices of "important" as well as the accuracy and completeness of the sorting should be watched. The main issue is their process—not teaching them to sort keys.

One measure of organization is the *Porteus Maze Test* (Porteus, 1933) which measures "planning capacity, prudence, and mental ability," and gives the subject an opportunity to realize errors, profit from the experience, and readapt the method used. The test allows starting again on each maze in which an error is committed, and it presents harder and harder mazes. Many learning opportunities are afforded. Spatially challenged individuals will have more difficulty with this task, and could benefit from an organizational assessment based on language. The therapist might try having clients read paragraphs and make up headlines using just the key idea, not the incidental facts.

Behavioral difficulties that are reported or observed should be examined carefully to determine if they are caused by transition difficulties or sensory disorders. If sensory processing appears to be an obstacle to academic learning, the *Sensory Profile* (Dunn, 1999) may help pinpoint the most likely contributing factors. The *Sensory Integration and Praxis Tests* (Ayres, 1989) may provide valuable information for treating the person with learning disabilities, although in many school settings it is not practical to use such lengthy evaluation procedures.

Finally, addressing social skills and behavior is essential because of its importance for adult adjustment and vocational readiness.

Family

Learning disabilities often follow a familial pattern, and one or more other members of the learning disabled person's family may share similar learning problems. LD adults in the family may feel they "made it" okay without intervention, and may not favor time or costs associated with extra services. On the other hand, their own painful experience in school may be the basis of avid cooperation with intervention specialists on behalf of their child, or demands for increased services. The needs of the family must be considered and incorporated into the evaluation process before development of a treatment strategy.

Home assignments must be made with thought and caution. When affected children have parents or siblings with learning problems of their own, homework may increase tensions at home. Delayed students are easily discouraged, often becoming defensive when parental help is offered. Many such children work much more cooperatively with one parent than the other, thereby adding to the mix of emotions in the household. Adding a sensory diet or handwriting practice to this equation may tip the balance of family harmony.

In addition, learning disabled students often take a longer than average amount of time to carry out their required academic homework assignments because of processing, handwriting, or organizational difficulty; so evening time for additional therapy "homework" tasks is at a premium.

Practice Setting

Occupational therapists work with learning disabled people in a variety of settings. One third of all American Occupational Therapy Association (AOTA) members practice in schools—including both public schools and private schools for children with learning or other handicapping conditions. They may be employees of the school or school district, or may be contracted to the school by an agency that hires private practitioners.

For example, a large portion of the school therapists' time is spent in classrooms observing for sensory or organizational problems as they occur, or interviewing teachers and aides about academic difficulties that might be related to underlying therapy issues. Therapists may first observe teachers teach, then collaborate on methods or materials that might help the LD student focus or learn more effectively (i.e., teachers' arm movements, use of colored chalk, visual aids, location of materials in the classroom, sensory tips, etc.). Therapists should review classroom treatment strategies that were effective in previous years and encourage their continuation with the next year's teachers.

School therapists should arrange to gain and give information by attending individualized educational program (IEP) and instructional support team (IST) meetings, or "back to school" nights with parents whenever possible. Therapists who contribute to the writing of the goal plan should indicate methods of facilitating *how* academic goals are reached (rather than clinical goals such as "improve bilateral coordination"). In some schools parents are invited to attend all or some therapy sessions in order to exchange information related to the home environment. Therapists should also investigate school policies regarding educational planning for the transition from high school into community living or advanced education, and should have therapeutic input into related team planning. School therapists who are employed by therapy contract services and not by the school district may have more difficulty accessing the principal and other administrative personnel for making suggestions or gaining information.

Therapists may treat persons with learning disabilities in non-school settings in which there is more latitude concerning whom they treat and the areas addressed. For example, a gifted student in a private school may be quite handicapped by a low-average ability in written expression and may seek private therapy to address this issue.

Sociopolitical

The Individuals with Disabilities Education Act (IDEA, 1997; Chandler, 2003) promotes the concept of evidence-based practice. It requires that objective procedures be used in educational settings, and that they be both rigorous *and* systematic.

The "No Child Left Behind" federal legislation initiative developed in 2001 outlined new guidelines and supports for promoting academic improvement using accommodations, modifications, and alternate ways of teaching. It opened the door for Congress to consider regulations to promote screening at age four to fade out the "wait to fail" system before providing specialized intervention for specific learning delays (National Center for Learning Disabilities staff, personal communication, February 12, 2003).

The Health Information Portability and Accountability Act (HIPAA) federal regulations regarding privacy and security which went into effect in April, 2003, for healthcare providers may serve as a reminder for all therapists regarding "patient identifiable information." Itinerant school therapists who take records home and transform their cars into well organized closets and filing cabinets *must* safeguard personal student files from being seen through car windows or by guests or family members in the home.

School programs are legally bound to follow the IEP for each student, so they keep careful records of relevant information. If a required therapy appointment is missed because of a class field trip, class standardized testing, or illness of the therapist or student, it must usually be made up at a later time. A series of missed appointments may need to be repaid by the therapist through visits to the student's home.

If possible, a school therapist should have access to communication with at least the building principal and hopefully also the school district director of special education to provide an accurate picture of the scope of services that the occupational therapist(s) can provide. In some school districts, even a 15-minute follow-up meeting monthly with these important administrators is sufficient to review the current effectiveness of strategies or plans agreed upon in previous discussions.

In some clinic and private practice settings, medical insurance reimbursement can be achieved for conditions that accompany learning problems (for example, motor coordination disorder). However, therapists may have difficulty achieving reimbursement for novel approaches to treatment of organizational skills and academic learning disorders if the insurer considers them "educational" in nature.

Lifestyle/Lifespan

A specific learning disorder is often first identified in the early grades of school, and it may continue into the adult years. Sometimes the first identification is made in high school or at the college level for students who have gotten by on hard work and using the strong portions of their intellectual abilities to compensate for weaknesses. At those higher school levels, an increase in academic expectation may result in a breakdown in previously effective coping strategies.

Because of the high school dropout rate of students with learning disorders, it is important for services to the learning disabled to be continued right through the high school years. An Individualized Transition Program is required for students who are 14 years of age or older and who qualify for special education services. It contains plans for successfully transitioning from school to work, additional training or higher education, and community living. This step in the educational process helps to assure that the student is moving beyond dependence on adults or helpful study buddies and into self-reliant accommodation for learning, remembering, and applying newly learned information.

Adults with learning disorders often experience difficulty with employment or social competencies. They may encounter anxiety, discouragement, and lack of confidence because of the variability of the strengths and weaknesses in their intellectual profile, especially if they have not become self-sufficient in their accommodations.

Clinical Decision Making Process

Defining Focus for Intervention

Once the referring complaint is considered along with the data collected from all sources, it is necessary to prioritize the information that has been gathered. Then, one looks carefully for the impact of underlying neurological information-processing considerations that may be uniquely addressed by the occupational therapist. The therapist may choose to initiate direct hands-on treatment. However, the school therapist, accustomed to working more frequently in collaboration with others or as a consultant to others, may initiate a broad base of change opportunities by suggesting new ways for the student to work with classroom teachers, aides, individual therapeutic support staff, or parents. Learning disabilities that have the most impact on academic progress are the initial focus of the school therapist's intervention.

It is the role of occupational therapy to support learning; not to create improvement in perceptual scores or fine motor coordination. For example, the school therapist may, after meeting with a child's math teacher, design a chart of number facts that will help the spatially competent learner see a visual relationship between number facts that he or she has otherwise had difficulty memorizing. Or, the therapist may encourage a teacher to have the classroom aid suggest an easy set of rainforest jigsaw puzzles to a perceptually impaired student for sharing with a shy classmate, thereby building confidence and competence in a weak area while furthering social interaction skills in the classmate. The therapist will maintain a brief ongoing monitoring schedule with the math and classroom teachers over the coming weeks and months to be certain that progress continues. The goal here is not to learn perception, but to use activity and the therapist's awareness of underlying neurological strengths and non-strengths to build academic competence.

Meanwhile, for the therapist in the non-school setting, the family's or individual's primary complaint will be the target of the initial focus of intervention. The non-school therapist may be working on organizational skills as requested by the family, and may begin by suggesting several new types of homework-recording plan books to try, and a new place to put homework that may remind the student to pass it in on time.

Establishing Goals for Intervention

Goals are developed from the referral complaint, formal evaluations, and informal interviews. Goals are related to the individual's learning needs, and relevant outcomes are in the academic and problem solving realms. The goals may list programs or supports needed to achieve results, and they emphasize the context of the learning disabled person's learning and activity—on the job, in the classroom, around the house, or on the sports field. Goals are stated in positive terms and reflect realistically high expectations.

Designing Theory-Based Intervention

The developmental frame of reference is helpful when working with learning disabled individuals, and assumes that an individual achieves mastery in all areas of development in a continuous process as individuals age and one skill is built upon another skill. If the developmental process is interrupted, there may be a gap in the process of development that undermines further development (Shortridge & Walker 1993). Of course, not all learning problems are developmental delays, and some emerge from neurological and physiological changes that never occur in the normally developing person. However, knowledge of the developmental frame of reference outlines those predictable sequences that usually occur as people learn new information, and can be extremely helpful in planning effective intervention. For example, during handwriting instruction, children benefit from first watching someone write an alphabet letter before trying to copy the letter. Only later does writing the letter from memory occur. A second example involves children's ability to perceive (visually) and reproduce (motorically) obliqueness at a later time developmentally than they are aware of verticality, horizontalness, and circularity. The second example also influences the sequence of instruction for handwriting, drawing, and playing tic-tac-toe. Knowing this type of sequence aids the therapist in setting realistic learning expectations.

The sensory integration frame of reference (Walker, 1993) assumes that the central nervous system receives, organizes, and uses information from the environment to plan and execute appropriate and effective responses. Some children have sensory modulation difficulty and cannot respond appropriately or consistently to sensory stimuli. As a result, they have difficulty attending and learning. Knowledge and insight in this area enables a therapist to provide sensory input, environmental adaptation, and learning strategies for children trying to learn in noisy and visually over-stimulating learning environments. Other principles of sensory integration can influence effective learning. When a student is learning to organizing a written response, watching another person's motor plan for writing a letter gives the new writer a model of the motor plan. Multisensory experiences, including touch and proprioception, can enhance learning. Writing letters from memory requires the further sensory challenge of visualizing the letter (ideation) while creating the motor plan for responding.

The model of human occupation (Miller, 1993) assumes that effective intervention addresses a person's roles, routines, habits, and motivation within his or her environment and the importance of mastering a variety of roles. Its emphasis on life roles is useful, as the child with learning disabilities is experiencing difficulty in a primary childhood role—that of student. The therapist should be as supportive and positive as possible in bringing about change for the student, and in providing information to the parent. Also, the therapist should use roles the child knows and in which the child excels to build confidence and new skills, such as introducing perceptual concepts through using aerial view diagramming of football plays to help the child interested in football. Ineffective study and learning habits and routines should be replaced with strategies effective for the student.

Service delivery in schools may take the form of *consultation* to the administration or *consultation* to teachers, classroom aides, or a child's individual therapeutic support staff. *Direct therapy* should be accompanied by communication with educational and family personnel (perhaps with a communication notebook that accompanies the child to school and home). The service delivery method may be to *monitor* progress from a distance, checking back at regular intervals to be sure progress is steady in areas that were previously the focus of direct therapy or consultation. The *collaborative model* of service delivery that is urged in IDEA encourages team work between therapists, families, and school personnel for consensual decision making regarding educational decision making.

Any classroom intervention recommendations must be reasonable and considerate in their expectations of busy teachers, who have the responsibility for maintaining order, educational environment, and scheduling for a whole class of students. Recommendations for home activities may need to be incorporated into the busy family routine. For example, the therapist may suggest that the child carry heavy bags of groceries in from the car, jump on a newly acquired trampoline, toss the family salad with clean hands, or play penny-passing or other palming dexterity activities during car rides. The therapist may also suggest the use of summers as a time to encourage extra emphasis on areas such as handwriting (including keeping vacation journal), visual perception (including commercially available graded activities), and initiation of a time consuming protocols, which involve frequent application of tactile and proprioceptive stimulation.

Evaluating Progress

To evaluate progress, the therapist must identify whether functional skills in learning and retrieving information and in applying the information to effective problem solving are increasing. Current performance levels must be compared to previous behavioral goals and objectives, standardized test results, or observation of current new problem solving abilities.

Measures of progress in learning must also evaluate independence in using compensation strategies, without dependence on hovering adult intervention. The student's rate of problem solving must also be explored to analyze whether the learning methods adopted are efficient enough to be realistically applied. The student's ability to generalize problem solving skills to new situations and experiences must be evaluated by exposure to novel applications. Being able to recite back answers or methods of problem solving is not the goal.

Determining Change in or Termination of Treatment

The therapist monitors the learning disabled person's goals regularly to identify goal areas achieved (or consistently not achieved). Plateauing may warrant discontinuation of treatment, although temporary plateauing sometimes occurs followed by growth spurts or setbacks. Just because a child achieves academic grade level in a subject, or an adult achieves a desired organizational goal, does not mean therapeutic support should be removed right away. The therapeutic underpinnings may still be necessary for a while to support the newfound independent achievements, and without them the individual may hit a stumbling block. It is also important to avoid discontinuation of therapeutic input around the time of a major transition, such as a new educational placement, receiving a new teacher, or delivery of a new baby in the family. Otherwise, the organizational or other therapeutic gains put in place may regress.

Termination of treatment occurs when learning disabled persons have been empowered to effectively, and over time, take charge of adaptations or compensations needed to help them succeed at learning demands appropriate to their age and potential.

Case Study

Description

Duncan is a fourth-grade student who reads several months below his grade level, but comprehends far above his grade. Spelling is good for words that are phonetically simple (banana, watermelon), but poor for irregularly spelled words (light, could). He can cut intricately, snap his fingers, dress and undress small action figures quickly, and trace simple pictures excellently on onion skin paper. He excels in oral reports.

Duncan's highly informative handwritten reports hanging on the bulletin board look messy, and fail to reflect his good dexterity for other activities. He hates reading aloud. He can recite number facts well and can explain to other students what the word problems mean, yet he often makes errors on his math tests and homework papers. He is lax about turning in his homework, though he always claims he has done it, and he frequently has trouble finding his pencil and the book he is looking for in his untidy desk. Duncan's good grades are beginning to slip with the increased challenges of fourth grade. The teacher suspects underlying perceptual deficits, but also wonders if he is really trying his best.

The occupational therapist administers the *Test of Visual Perceptual Skills–Revised,* the *Developmental Test of Visual Motor Integration,* and the pegboard (fine motor) section of

The Wide Range Assessment of Visual Motor Abilities. The therapist finds that Duncan excels in the pegboard task, but scores in the 22nd percentile in the VMI. The TVPS-R identifies considerable difficulty with memory for visual sequences and individual stimuli, visual-spatial relations, and visual figure ground. The therapist notices during the testing no evidence of inattention, noncompliance, casualness, or slipshod effort. However, he notices that when Duncan looks at the test answers, his scanning is erratic and inefficient, and by the end of the long TVPS-R he is rubbing his eyes. She asks him to read aloud two paragraphs, and notes that on two occasions he skipped a line in the reading. He shows no evidence of strategies to help him with the memory tasks, and begins guessing wildly as the tasks become harder.

Long- and Short-Term Goals

In the long-term, Duncan will be able to:

1. Increase memory for irregularly spelled words.
2. Improve ocular-motor control.
3. Increase awareness of part versus whole of visual stimuli.
4. Improve spacing and figure ground aspects of written math and handwriting.
5. Organize desk, homework, and personal belongings according to a consistent plan he has established for himself.

In the short-term, Duncan will be able to:

1. Correctly solve familiar math problems independently on full printed pages containing no more than six problems, with 95% accuracy in each of four sessions (using enlarged photocopies). Increase to 8, 10, and then 12 problems per page.
2. Independently place a frame around each math problem and solve it correctly with 95% accuracy in each of four sessions.
3. Copy math problems from book or chalkboard with correct spacing in $^1/_2$-inch graph paper squares with 90% accuracy, then decrease the size of the squares.
4. Copy math problems from book or chalkboard with correct spacing on lined paper, independently using highlighter to emphasize correct spacing, with 90% accuracy.

Therapist Goals and Strategies

1. Establish and maintain initial collaborative relationship with the classroom teacher and aide.
2. Meet individually with Duncan several times to help him improve memory by (1) training visualization ability, (2) applying sensory strategies like use of color highlighting or sandpaper tracing to stress letter groupings (such as *-ight, -ould, -eight*), and (3) using kinesthetic tracing above the word or sub-vocalization, etc. Then consult with educational personnel and demonstrate memory method(s) found to be most effective. Monitor their progress together.
3. Refer Duncan for a developmental vision specialist screening. (This occupational therapist works in a school, so it is necessary to verify the district policy before making such a referral outside the school). The therapist also initiates a variety of

marble rolling activities, throwing to moving targets, and throwing to stationary targets while the child is swinging on suspended equipment.

4. Use a favored activity of his—tracing—to clarify awareness of "the whole" and "the parts" of increasingly complex pictures while still keeping outlined items separate.
5. Meet individually with Duncan several times to help him create a plan for organizing his belongings and demonstrate his effectiveness in using it. Then, consult with educational personnel to demonstrate the child's own plan, and follow up by monitoring for success.
6. Arrange for Duncan to write a letter to a teacher or relative on lined paper having a red margin line drawn 3/4-inch in from the beginning and end of all lines. Grade up to lighter lines, and then absent lines, encouraging Duncan to visualize their presence. Similarly facilitate matching verticality of letters, accuracy of touching horizontal lines, and space between words.

Activity

Encourage Duncan to create a poster by (1) tracing only the mountain portion of a busy landscape picture, then (2) tracing only appropriate mountain/forest animals from another complex picture of overlapping and touching animals. Duncan should complete this figure ground activity with a hand-lettered descriptive label written within the margins.

Treatment Objectives

1. Visually discriminate foreground from background characteristics.
2. Begin and end writing within $^1/_2$-inch of left and right margin lines of writing.

Resources

The following resources can be helpful for gathering clinical data:

Contract therapists
District employees
Private/clinic therapists
Test of Visual Perceptual Skills–Revised
Motor-Free Visual Perception Test–Revised
Wide Range Assessment of Visual Motor Abilities
Raven's Progressive Matrices
Beery-Buktenica Developmental Test of Visual-Motor Integration (VMI) Fourth Edition
Bruininks Oseretsky Test of Motor Proficiency
Porteus Maze Test
Sensory Integration and Praxis Tests

The following resources can be helpful for gathering family data:

Family history
Public vs. private vs. home schooling decisions

Tensions regarding homework schedule and content
IEP/IST
Education law centers

The following are common practice settings:

Academic goals of schools
Special education
Collaboration with other professionals
Consultation, monitoring, direct hands-on treatment, groups
Interaction with teachers and administrators
Clinics
Private practices

Internet Resources

AOTA backpack awareness information:
www.aota.org/backpack/

IDEA regulations:
www.ideapractices.org/idearegsmain.htm

International Dyslexia Association:
www.interdys.org

Learning Disabilities Association of America:
www.ldanatl.org

National Center for Learning Disabilities:
www.ncld.org

National clearinghouse on post-secondary education for individuals with disabilities:
www.heath.gwu.edu

Published Resources

Durheim, M. (2003). A Parent's Guide to Section 504. *Attention!,* 10(1), 36–41.

Hanft, B. & Marsh, D. *Getting a Grip on Handwriting: A Self-Guided Video and Manual.* Bethesda, MD: AOTA.

Parker, F. (2003). How to Select the Right College. *Attention!,* 10(1), 28–35.

Thompson, S. (1997). *The source for nonverbal learning disorders.* East Moline, IL: LinguiSystems.

References

Adams, W., & Sheslow, D. (1995). *Wide range assessment of visual motor abilities.* Wilmington, DE: Wide Range, Inc.

American Psychiatric Association. (2000). *Diagnostic and statistical manual of mental disorders* (4th ed., text revision). Washington, DC: Author.

Ayres, A. J. (1989). *Sensory integration and praxis test.* Los Angeles: Western Psychological Services.

Beery, K. (1997). *Beery-Buktenica developmental test of visual-motor integration* (*VMI;* 4th ed.). Parsippany, NJ: Modern Curriculum Press.

Bruininks, R.H. (1978). *Bruininks-Oseretsky test of motor proficiency.* Circle Pines, MN: American Guidance Services.

Chandler, B. (2003, May 5). Evidence-based practice in the schools. *Advance for Occupational Therapy Practitioners, 19*(9), 7.

Collarusso, R. P., & Hammill, D. D. (1995). *Motor-free visual perception test–revised.* Novato, CA: Academic Therapy Publications.

Dunn, W. (1999). *Sensory profile.* San Antonio, TX: Psychological Corporation.

Focus on brain imaging research. (2003, Winter). *Focus: The Newsletter of the Greater Philadelphia Branch of the International Dyslexia Association,* Winter, 3-4.

Gardner, M. F. (1996). *Test of visual perceptual skills–revised.* Novato, CA: Academic Therapy Publications.

Gorman, C. (2003, July 28). The new science of dyslexia. *Time, 162(4),* 52–59.

Hart, A. C., & Hopkins, C. A. (2002). *International Classification of Diseases, 9th Revision.* Salt Lake City, UT: Ingenix St. Anthony Publishing.

Individuals with Disabilities Education Act (IDEA) Amendments of 1997 (P. L. No. 105-17). U. S. C., 1400.

Miller, R. J. (1993). Gary Kielhofner. In R. J. Miller & K. F. Walker (Eds.), *Perspectives on theory for the practice of occupational therapy* (pp. 179–208). Gaithersburg, MD: Aspen Publishers.

Muhlenhaupt, M. (1998). Does Johnny need OT in school? *OT Practice, 3(11),* 26–28.

National Center for Learning Disabilities. (2003). *LD at a glance.* Retrieved 5-12-2003, from http://ld.org/LDInfoZone.

Porteus, S. D. (1933). *Porteus mazes.* San Antonio, TX: The Psychological Corporation.

Raven, J. C., & Raven, J. (1991). *Raven's progressive matrices.* Oxford, England: Oxford Psychologists Press, Ltd.

Shortridge, S. D., & Walker, K. F., (1993). Lela A. Llorens. In R. J. Miller & K. F. Walker (Eds.), *Perspectives on theory for the practice of occupational therapy* (pp. 65–90). Gaithersburg, MD: Aspen Publishers.

Thompson, S. (1997). *The source for nonverbal learning disorders.* East Moline, IL: LinguiSystems.

U. S. Department of Education. (2001). *Twenty-third annual report to congress on the implementation of IDEA.* Washington, DC: Author.

Walker, K. F. (1993). A. Jean Ayres. In R. J. Miller & K. F. Walker (Eds.), *Perspectives on theory for the practice of occupational therapy* (pp. 103–138). Gaithersburg, MD: Aspen Publishers.

Neurological Disorders 12

Arley Johnson, OTR/L
James Foster, MS, OTR/L

Occupational therapists commonly treat several neurological disorders. These include multiple sclerosis, amyotrophic lateral sclerosis (ALS), and Guillain-Barré syndrome. The focus of this chapter will be multiple sclerosis and amyotrophic lateral sclerosis. A brief discussion of Guillain-Barré will also be provided.

Multiple Sclerosis: Synopsis of Clinical Condition

Multiple sclerosis (MS) is a neurological disease characterized by progressive demyelinization of nerve fibers of both the brain and spinal cord (Anderson, Anderson, & Glanze, 1994). Because myelin conducts impulses along nerves, demyelinization of nerve fibers results in blocked or delayed nerve impulses.

Prevalence and Etiology

Over 300,000 Americans currently suffer from the disease, with nearly 200 new cases being diagnosed every week (National Multiple Sclerosis Society [NMSS], 1996). Multiple sclerosis most often strikes people in their twenties or thirties, and women develop it twice as often as men (NMSS, 1996). The sequence of progression is difficult to predict. After presentation of the early signs, symptoms continue to present and subside throughout life with periods of exacerbations and remissions. Because other neurological conditions such as cerebral vascular accidents and brain tumors present with similar symptoms, MS is difficult to diagnose. To make a definitive diagnosis, two main factors must be present. First, there must be evidence of multiple patches of scar tissue within the central nervous system, detected via magnetic resonance imaging (MRI). Second, there must have been a minimum of two separate exacerbations of the disease (Franklin, Heaton, Nelson, Filley, & Seibert, 1988). A definitive diagnosis often takes months or years.

The cause of MS is not known at this time (Multiple Sclerosis International Federation, 2002). There are, however, several working theories. One theory is that MS is a virus which lies dormant in the body, or could be triggered by another virus such as measles or herpes (Multiple Sclerosis International Federation, 2002). Another theory suggests that MS is an autoimmune disease in which the body attacks its own cells and tissue, or, in the case of MS, its own myelin.

Common Characteristics and Symptoms

One of the first signs of the disease is paresthesia, or tingling, in the extremities or on one side of the face. Additional early signs include muscle weakness; vertigo; and visual disturbances such as nystagmus, diplopia, and partial blindness. As the course of the disease progresses, there may be extreme emotional lability, ataxia, abnormal reflexes, cognitive disabilities, intention tremors, swallowing deficits, and urinating difficulty. (Multiple Sclerosis International Federation, 2002).

Once the disease is diagnosed, it can be classified into one of four major categories: relapsing-remitting, benign, secondary progressive, and primary progressive (Multiple Sclerosis International Federation, 2002). Relapsing-remitting MS occurs in 25% of patients and presents with unpredictable exacerbations during which new symptoms appear or existing symptoms become more severe. This lasts for days or months and there is a partial or total remission. Benign MS exists in approximately 20% of patients and presents with one or two exacerbations with complete recovery. Secondary progressive MS exists in approximately 40% of patients and presents in individuals who initially have relapsing-remitting multiple sclerosis, and then subsequent progressive disability later in the course of the disease. Primary progressive MS is present in approximately 15% of individuals and is characterized by slow onset and steadily worsening symptoms, with an accumulation of deficits and disability. However, these classifications are also difficult to assign, as there tends to be some residual disability after exacerbations and a cumulative effect over time (Bhasin, 1989). Consequently, patients who are assigned to one classification at the beginning of their disease often are reclassified into other categories as it progresses. There are several precautions for those diagnosed with MS. For those who are affected with cognitive deficits, constant supervision may be required since short-term memory, attention span, problem solving, and reaction time can be impaired. There are also precautions in terms of avoiding extreme heat, cold, humidity, and stress as they can bring on or worsen exacerbations.

Target Areas for Intervention

Occupational therapy for individuals with MS focuses on self-care and transfers. Occupational therapists utilize compensatory techniques, activity analysis, environmental accommodation, and energy conservation to assist individuals to compensate in these areas. In addition, the occupational therapist plays an important role during family training in terms of educating the caregiver regarding the strengths and deficits associated with the individual with MS.

Contextual Considerations

Clinical

The occupational therapist should evaluate the patient with MS in the following areas: extremity strength; range of motion and coordination; visual acuity and tracking; cognitive abilities such as memory, problem solving, and insight into his or her own deficits; social disposition; level of self-care independence; balance during functional mobility activities; and, most importantly, previous functional status. The previous functional status will assist in goal setting.

In terms of treatment goals, the occupational therapist should concentrate on maintaining passive and active joint range of motion, preventing spasticity or joint contractures, improving coordination and standing balance during functional activities, and maximal independence in self-care activities using assistive devices as needed (Crepeau, Cohn, & Schell, 2003). The ability to achieve these goals is highly dependent on the previous functional level of the person and the MS category in which they have been diagnosed.

Family

MS has implications for the client's spouse, children, friends, parents, and colleagues (Multiple Sclerosis International Federation, 2002). Physical assistance may be necessary to aid the individual with MS with self-care and functional mobility, and emotional support may be necessary to cope with the degenerative nature of the disease. Financial assistance may be required as MS affects an individual in the prime of life. If cognitive deficits are present, 24-hour supervision may be required, as safety awareness and memory may be impaired and the individual may be at risk for falls. Patient and family education must also be involved in terms of understanding and accepting the progressive course of the disease.

Practice Setting

Rehabilitation services are frequently advocated as a means of intervention for MS patients during times of inpatient hospitalization. Inpatient rehabilitation has been linked to reduced disability in patients with progressive MS (Freeman, Langdon, Hobart, & Thompson, 1997). In addition, cognitive status can affect the types of treatment a patient will receive, as well as the amount of training the patient's family will require. Home care services are also warranted to personalize treatment within the individual's home environment.

Sociopolitical

MS is a costly disease. It attacks individuals during their period of greatest potential and productivity. The mean age of MS onset is between 29 and 33 years of age, with actual diagnosis several years after the first appearance of symptoms (Aronson, Goldenberg, & Cleghorn, 1996). The unpredictable nature of the disease process limits the ability to maintain consistent employee roles.

The annual cost of MS, per individual, including personal services, alterations to home, vehicle, purchase of special equipment, and earnings loss was nearly $35,000 in 1994. This translates into a national annual cost of $9.7 billion (Whetten-Goldstein et al., 1996). Mean total lifetime cost, per MS patient, was $2.5 million in 1994 (Whetten-Goldstein et al., 1996).

Lifestyle/Lifespan

The lifespan for individuals with MS varies with the classification with which they are diagnosed. It is difficult to predict accurately the course of MS for any individual. The first five years give some indication of how the disease will progress for that person (Multiple Sclerosis International Federation, 2002). Approximately 45% of individuals with MS are not severely affected and can live normal and productive lives (Multiple

Sclerosis International Federation, 2002). Life expectancy of individuals with multiple sclerosis is near normal (Multiple Sclerosis International Federation, 2002).

Clinical Decision Making Process

Defining Focus for Intervention

The focus for occupational therapy intervention and treatment planning is based on three factors: (1) baseline functional level prior to the occupational therapy evaluation, (2) cognitive status, and (3) medical history and disease classification of MS.

1. Since MS is a progressive disease, it is important to identify baseline function. An individual with MS who has required moderate assistance for self-care and has used a wheelchair for five years will not likely reach independence in self-care and functional mobility.
2. The rate and extent of progress is often dependent upon cognitive status. Deficits in memory and attention span will diminish the ability to comprehend and follow instructions. If there are deficits in problem solving new information, the ability to adjust to unfamiliar situations will be impaired.
3. Past medical history can provide insight regarding the prognosis for progress. The MS classification and answers to the following questions will impact the goal setting and treatment planning process. How long has it been since multiple sclerosis was diagnosed? What were previous exacerbations like? How frequent have they been? How severe have the exacerbations been? Has the individual recovered to pre-admission functional level or are exacerbations followed by progressive deterioration? For example, someone who was diagnosed with multiple sclerosis 10 years ago and has had five exacerbations, all requiring hospitalization and resulting in declining functional level, would probably be classified within the primary progressive classification. Continued maintenance and family training should be initiated. However, if the individual was diagnosed five years ago and this is the first exacerbation, with mild weakness of their lower extremities, it would be realistic to set goals to attain the functional level that existed prior to admission.

Establishing Goals for Intervention

Within the acute inpatient setting, intervention goals usually address activities of daily living and functional mobility. These goals are set, with the patient's involvement, based upon a thorough evaluation of the occupational profile. The occupational profile delineates the individual's needs, problems, concerns about occupations, and daily life activity performance (AOTA, 2002). The second step of the evaluation process focuses on occupational performance. What are the functional performance levels in work tasks, activities of daily living, homemaking, leisure activities, and functional mobility? Considerations should be made for fatigue, temperature, mood, stress level, and time of day, as all of these factors can influence functional performance on a daily basis.

Within the outpatient or home care setting, goals are often set with the maintenance of current functioning in mind. In addition, the home care setting allows the occupational therapist to more specifically design goals within the person's own environment. For example, the goal of independently performing a tub transfer with a tub bench is more realistic when actually performing the task in the person's own bathroom.

Designing Theory-Based Intervention

The rehabilitation frame of reference emphasizes compensation for disabilities that cannot be remediated. Compensation frequently takes the form of adaptations that address self-care tasks and environmental control and mobility (Crepeau, Cohn, & Schell, 2003). Specifically, intervention strategies that are characteristic of the rehabilitation frame of reference and cogent to treatment planning for persons with MS include: adaptive devices, upper extremity orthotics, environmental modification, wheelchair modification, ambulatory devices, adaptive procedures, and safety education (Crepeau, Cohn, & Schell, 2003). The notion that motivation for independence cannot be separated from the individual's cognitive ability, emotional disposition, financial status, and family support is central to the rehabilitation frame of reference (Kemp, 1990). The biomechanical frame of reference maintains that purposeful activities can be used to foster range of motion, strength and endurance.

The rehabilitative frame of reference assists with goal setting for the person with MS by employing the use of assistive devices to accomplish goals. For instance, independence in lower extremity dressing, hindered by poor trunk mobility, is fostered by the use of a dressing stick. Independence in functional mobility from a wheelchair to a commode, hindered by decreased lower extremity strength, can be accomplished with use of swing-away wheelchair arms and a transfer board. Independence in feeding, hindered by poor gross motor coordination of the upper extremities, can be accomplished by utilizing a built-up handle.

The biomechanical frame of reference assists with goal setting by addressing the performance of motor skills, such as posture, coordination, and strength. Therefore, the goal of being independent in meal preparation at standing level will be accomplished through increased lower extremity strength. The goal of independence in feeding can be accomplished through increased fine motor coordination in the upper extremities. Rood and Brunstrum use a variety of sensory and positional techniques to facilitate functional movement through neurodevelopmental approaches, such as neurodevelopmental treatment (NDT) and proprioceptive neuromuscular facilitation (PNF; Crepeau, Cohn, & Schell, 2003).

Evaluating Progress

Progress can be evaluated by assessing the goals that are reached and the time period within which they are reached. Within the acute inpatient rehabilitation setting, individuals with MS are generally given two to four weeks to reach their goals. If treatment has slowed to the point where progression towards goals is no longer occurring, the rehabilitation team must begin to investigate discharge planning. This is a process that is accomplished by the rehabilitation team, made up of the occupational therapist, physician, physical therapist, nurse, psychologist, social worker, family members, and the individual with MS. Areas of discussion will include family resources for care at the current functional level within the home environment. If the individual's family cannot provide a safe and supportive environment, long-term placement options must then be explored. When the rate of goal accomplishment slows or plateaus in outpatient or home care settings, therapies are usually changed or terminated.

Case Study

Description

T is a 31-year-old female who was diagnosed with MS two years ago and has had five exacerbations, all requiring hospitalization and two requiring inpatient rehabilitation. Currently, she is hospitalized with the onset of dizziness, double vision, numbness on the left side of her body, and poor coordination of her left upper extremity. T lives with her very supportive parents in a two-story home. She ambulates short distances (approximately 50 feet) with a rolling walker and is independent with all activities of daily living. Durable medical equipment that T owns include a rolling walker, standard wheelchair, tub transfer bench, and 3-1 commode. She also owns various assistive devices such as a reacher, a dressing stick, a long shoe horn, a long handled sponge, and a sock donner.

T was hospitalized within the acute floor of the hospital, administered three days of intravenous steroids, and transferred to the inpatient rehabilitation unit. Upon admission, T was evaluated to be oriented to the person, place, time, and reason for hospitalization. T's left upper and lower extremity strength was 4/5. Her gait was determined to be ataxic. A mild intentional tremor was also noted in T's left upper extremity, which was her dominant side. Sensation of all extremities was grossly intact, plus speech and swallowing was noted to be grossly intact. Her sitting balance was good both in static and dynamic situations, however, her standing balance was fair both statically and dynamically. A summary of her self-care and transfer status with related goal projections follows:

Table 12.1
Multiple Sclerosis Self-care Summary

Performance Area	Admission	Short-Term Goal (7–10 Days)	Long-Term Goal (10 Days To 3 Weeks)
Feeding	Minimum assistance	Supervision	Independent
Grooming	Minimum assistance	Supervision	Independent
Bathing	Minimum assistance	Supervision	Independent
Upper extremity dressing	Minimum assistance	Supervision	Independent
Lower extremity dressing	Moderate assistance	Minimum assistance	Independent
Toileting	Moderate assistance	Minimum assistance	Independent
Bed transfer	Minimum assistance	Supervision	Independent
Toilet transfer	Minimum assistance	Supervision	Independent
Tub transfer	Minimum assistance	Supervision	Independent

Long- and Short-Term Goals

T's long-term goal is to complete lower extremity dressing using a rollator walker to retrieve clothing from a closet, and selected adaptive equipment (reacher, dressing stick, long handled shoe horn, and sock donner) to dress.

In the short-term, T will retrieve clothing from the closet using a rollator walker for support.

Therapist Goals and Strategies

The therapist's goals include:

1. Decrease intentional tremors in left (dominant) upper extremity.
2. Increase strength on left side (upper and lower extremities).
3. Increase standing balance and tolerance.

The therapist's strategies include:

1. Provide therapeutic exercise activities using graded wrist weights to increase upper extremity strength.
2. Apply light resistance to left upper extremity during activity to attempt to reduce intention tremor and improve control.
3. Integrate proprioceptive neuromuscular facilitation (PNF) patterns into activity to promote strength and control of movement in the left upper extremity.
4. Provide and retrain in the use of assistive devices for activities of daily living.
5. Design activities that will challenge T's balance while supported by a rollator walker.

Activity

Morning Routine

During her self-care routine in the morning, T will practice using the assistive devices that she requires for lower extremity dressing (sock donner, dressing stick, long handled shoe horn, and reacher). She will dress while sitting at the edge of her bed. It is anticipated that learning to reintegrate these pieces of equipment into her routine should be fairly easy for T. She is familiar with the equipment and has been using it prior to admission. A challenge to T's independence is her remastering the use of the rollator walker to support her retrieving clothing from her closet in preparation for dressing. This task is complicated by her fair standing balance (static and dynamic) and the weakness and intention tremor present in her left upper extremity. An activity that challenges T's standing balance and requires her to use the rollator walker for support is indicated. Additionally, an activity that requires her to place objects will challenge and develop the strength and control in T's left upper extremity.

Decorating a "Holiday Tree"

In preparing for T to decorate a "holiday tree" the therapist assembles the following: a small (three- or four-foot) artificial tree, an assortment of holiday decorations that have been fitted with wire loops (two inches in diameter) to replace traditional ornament hooks, and a one pound wrist weight.

To begin the activity, T will be seated in a chair, the tree placed on the table to her right and the box of ornaments placed on a surface (12 inches high) on her left. Placement of the tree and ornaments in these positions facilitates the use of a proprioceptive neuromuscular facilitation (PNF) pattern. The one-pound wrist weight, applied to T's left wrist, provides stability and helps to reduce attention tremors. T is encouraged to reach for the ornaments and decorate the tree covering the front and sides. For this phase of the activity, T will be moving in the PNF pattern using the wrist weight for stability. The nature of the activity requires that she reach and place objects using upper extremity control. This will prepare her to place and retrieve objects from a closet for dressing.

To decorate the remainder of the tree T will stand supported by her rollator walker. This time, the tree will be placed on the table to her left and the ornaments to her right at chair level. She will use the one-pound wrist weights on her left hand. Placement of the tree and ornaments in this position requires T to use another PNF pattern. Again, the one-pound weight may help to reduce attention tremors by providing distal stability. Use of the rollator walker in the completion of this tree trimming activity will support T's use of this device to retrieve clothing from a closet for dressing.

Resources

The following resources can be helpful for gathering clinical data:

Functional Independence Measure

Manual Muscle Testing

The following resources can be helpful for gathering family data about MS:

Interview with patient and family

Home visit

The following are common practice settings:

Inpatient hospitalization, acute rehabilitation

Outpatient services

Home care

The following resources can be helpful for gathering sociopolitical data about MS:

Interview with patient and family

ADA (Americans with Disabilities Act)

Internet Resources

Archives of Neurology:
www.archneur.ama-assn.org

Centers for Medicate and Medicaid Information:
www.cms.hhs.gov

Mswatch.com (online community for people with MS)

Multiple Sclerosis International Federation:
www.msif.org

National Multiple Sclerosis Society:
www.nationalmssociety.org

Amyotrophic Lateral Sclerosis: Synopsis of Clinical Condition

Amyotrophic lateral sclerosis (ALS), also known as motor neuron disease (or Lou Gehrig's, or Charcot's disease) is a progressive degeneration of motor neurons in the spinal cord, brainstem and motor cortex (Adams & Victor, 1993). There are three clinical subtypes of ALS: primary amyotrophic lateral sclerosis (PLS), progressive muscular atrophy (PMA), and progressive bulbar palsy (PBP). Each subtype presents with a different affected area and clinical presentation, to be discussed later.

There are three forms of ALS: sporadic, familial, and Mariana Island. Sporadic ALS (SALS) is the most common and demonstrates a random pattern of incidence throughout the world. Familial ALS (FALS) accounts for five percent of those diagnosed with ALS, the victims having inherited an autosomal dominant trait (Adams & Victor, 1993). Mariana Island ALS represents a very small and unusual cluster of people diagnosed with ALS in Guam with muscle weakness accompanied by dementia and Parkinsonism.

Prevalence and Etiology

ALS is a common disease, which affects approximately 1 to 2 persons per 100,000 of the population annually. Males are affected more than females in a ratio of 2:1 with the onset age of symptoms between 50 and 70 years old (Adams & Victor, 1993). Life expectancy from onset of symptoms range from two to four years, with respiratory failure being the primary cause of death.

The etiology of ALS is unknown in SALS, however, some theories suggest that metal poisoning, metabolic disturbances, trauma, viral, and autoimmune factors play a vital role in the development of the disease. The pathophysiology of the disease is characterized by destruction of the motor neurons of the anterior horn and degeneration of the white matter of the anterior and lateral columns, which mostly affect the corticospinal tract. Degeneration of the ganglion cells of the motor nuclei and pyramids of the medulla is seen in microscopic examination. The primary area of motor neuron destruction varies according to the type of ALS. For example, the primary area of destruction in PBP occurs in the corticobulbar tracts and motor nuclei of the medulla, while in PLS the destruction affects the cortical motor neurons of the anterior horn. There is no cure for ALS, however there are pharmaceutical drugs, such as Rilutek® and Myotrophin™ that have been effective in delaying the progression of the disease. Most of the medical care for those with ALS focuses on treatment of the side effects of having this disease such as pneumonia, respiratory failure, and dysphagia.

Common Characteristics and Symptoms

The signs and symptoms upon presentation vary based on the type of ALS and progression. Generally, individuals may present with tongue and facial weakness, limb weakness, fasciculations (muscle twitching at rest), spasticity, muscle atrophy, slurred speech, and weight loss. Cognitive changes are extremely infrequent and the individual remains cognitively intact. Functionally, the individual may complain of frequent tripping or falls, impaired fine motor dexterity, and possibly difficulty with swallowing and breathing.

The progressive nature of ALS causes continuous changes in physical status and medical precautions. Some of the main issues to monitor are frequent falls; swallowing and breathing difficulties leading to aspiration of liquids and foods; pneumonia; and psychological issues regarding anxiety, denial, hopelessness, depression, and dying.

Contextual Considerations

Clinical

The individual with ALS will present with muscle weakness, signs of anxiety, and depression. As the disease progresses, more pronounced weakness will be evident with increasing difficulty of maintaining instrumental activities of daily living (IADLs), chewing, swallowing, walking, and breathing. Mechanical ventilation may become necessary as the disease affects the diaphragm and intercostal musculature. Many of the medical complications related to ALS will continue to challenge the individual and family.

Psychosocially, the individual will present with a multitude of issues including anxiety, anger, and hopelessness, plus fears of isolation, pain, dependence, and death (Umphred, 1997).

Family

The family will need to understand the prognosis of the disease, cope with the changing roles and tasks of family members throughout the process, and acknowledge the change in their own roles and tasks. Shifts of responsibilities and expectations among family members are common, and the need for high-intensity assistance can tax family resources. Referral to support groups or counseling may alleviate the effects of these abrupt changes, and allow the family to develop effective coping strategies.

Practice Setting

Those individuals affected with ALS are usually encountered by the occupational therapist in the inpatient acute care setting. Difficulty with ADLs, IADLs, and functional mobility due to muscle weakness indicate the need of a referral to occupational therapy. Inpatient acute rehabilitation will follow the acute medical intervention. Treatment will expand into the home setting due to the need for follow-up care, family training, and environmental adaptations. During the late stages of ALS, hospice care may be indicated for palliative care of the individual and family.

Clinical Decision Making Process

Defining Focus for Intervention

Because of the progressive nature of this disease, treatment should focus on instruction and training of ADL compensatory strategies to maintain independence, and maintaining existing strength and endurance. Some of these strategies will include work simplification and energy conservation, self-care adaptations to promote safety, and compensation for limb weakness and balance deficits caused by weakness.

Establishing Goals for Intervention

Occupational therapy goals are established based on an understanding of the disease process and the physical and psychological presentation during evaluation of task performance and patient interview.

Designing Theory-Based Intervention

Due to the progressive nature of the disease, occupational therapy intervention is focused on adaptation and optimization of residual abilities rather than the remediation of the disability. The rehabilitation frame of reference will be used to develop interventions that include the use adaptive equipment and compensatory techniques to maintain independence. Additionally, the biomechanical frame of reference will serve as a guide in the design of activities that maintain joint and muscle integrity and range of motion.

Evaluating Progress

Progress is difficult to achieve in ALS because of its rapid progression and consequent deterioration of function. Occupational therapy intervention should be continued with the patient until the later stages of the disease when dependence in ADLs and functional mobility is identified. At that point, family training becomes the focus of intervention. Caretaker independence in carrying out passive range of motion and handling techniques becomes the desired outcome, as well as psychological support for the individual.

Case Study

Description

Linda is a 52-year-old woman who lives in a two-story house with a strongly supportive husband. She has been living with ALS for two years. She is presently unemployed, but was working as a bank teller a year ago. Her major life roles are those of being a wife, grandmother, friend, and confidant. Her leisure interests include reading, writing, singing, talking on the phone to her friends, and spending time with her granddaughter. Linda is a very charismatic and insightful person and loves to talk with everyone. Linda has made it a point to educate herself about ALS, but does not discuss the prognosis of the disease with her therapists or other healthcare team members. During this admission, she has noticed a change in her lower extremity strength, her writing abilities, and occasional slurred speech. Her shoulder and interphalangeal joints bilaterally are somewhat painful with passive range of motion and unable to achieve full passive range of motion in shoulder flexion and abduction and interphalangeal flexion. Linda reports the active and passive range of motion of both upper extremities has been decreasing over the last three months.

Table 12.2
Amyotrophic Lateral Sclerosis Self-care Summary

Performance Area	Initial Evaluation	Short-Term Goal 5 Days	Long-Term Goal 10 Days
Feeding	Moderate assistance	Minimal assistance with adaptive devices and compensatory strategy for upper extremity support in 30 minutes.	Supervision with adaptive devices and compensatory strategy for upper extremity support in 15 minutes.

(Continued)

Table 12.2 (*Continued*)

Performance Area	Initial Evaluation	Short-Term Goal 5 Days	Long-Term Goal 10 Days
Grooming	Moderate assistance	Minimal assistance with adaptive devices to brush hair in 3 minutes.	Minimal assistance with adaptive device to brush hair in 1 minute.
Upper Extremity Dressing	Maximum assistance	Moderate assistance to thread shirt over both arms in 2 minutes.	Moderate assistance to thread shirt on both arms and over head in 2 minutes with assistive device.
Lower Extremity Dressing	Maximum assistance	Moderate assistance to thread legs into sweatpants with assistive device while seated.	Minimal assistance to don sweatpants with assistive device.

She reports she can still dress, bathe, and groom independently, and has developed slight difficulty with feeding utensils because of hand weakness. She ambulates with a pair of forearm crutches and uses a tub chair for bathing, and a raised toilet seat. Her husband performs all household cleaning and maintenance and prepares and cooks all of her dinners. A home health aide assists with breakfast and lunch preparation. A summary of her self-care status and goal projections follow. Note the inconsistencies of self-care level of assistance during initial evaluation.

Long- and Short-Term Goals

As a long-term goal, Linda will complete feeding with supervision and adaptive equipment in 15 minutes while using a compensatory strategy for upper extremity support.

The short-term goal is for Linda to complete feeding with minimum assistance and adaptive equipment in 30 minutes while using a compensatory strategy for upper extremity support.

Therapist Goals and Strategies

The therapist's goals include:

1. Improve passive and active range of motion and reduce joint pain.
2. Educate family in passive range of motion.
3. Provide compensatory strategies for upper extremity weakness during self-care tasks.

The therapist's strategies include:

1. Provide built-up utensils and handles-on objects.
2. Teach use of proximal upper extremity support on elevated surface to compensate for shoulder weakness during tasks.
3. Illustrate use of adapting environment for activity.

Activity

Morning Routine

During her morning self-care routine, Linda completes feeding using a large lightweight mug with handles and built-up utensils. She sits at a bedside table that is raised to the height of her chest. While eating, Linda supports her elbows on the table. The support of the table allows Linda to compensate for the lack of strength and endurance in her shoulders. Linda is also practicing the use of adaptive equipment and techniques for dressing and grooming. Any activity that is designed for Linda should incorporate lightweight materials, use equipment that has large handles or could be adapted to have large handles, and be able to be positioned on a raised bedside table. It should be short in duration and provide Linda with the opportunity to engage in her leisure interests. Focusing an activity in the leisure domain will allow Linda to see how the compensatory strategies and adaptive equipment utilized in self-care can be translated to support her leisure skills.

Activity

Book With Grandchild

To prepare to engage Linda and her granddaughter in the activity, the therapist will assemble a bedside table, an activity book, a set of colored markers, and foam to build up handles. Linda and her granddaughter will be on the same side of the bedside table. Linda is seated with the bedside table raised to chest height. The granddaughter may sit or stand. A set of markers and the activity book is placed between them. Linda places her elbows on the table to provide proximal support. Linda's granddaughter is instructed to insert markers into foam grips. Linda and her granddaughter take turns completing selected puzzles and pictures in the activity book. As Linda completes this activity she is reinforcing the skills and adaptive strategies that she will need to attain her long-term feeding goal while at the same time spending important quality time with her family.

Resources

The following resources can be helpful for gathering clinical data about ALS:

Functional Independence Measure™ (FIM)

Moberg Pick-Up Test

Jebsen Test of Hand Function

The following resources can be helpful for gathering practice setting data about ALS:

Inpatient: acute care, acute rehabilitation

Home care

Hospice

The following resources can be helpful for gathering sociopolitical data about ALS:

Interview with patient and family

ADA (Americans with Disabilities Act)

Exploring the following topics can elicit helpful information:

Fear of dying

Patient/family transitions of roles and tasks

Internet Resources

ALS Survival Guide:
www.lougehrigsdisease.net

ALS Association:
www.alsa.org

Guillain-Barré Syndrome: Synopsis of Clinical Condition

Guillain-Barré syndrome (GBS) is also known as acute inflammatory polyneuropathy, idiopathic polyneuritis, acute inflammatory polyneuritis, Landry's paralysis, Landry-Guillain-Barré syndrome, or autoimmune neuropathy. It involves a syndrome of acute weakness of the extremities in which the body's immune system attacks part of the peripheral nervous system (Umphred, 2001).

Prevalence and Etiology

This disease affects people worldwide regardless of age, ethnicity, race, or gender. It has no seasonal or epidemic incidence and it affects approximately 1 to 2 persons of every 100,000. It has been documented in both children and adults (Umphred, 2001).

The etiology of GBS is unknown; however, viral infections, respiratory infections, and gastrointestinal bacterial infections usually precede symptoms by one to three weeks. Approximately 50% of GBS patients will have a recent history of viral infection within the last two to four weeks. In rare instances, surgery, vaccinations, pregnancy, cancer, and lymphoma will initiate the disease process. These listed conditions trigger an immune response against the myelin sheath of the peripheral nerves. One theory of causation implies that the viral infection has changed the nature of the cells in the peripheral nervous system, which are then treated as foreign bodies. Another theory suggests the immune system becomes less discriminatory, allowing for lymphocytes and macrophages to attack the axonal myelin sheath. Also, it is believed the invading antigen has antigenic similarity to the myelin antigens (Umphred, 2001).

Common Characteristics and Symptoms

The initial clinical presentation of this syndrome will be somewhat symmetrical muscle weakness and paraesthesias of the lower extremities with ascending weakness to the upper extremities and trunk musculature within hours, days, or up to four weeks. Decreased or absent reflexes, increased presence of protein in the cerebral spinal fluid, slow nerve conduction velocity, and accompaniment of the rapid onset of symmetrical weakness are good indicators of GBS. Cranial nerve impairment can lead to dysarthria, dysphagia, and ptosis. Complaints of generalized pain especially at the joints and tenderness at the muscle bellies are common. The intensity of weakness can increase to the point of leaving those severely affected with total paralysis. Within two weeks of the onset of symptoms, most people will have reached the most severe level of weakness they will encounter during this course. Complications and precautions of GBS may be abnormal heart rate and blood pressure, deep vein thromboses, infections, and insufficient respiration indicating the need for possible mechanical ventilation. Skin decubiti, hemodynamic instability, increased risk of falling, and range of motion limitations such as adhesive capsulitis are other precautions for the occupational therapist to recognize during treatment.

The medical treatment for GBS lessens the severity of the illness and facilitates recovery. Plasmaphoresis and high-dose immunoglobulin therapy are the current choice for treatment. These two interventions are generally successful, although the cause is unknown.

Recovery time varies based on the amount of axonal damage that has occurred. Usually axonal damage is mild after GBS, often leading to complete recovery. Sixty-seven percent of those with GBS will present with no residual weakness three years after onset. However, if axonal degradation has occurred, complete recovery will be limited (Goodman, Boissonnault, & Fuller, 2003).

Target Areas for Intervention

The role of the occupational therapist when treating those afflicted with GBS is to facilitate the victim's ability to achieve maximal independence in all areas of occupation performed prior to onset of disability.

Most commonly, the biomechanical and rehabilitative frames of reference are employed in the treatment of individuals with GBS. The two approaches are used together because while the victim is learning ADL strategies to compensate for temporary muscle weakness, he or she must continue to perform activities to improve motor skills. During the initial phase of intervention, the occupational therapist will identify problem areas of occupation and performance skills. Assessment of body position, activities of daily living, and communication are pertinent skills to evaluate in this population. Treatment intervention focuses on proper instruction in the use of compensatory strategies for ADLs, splinting, and activities to improve motor skills. Ongoing assessment of the psychosocial impact of the disease process on the patient and family should be addressed. The abruptness of this disease can adversely affect the patient's ability to engage in life roles and tasks, and cause family disruption.

References

Adams, R., & Victor, M. (1993). *Principles of neurology,* New York: McGraw-Hill.

Anderson, K. N., Anderson, L. E., & Glanze, W. D. (1994). *Mosby's medical, nursing, and allied health dictionary.* St. Louis, MO: Mosby.

Aronson, K. J., Goldenberg, E., & Cleghorn, G. (1996). Socio-demographic characteristics and health status of persons with multiple sclerosis and their care givers. *MS Management, 3(1),* 1–17.

Bhasin, C. A. (1989). Occupational therapy in the management of multiple sclerosis. *AOTA Physical Disabilities Special Interest Section Newsletter, 12(4),* 1–4.

Crepeau, E., Cohn, E. & Schell, B. (2003). *Willard and Spackman's occupational therapy* (10th ed.). Philadelphia: Lippincott.

Franklin, G. M., Heaton, R. K., Nelson, L. M., Filley, C. M., & Seibert, C. (1988). Correlation of neuropsychological and MRI findings in chronic/progressive multiple sclerosis. *Neurology, 38(12),* 1826–9.

Freeman, J., Langdon, D., Hobart, J., & Thompson, A. (1997). The impact of inpatient rehabilitation on progressive multiple sclerosis. *Annals of Neurology, 42,* 236–244.

Goodman, C., Boissonnault, W., & Fuller, K. (2003). *Pathology: Implications for the physical therapist* (2nd ed.). Philadelphia: Saunders.

Kemp, B. (1990). *The psychosocial context of geriatric rehabilitation.* Boston: Little Brown & Co.

National Multiple Sclerosis Society. (1996). *What is multiple sclerosis?* New York: Author.

Occupational Therapy Practice Framework Domain and Process. (2002).

Umphred, D. A. (2001). *Neurological rehabilitation* (4th ed.). St. Louis, MO: Mosby.

Whetten-Goldstein, K., Sloan, F., Conover, C., Viscusi, K., Kulas, B., & Chesson, H. (1996). The economic burden of multiple sclerosis. *MS Management, 3(1)*, 33–37.

Amputations

13

James Foster, MS, OTR/L

Synopsis of Clinical Condition

Prevalence and Etiology

Limb loss occurs as a result of many different causes. There are approximately three million amputees in North America, with an estimated 3,000 new amputees each week and 170,000 each year (Alberta Amputee Sport and Recreation Association, 2002). Leg amputations make up 90% of all cases. At 77%, males make up an overwhelming majority of cases. Approximately 50% are between the ages of 21 and 65 (AASRA, 2002).

The primary cause of amputations in North America is vascular and circulatory disease, with diabetes the primary cause of 50% of amputations (AASRA, 2002). Other causes of amputation include bone cancer, trauma, and congenital deformities (Edelstein, 2001). Improvements in the early detection and treatment of bone cancer will be accompanied by an increase in amputations, with surgeons attempting to remove the shortest amount of limb while still maintaining vascular integrity to the residual limb.

Common Characteristics and Symptoms

Each type of amputation is characterized by an array of characteristics, symptoms, and challenges. From distal to proximal, lower extremity amputations can be classified into those at the toe, trans-metatarsal (TMA), below-the-knee (BKA), knee disarticulations, above-the-knee (AKA), or directly at the hip (hip disarticulation). BKA is the most common of all amputations at 55% (Muilenburg and Wilson, 1996).

Upper extremity amputations can be digit amputations, wrist disarticulation, below the elbow, elbow disarticulation, above the elbow, and shoulder disarticulations. Generally, the closer to the body that the amputation occurs, the more stability that must be provided by a prosthetic.

Target Areas for Intervention

Upper and lower extremity rehabilitation can be broken down into three stages: pre-prosthetic, prosthetic, and post-prosthetic. Target areas for occupational therapy intervention vary with the location of the amputation and the stage of rehabilitation. The occupational therapist has an important role within the pre-prosthetic and prosthetic stages.

In the pre-prosthetic stage for lower and upper extremity amputation, the occupational therapist concentrates on limb desensitization, edema control, and limb shaping.

Treatment is also directed toward maintaining range of motion and positioning of the limb to achieve full active range of motion of the remaining joint or joints.

The prosthetic stage for the occupational therapist includes teaching the patient to put on and take off the prosthetic and the under-stockings, in addition to performing functional activities with the new limb.

The post-prosthetic stage includes fitting for a final prosthetic and higher-level prosthetic use.

Contextual Considerations

Clinical

During the pre-prosthetic stage, the focus for treatment is: limb and incision inspection, limb wrapping, limb desensitization, and positioning. The pre-prosthetic stage generally lasts two to four months in which approximately two to four weeks are spent hospitalized or in acute inpatient rehabilitation. The preferred scenario exists if a temporary prosthetic is applied to the residual limb within two to four weeks of the original surgery. However, many times, due to financial and medical constraints, this rarely occurs.

The patient should be educated to inspect the incision and residual limb two to three times daily. This process can be assisted using an inspection mirror to view distal and posterior aspects of the limb. The patient should look for areas around the incision that blacken or become pale, either of which can suggest vascular changes or necrosis within the limb. Incisions that are not healing are also to be noted, as well as amounts and color of any drainage. Sutures of the incision will be removed when the incision is fully healed, usually within two to four weeks. Sutures may be partially removed, as the wound may not uniformly heal throughout the entire incision.

There is much debate over the use of rigid versus soft post operative residual limb dressings (Smith, et al. 2003). Examples of rigid and semi-rigid dressings include plaster casting material, Unna's paste dressing, and bivalved splints. The benefits of these dressings include good contracture prevention and good shaping. The disadvantages include poor ability to monitor the incision and increased probability of pressure sores if applied incorrectly.

Examples of soft dressings include Ace Wrap™, and Tubigrip™. Advantages of soft dressings include good shaping , allowance of daily incision inspection and ease of application. Disadvantages include difficulty for some patients to apply and much variance in pressure with application. This chapter will discuss application of soft dressings as it is this type of dressings that indicate the most hands on involvement for the patient.

Limb-wrapping can occur at the same time the patient is inspecting the limb. Limb-wrapping is necessary to control edema, to shape the limb, and to provide sensory input and pressure to the limb. During the acute stage, the residual limb should be covered with both an inner and outer wrapping. The inner wrap should consist of absorbent gauze such as sterile 4X4 and Kling Wrap™ or Kerlex™, to collect any drainage and keep it from soaking the outer wrap. The outer wrap should initially be Ace Wrap™ and should be applied in a figure-8 method, utilizing a diagonal pattern. For the BKA patient, the Ace Wrap™ can be anchored above the knee to avoid dressing slippage.

The wrap should be tighter at the distal end of the limb and looser at the proximal aspect to allow for circulation proximally. Special attention must be paid to the medial and lateral distal edges of the limb and incision. Fleshy folds (referred to as "dog ears") can occur at these areas, and need to be flattened via the wrapping process for the proper shaping to occur.

Generally, the wider the residual limb, the more difficult it is to wrap and for the wrap to remain in place. This is especially true for AKA cases, which can leave wide and short residual limbs. In these cases an Elastinet™ covering over the Ace Wrap™ will help keep the wrap in place. The Elastinet™ covering can also incorporate a belt to wrap around the waist and then tie off at the distal end of the limb.

The wrap should be secured to itself using medical tape and not the metal clips that usually accompany the wrap. Many amputees have decreased sensation in the residual limb and may not feel the metal clip against their skin. The patient should also be instructed to wear the wrapping 24 hours a day unless performing self-care.

The patient should be instructed via a physical demonstration in addition to illustrated handouts. An "artificial limb" can also be fabricated from sheets and rounded at the edges to provide the patient another medium to practice wrapping. The residual limb should be unwrapped and wrapped two to three times a day, as the wrap's elasticity decreases after several hours. If drainage is present on the inner wrap, it should be replaced every time the limb is wrapped. The outer wrap should be discarded and replaced every three to four days as it loses its elasticity.

Circumferential measurements should be made to track the effectiveness of the wrapping in terms of edema management. These measurements should be shared with the patient to demonstrate the importance of limb wrapping.

Limb wrapping also provides constant pressure to the limb. This is beneficial for several reasons. First, consistent and equal pressure on a wound or incision promotes healing and prevents scar formation. Second, it provides sensory and tactile input to the limb. This is necessary as initially the limb will be painful and sensitive to touch, but it must be desensitized in order for the patient to tolerate the use of a prosthetic.

As noted previously, the wrap of choice should initially be Ace Wrap™. Many patients, however, have difficulty utilizing the figure-8 method because of issues related to their vascular disease. Poor vascular flow to the peripheral extremities can result in poor sensation of the upper extremities and consequently affect fine motor coordination during limb wrapping. Many individuals with compromised vascular systems also have poor visual acuity and cannot see the end of the limb or fully appreciate the figure-8 technique required for proper wrapping.

For these reasons, it may be easier to apply Tubigrip™ stocking to the limb. This can be done by measuring the limb for the correct width stocking and applying with a Tubigrip™ applicator, proximally to distally, to avoid sheering of the incision. A double layer should be utilized with a twist between layers at the distal end of the limb. The second layer should also be shorter to provide increased pressure at the distal aspect of the limb. The Tubigrip™ should be replaced every three to four days as it too will loose its elasticity.

When the incision is able to sustain minimal sheering force, a limb shrinker or limb sock can be utilized. This item is a sized, elastic sock that can be donned and doffed over the residual limb. Again, this should not be applied until the physician and rehab team decide the incision can sustain the sheering force that will occur when applying the shrinker. This will be discussed more during the prosthetic and post-prosthetic stages.

Limb desensitization is important in order to allow prosthetic usage in the future. Desensitization begins by having the patient envision placement of the prosthetic over the limb. The patient should be instructed to physically feel and palpate the residual limb. This is important not only for sensory purposes but also for self-image purposes. For this reason, the patient may have emotional difficulty accomplishing self-palpation of the limb. Tapping of the limb can be done with foam-handled instrument called a "limb tapper." The patient should be instructed to carry the tapper with him or her at all times.

Alcohol-free and fragrance-free lotions can also be used to provide tactile input to the limb. During this process, deep massage and pressure should be applied to accomplish skin mobilization. This will prevent any skin-to-muscle adhesions, which can occur after surgery.

These processes of sensory input and skin mobilization should last 10 to 15 minutes and should take place two to three times daily.

Amputee patients may also experience phantom sensation and phantom pain. Phantom sensation is a non painful sensation or awareness that gives form to a body part with specific dimensions, weight or range of motion (Gailey, 1994). Examples of phantom sensations include touch, pressure, cold, wetness, or movement. One movement in particular that amputees report is that of bed mobility especially during supine ot sit while the patient is bringing his or her residual limb over the end of the bed.

Phantom pain is a painful sensation experienced below the residual limb. Examples of phantom pain are dull aching, burning, and knife like stabbing. Etiology of both phantom sensation and pain are debated within literature pointing towards the homunculus for the leg remaining in the brain and production of abnormal neurologic signature patterns (Melzack, 1992). Treatment methods such as use of heat, proprioceptive imput, use of prosthesis, and stretching have been researched and not consistently shown to be effective (Sherman, 1989).

Positioning issues must also be addressed within the pre-prosthetic stage. These issues are especially evident for BKA and below elbow amputations, as range of motion of the knee and elbow will be critical during the prosthetic and post-prosthetic stages.

The patient should be educated to maintain full extension of the knee and elbow joints when not ambulating or utilizing residual limbs. When extension is not maintained, a flexion contracture can occur. Range of motion exercises can be utilized, in addition to heat combined with a sustained passive stretching of the contracted joint.

For a lower extremity, full extension can be assisted through several means. If the patient will be immobile or supine during a lengthy hospitalization, a dorsal knee extension splint can be fabricated from thermoplastic splinting material and applied to the limb while in bed or in a chair. Serial casting of the knee joint in extension can be utilized in more extreme cases; however, this makes it difficult to address sensory and shaping issues. While supine in bed, the patient should be instructed to never place a pillow under the knee, as this will only encourage a flexion contracture. When the patient is in a wheelchair, an amputee leg-rest should be utilized to maintain knee extension if a prosthesis is not being worn.

For elbow contractures, an anterior extension splint can be fabricated from thermoplastic splinting material and applied to provide force and encourage elbow extension. The splint may need to be modified as more extension is gained. Goniometer measurements should be utilized on a daily basis and shared with the patient to encourage proper positioning of the residual limb.

Goals of independence in functional mobility and self-care are also addressed within the pre-prosthetic stage. Independence in functional mobility and lower extremity dressing may prove to be especially challenging to the lower extremity amputee due to decreased standing balance. Generally, the higher the amputation, the more standing balance deficits will exist. This is true because longer limbs allow for increased righting reactions. AKA amputees do not have much limb to assist in righting reactions. Independence in these areas may require the use of assistive devices such as a rolling walker, auxiliary crutches, tub seats, or tub transfer benches.

Upper extremity amputees will require instruction in one-hand techniques for a variety of self-care tasks, such as manipulating clothing fasteners, cooking, and eating. If the dominant extremity has been amputated, the challenge presented by this aspect of treatment is increased.

The prosthetic stage consists of application of a temporary prosthetic and ultimately a permanent prosthetic. During the prosthetic stage, a prosthetist creates a mold of the residual limb once the incision is fully healed, and the limb is completely shaped with little or no edema present. This generally occurs two to four months after the amputation surgery. A positive plaster mold is created from a negative cast of the limb and then hardened. Thermoplastic material is heated and draped over the plaster mold and shaped to the form of the mold to create a socket. Prior to delivery of the temporary prosthesis, the prosthetist will often perform a home visit to check the fit of the socket and gauge the amount and thickness of limb socks that will be required.

For a lower extremity prosthesis, a lightweight metal pole (also know as a pylon) is connected to the socket with a foam or plastic foot attached to the end. For an upper extremity prosthesis, the socket is attached to a hook-like terminal device with a pull cable looped around the opposite shoulder that serves to open and close the hook for grasping.

The occupational therapist, along with the prosthetist, physical therapist, and physician, instruct the patient on how to put on and take off the temporary prosthetic. For upper extremity amputees this is generally accomplished in an outpatient therapy setting, but for lower extremity amputees this may involve inpatient hospitalization. The patient must also gain tolerance to wearing the prosthetic. A wearing schedule should be set, with the patient wearing the prosthetic no longer than 30 minutes to three hours by the end of the first week. After the first week the schedule should consist of two 2- to 3-hour wearing sessions. Prosthetic limbs should not be worn overnight when the patient is sleeping as prolonged wear can compromise skin integrity. After the second week the prosthetic can be worn as tolerated, with multiple inspections for areas of redness. It is not uncommon for changes in the foam insert or thermoplastic socket to be made by the prosthetist. This usually includes certain areas to be "blown out" to relieve pressure points.

It also must be stressed to the patient that the limb shrinker must continue to be worn when the prosthetic is not. Without shrinker use, there will be much variability in edema and shape of the limb, affecting prosthetic use and fit.

There is generally a cotton limb sock or socks under the socket that serves several purposes. First, it absorbs the sweat or moisture within the area. Second, the number and thickness (also known as ply) of the socks can be changed to improve the fit of the limb within the socket. The size of the residual limb is dynamic within the first several months of prosthetic use due to changing edema levels within the limb. The prosthetic user and the rehab team must constantly evaluate the fit of the limb within the socket and change the ply of the socks as warranted. For lower extremity BKA amputees, there is often a light foam, custom-molded insert that is either used in addition to the cotton sock or instead if the cotton sock.

To avoid constant changing of the limb socks, or irritation from the cotton socks, some prosthetists suggests use of an inner Alpha Gel Sock™, which is a sock that is made of gel and will change with the shape of the limb. These socks do have drawbacks, including the trapping of moisture within the liner. Also, they are much more expensive than a cotton limb sock.

Function with the lower limb prosthetic is accomplished through high-level standing balance activities, such as cooking at the stove, or putting on and removing the prosthetic for bathtub transfers. The new prosthetic user must also achieve independence in self-care and functional mobility with the prosthetic. For some, this mobility can be accomplished through outpatient therapy; but others accomplish these goals, in addition to independence in ambulation and stairs, within an acute inpatient rehabilitation setting. One must consider that most patients were functioning at a level of supervision to independent at home for one to two months while their incision was healing. So the goal is not to achieve independence in self-care and functional mobility, but to achieve independence in self-care and independence with the prosthetic.

Upper extremity amputees often develop prosthetic functionality in an outpatient setting. The decision to use a hook or a cosmetic hand is made during the prosthetic stage of rehab. Prosthetic hands can be utilized for fine motor tasks, although they are mainly used for cosmetic purposes.

The post-prosthetic stage involves fitting for a permanent prosthetic, and is generally accomplished on an outpatient basis with the assistance of a physical therapist and prosthetist. The main issues that concern prosthetic wearers during these latter stages are comfort and function (Nielsen, Psonak, & Kalter, 1989). The patient should have his or her permanent upper extremity prosthetic within one year of their original surgery.

Family

There are several considerations concerning the family of an amputee throughout all of the prosthetic stages. The family members should be enlisted in education programs during the pre-prosthetic stage so they feel involved from the very beginning. Tasks such as limb wrapping and limb desensitization may fall upon a primary caretaker if the patient is not able to complete these tasks independently. The patient requires emotional support and encouragement from the family. Roles and hobbies that were performed prior to amputation may need to be adjusted or altered to fit the patient's new functional status.

Practice Setting

The practice setting for occupational therapy treatment of the amputee varies for upper and lower extremity amputations. The pre-prosthetic stage for both types of amputee will include some inpatient hospitalization. The lower extremity amputee's hospitalization length will likely be longer and may include inpatient acute rehabilitation during the prosthetic stage. The upper extremity amputee will likely achieve most goals in an outpatient setting during both the prosthetic and post-prosthetic stages.

Sociopolitical

Medicare will reimburse a patient for a new prosthetic every year, or when medically necessary. This is covered under Medicare B and will cover 80% of the cost included costs for related equipment such as inserts limb socks and limb shrinkers (Medicare.gov, 2003). Private pay insurance companies differ in their coverage for a prosthetic. The worst-case scenario is that private companies will only cover one prosthetic per lifetime. If a patient is of working age, the state Office for Vocational Rehabilitation (which assists disabled persons' return to work) can assist in providing funding for a prosthetic.

The frequency of prosthetic replacement depends on several factors, such as the activity level of the patient, the way the prosthetic is utilized, and the complexity of the actual prosthetic. The moving parts of a prosthetic (such as knee and elbow joints) will eventually break down. Also, the insert within a lower extremity requires replacement on a yearly basis. The timely processing of all claims for reimbursement is essential since delays in receipt of the prosthetic will interfere with the therapeutic process. The prosthesis should be delivered to the patient within his or her home setting as Medicare and most private insurances will not reimburse for medical equipment delivered during an inpatient hospitalization.

It is important for the occupational therapist to collaborate with the prosthetist. It is important that the prosthetist understands the patient's functional goals, since the prosthetist is usually responsible for submitting reimbursement claims to Medicare and private pay insurances.

Lifestyle/Lifespan

The needs of an amputee vary throughout the life span. Prosthetics for both the upper and lower extremity can be created or adjusted for almost any need imaginable. Advancements in lightweight graphite and metals continue to advance athletic and active prosthetic technology. These high technology prosthetics, however, are much costlier than the prosthetic required for basic ambulation needs. In addition, these prosthetics for the active user need replacement more often because to their increased usage.

Clinical Decision Making Process

Defining Focus for Intervention

Occupational therapy intervention is based the prosthetic stage and the patient's premorbid disposition, cognitive ability, social support systems, and the physical arrangement of the individual's living quarters. Also, for persons with upper extremity amputations, limb dominance is an issue. In addition, the patient's expectations with regard to post-amputation activity resumption must be taken into consideration when establishing goals for treatment.

During the post-prosthetic stage for upper extremity amputations, a definitive, or permanent prosthetic will be applied. This may include delivery of both a cosmetic hand

and a terminal hook device. Most upper extremity prosthetics include interchangeable terminal devices. Focus will be on utilizing the prosthetic for fine motor tasks and instruction for when to utilize each device.

Establishing Goals for Intervention

Occupational therapy goals are set together with the patient. During the pre-prosthetic stage for lower extremity amputation, goals concerning limb care, functional mobility, and self-care are generally made. The level at which the patient will be able to perform these tasks depends on many factors, including the patient's cognition, standing balance, fine motor coordination, and visual acuity. The availability of assistance, the home environment, and premorbid functioning will determine goals with regard to ambulation and mobility. If a wheelchair is necessary, a goal of independence in wheelchair mobility will be set. If the patient is cognitively impaired, and has the social support to allow the patient to return home, family training in safe transfer methods will also be an important goal. For patients who are anxious to return to previous roles, such as head of household, goals are set to practice these roles within the rehabilitation setting. The patient should be encouraged to participate in these roles soon after discharge from the hospital.

The upper extremity amputee will also need to achieve goals in limb care during the pre-prosthetic stage, with a focus on many of the same factors as the lower extremity. The main difference is whether the dominant hand has been amputated. This will dictate whether dominance transferal training will occur. One-handed techniques will not be as challenging if the dominant hand can be utilized for fine motor tasks.

During the prosthetic stage, patient education about the appropriate thickness or "ply" of limb sock, and how and when to change the sock is necessary. A goal will also be set for increased wearing tolerance. This goal will greatly depend on the patient's skin integrity and his or her compliance with limb wrapping or use of the limb shrinker since the surgery.

For lower extremity amputees, a goal will also be set to reach independence in functional mobility and self-care with the prosthetic. This may or may not occur within an inpatient setting, and the patient may already be independent in functional mobility and self-care without the prosthetic. If the latter is true, the goals will likely be achieved quickly.

For upper extremity amputees, the goals during the prosthetic stage will likely be achieved within an outpatient setting. It is important to note that the longer the patient is without a prosthetic, the more he or she will get accustomed to not needing it. It is important that clear and precise goals are set with the patient long before delivery of the upper extremity prosthetic.

Designing Theory-Based Intervention

There are several frames of reference utilized with the amputee patient, including biomechanical, rehabilitation, and the model of human occupation.

The biomechanical frame of reference states that purposeful activities can be utilized to treat loss of range of motion, strength, and endurance (Hopkins & Smith, 1993). Within the function-dysfunction continuum the domain of concern includes edema control, passive range of motion, strength, and high level endurance. These are all areas addressed with amputees via independence in certain areas of occupation.

The rehabilitation frame of reference addresses underlying deficits that cannot be remediated or compensated. Domains of concern included within this frame of reference are activities of daily living, work, and leisure tasks, which are all areas affected by a limb amputation. This frame of reference stipulates rehabilitation methods such as adaptive devices, ambulatory devices, wheelchair modification, environmental modification, adaptive procedures, and safety education (Hopkins & Smith, 1993).

The model of human occupation is appropriate for amputees utilizing the volition, habituation, and performance subsystems. Values and interests are assessed during the pre-prosthetic stage for amputees. Roles and habits are kept in mind when designing and selecting the proper prosthetic or prosthetics for the patient.

Evaluating Progress

Progress can be evaluated by assessing the goals that are accomplished and appreciating the time periods involved. The most important goal to be accomplished within the pre-prosthetic stage is independence in limb care. Often, the ability to reach independence in limb care is a predictor of future success in the prosthetic and post-prosthetic stages. Another important goal within the pre-prosthetic stage is for the patient to return home able to perform functional mobility and independent self-care. The level at which the patient returns home will not be the permanent level of function. Once the prosthetic training occurs, the level will likely change and possibly improve.

Determining Change in or Termination of Treatment

Once goals are achieved within the pre-prosthetic stage, the patient is generally discharged until the prosthetic is available for use.

During the prosthetic stage, once the patient with a lower extremity amputation is independent in ambulation, or an upper extremity amputee is independent with high level fine motor tasks, the patient will be discharged from all therapies.

Between the pre-prosthetic and prosthetic stages the rehab team and prosthetist will decide if the patient is a good prosthetic candidate. Factors that assist in this decision include the patient's compliance with limb care, his or her level of performance in functional mobility, and family support. If the team believes that the functional level will not be improved or may worsen with the prosthetic, the team may decide not to proceed into the prosthetic stage.

Case Study

Description

KR is a 30-year-old female with a history of intravenous drug use, endocarditis, hepatitis B and C, chronic liver disease, and sepsis. She was admitted to the hospital with complaints of bilateral leg pain. Upon examination, KR demonstrated gangrenous bilateral calf and foot areas. It was later determined that the patient had developed multiple septic emboli to her lower extremities. She had also been non-compliant with past drug rehabilitation and antibiotic therapy for her endocarditis. Approximately two weeks after admission the patient underwent amputation of the right leg below the knee and left leg below the knee.

Originally, all wounds were left open. The lower extremity amputations underwent a skin graft closure approximately two weeks after the original surgery.

Occupational therapy and all rehab services initiated therapy three days after surgery. The patient was in a considerable amount of pain and was only able to demonstrate bed mobility and bilateral upper extremity active range of motion. Both of her lower extremity amputations had flexion contractures and were covered in soft dressings. The remainder of her self-care and functional mobility activities were not tested due to complaints of pain and fatigue. These areas were ultimately assessed within the first week and goals were set. KR's sitting balance in bed was fair. In addition, there was a considerable amount of patient education in terms of her long-term rehabilitation needs and the settings within which that they would be accomplished.

KR's social situation was an obstacle to achieving her rehabilitation goals. KR was homeless and estranged from her family. KR also had a six-year-old son who was living with his father. The months leading up to her hospitalization had been spent in shelters or on the streets, and she had no medical insurance coverage. Her admission status and goals projections for activities of daily living and functional transfers are summarized below.

Table 13.1
KR's Admission Status and Goals Projections

Performance Area	Admission	Short-Term Goal	Long-Term Goal
Feeding	Independent	Independent	Independent
Grooming	Max A	Min A	Independent
Bathing	Mod A	Min A	Independent
Upper extremity dressing	Min A	Independent	Independent
Lower extremity dressing (including limb care)	Max A	Min A	Independent
Toileting	Mod A	Min A	Independent
Bed transfer	Mod A	Min A	Independent
Toilet transfer	Mod A	Min A	Independent
Tub transfer	Dependent	Mod A	Independent
Tub transfer	Dependent	Mod A	Independent

As part of her comprehensive OT program, KR will be educated in limb wrapping, skin inspection, and limb desensitization. These requisite components of her program will remain in place and integrated into her day as the healing process progresses. Fabricated knee extension splints will be checked on an ongoing basis and adjusted to reduce her contractures and facilitate full knee extension bilaterally. In choosing and designing an activity for KR, the therapist notes that she will be completing all activities from a wheelchair throughout the pre-prosthetic stage. Using a wheelchair, in combination with sitting unsupported at the edge of the bed, is the way she will approach her morning self-care routine. Specifically, the night before, KR will use her wheelchair to secure her clothing for the next day and place it within easy reach of her bed. She will then be able to dress in the morning prior to transferring to the wheelchair. In the early stages of rehabilitation, the transfer will be a challenge for KR, and grooming, hygiene, and toileting will require the assistance of the staff.

A key component of KR's ability to be successful at developing independence in the wheelchair and sitting at the edge of the bed will be sitting balance. As a new bilateral lower extremity amputee, KR has experienced a change in her center of gravity and an alteration of her sense of balance. She adapts by using her upper extremities to support sitting. Using her arms to maintain balance will severely impact her efforts to be independent. A new sense of her center of gravity and balance will be important to her independence.

Because the primary focus is to assist KR in developing sitting balance, a simple activity that is easy to understand, which allows KR to concentrate on keeping her balance, and that can readily be graded to challenge her, is best. As her sitting balance improves, KR will become more confident she will be able to move forward with more complicated tasks.

Long- and Short-Term Goals

KR's long-term goal is to be able to dress independently while seated unsupported in bed.

In the short-term, KR will be able to securely reach for a shirt from a closet without losing her seated balance.

Therapist Goals and Strategies

The therapist's goals include:

1. Reduce flexion contractures in the knees bilaterally.
2. Improve sitting balance to allow both upper extremities to be free to engage in activity from a wheel chair level, or seated at the edge of the bed.

The therapist's strategies include:

1. Fabrication of knee extension splints bilaterally. Splints will be constructed from thermoplastic materials and be designed to facilitate full knee extension.
2. Design of functional activities of daily living, independent activities of daily living, and leisure activities that can be graded to challenge KR's sitting balance.

Activity

Ball toss: O-U-T

KR is positioned sitting unsupported on a mat. The therapist stands in a three-foot square outlined on the floor. A large beach ball is tossed between KR and the therapist. Each time a person misses he or she receives a letter: O- U- T. The first person to miss three throws and spell OUT loses the game. The activity of catching and throwing is familiar to KR. Use of a large beach ball facilitates KR using both upper extremities in the game. This requires her to rely on her developing sitting balance. The therapist challenges KR's sitting balance in all directions by targeting the ball.

Treatment Objective

KR will achieve simultaneous bilateral upper extremity extension without loss of seated balance.

Resources

The following resources can be helpful for gathering clinical data about amputation:

Functional Independence Measure™ (FIM)

Financial resources

Informal interviews with patient and family

The following resources can be helpful for gathering family data:

Patient and family interview

Home visit

The following are common practice settings:

Acute: inpatient hospital

Pre-Prosthetic: acute inpatient rehabilitation hospital

Lower extremity: inpatient hospital or acute rehabilitation hospital

Upper extremity: outpatient setting

Prosthetic:

- Lower extremity: either inpatient or outpatient setting
- Upper extremity: outpatient setting

Post-prosthetic:

- Upper and lower extremity: outpatient setting

The following resources can be helpful for gathering sociopolitical data:

Amputee-online.com

Americans with Disabilities Act

Amputee-coalition.org

Medicare.gov

Office of Vocational Rehabilitation (or equivalent local agency)

The following resources can be helpful for gathering lifestyle/lifespan data:

Amputee-online.com

American Association of Retired Persons (AARP)

Amputee Golf Association

References

Alberta Amputee Sport and Recreation Association. *Frequently asked questions about amputees.* Retrieved 11/10/2002, from www.aasra.ab.ca/faq.htm

Edelstein, J.E. (2001). Prosthetic assessment and management. In S.B. O'Sullivan & T.J. Schmitz, *Physical rehabilitation: Assessment and treatment.* Philadelphia: FA Davis.

Gailey, R. (1994). *One step ahead: An integrated approach to lower extremity prosthetics and amputee rehabilitation.* Advanced Rehabilitation Therapy, Inc.

Hopkins, H., & Smith, H. (1993). *Willard and Spackman's occupational therapy.* Philadelphia: Lippincott.

Medicare, artificial limbs and eyes coverage. Retrieved 1/3/2003, from www.medicare.gov.

Melzack, R. (1992). Phantom limbs. *Scientific American,* April, 120-126.

Muilenburg, A & Wilson, A. (1996) *The immediate post surgical period- A manual for below-knee amputees.* www.oandp.com Retrieved 4/14/2004.

Nielsen, C., Psonak, R., & Kalter, T. (1989). Factors affecting the use of prosthetic services. *Journal of Prosthetics and Orthotics, 1*(4), 242–249.

Sherman, R.A. (1989). Stump and phantom limb pain. *Neuro Clinics 7*(2), 249-264.

Smith, D., McFarland, L., Sangeorzan, B., Reiber, G., Czerniecki, J. Postoperative dressing and management strategies for transtibial amputations: A critical review. *Journal of Rehabilitation and Development, 40*(3), 213–224.

Orthopedics: Fractures and Joint Replacements

14

Jonathan Niszczak, MS, OTR/L
Abu Panackal, BS, OTR/L

Synopsis of Clinical Condition

Orthopedics is the specialty concerned with the preservation, restoration, and development of the form and function of the musculoskeletal system, extremities, spine, and associated structures by medical, surgical, and physical methods (Cyriax, 1982). Medical conditions addressed in the field of orthopedics include fractures, strains and sprains, tendon or ligament repairs, joint replacements, and numerous associated soft tissue injuries.

Prevalence and Etiology

During the aging process, loss of bone density and calcium increases the chance that falls will result in fractures, especially in the spine, forearms or wrists, and femurs (the site for most hip fractures). Fractures affect roughly 6.8 million Americans each year, with a higher prevalence in men below age 45 and women above age 45. Fractures commonly occur in the extremities. The most common fracture to the upper extremity is a distal radius fracture or Colles fracture. The most common fracture to the lower extremity is the hip fracture, resulting in roughly 300,000 cases per year in the United States (orthopedics.about.com).

Hip and knee replacements are the most common joint replacement surgeries performed, frequently resulting from degenerative diseases (i.e, degenerative joint disease, arthritis, and osteoporosis.) Joint replacements performed in the upper extremities are most commonly performed at the wrist (the proximal row more than the distal row), and at individual metacarpals (MCPs) and individual phalanges (PIPs), usually as a result of rheumatoid arthritis. The shoulder (i.e., the glenohumeral joint) and the elbow (i.e., the humeral-ulnar joint) also can be replaced but are less frequent than the wrist and phalanges. Although joint replacements in the shoulder and elbow can result from degenerative conditions, a history of trauma (i.e., a fall on the outstretched extremity) is usually involved. Joint replacements are not permanent, usually lasting 10 to 15 years.

This chapter will focus on orthopedic conditions as they affect the hip, knee, wrist and hand, elbow, and shoulder, and related occupational therapy interventions.

Common Characteristics and Symptoms

Fractures

Fractures are classified as diaphyseal (a fracture in the mid-portion of the bone), metaphyseal (a fracture within close proximity to the flare of the bone at the articular joint surface), and articular (a fracture within the joint surface at the end of the bone).

Fractures are also classified by the involved joint, the angle of fracture, the number of fragments produced in the bone and whether they are closed or open. Fracture angles are described as transverse, oblique, longitudinal, or stellate (star-like). Simple fractures result in two major components, and comminuted fractures produce multiple fragments. Fractures that are contained within the bone or joint are considered closed, and those that protrude through the soft-tissues and skin are considered open (Rockwood, 1984; Hunter, Mackin, & Callahan, 1995).

Closed fractures are those fractures that are relatively stable and only require an orthosis (i.e., a splint or cast) to maintain good, anatomic positioning of the joint to allow natural healing to occur. Fractures can also be repaired utilizing many different surgical means. Common internal fixation includes Kirschner wires (i.e., K-wires), circlage wires, tension band wires, screws (lag and pressure), intrarmedullary rods and nails, and plate and screw combinations (Kauer, 1980). However, some complex fractures with multiple fracture sites and unstable fixation may require external fixation as well. External fixators (most commonly intermedullay pins) provide a stable force to oppose strong muscle compressive forces across the injured joint and allow healing to occur by pulling on ligamentous attachment points (known as ligamentotaxis) and maintaining good anatomic joint position for healing (Rockwood, 1984).

Healing of fractured bones typically takes four to six weeks. Healing time can be protracted by complications such as diabetes, poor nutrition, more compound injuries, and vascular insufficiency (Cyriax, 1982).

Weight-bearing activity contributes to the healing process and helps the bone re-model through callous formation. Patients are assigned weight bearing status based on the mechanism of injury and surgical repair. The healthcare professional promotes strict patient compliance to the weight bearing status during mobilization. Continued communication between the patient, therapist, and physician regarding the progress of the healing process, compliance with weight bearing restrictions, and effective pain management facilitates patient independence in ADLs, and helps to reduce the length of hospital stay.

The Wrist and Hand

The Colles fracture is one of the most common fractures of the upper extremity. It is defined as a fracture involving the distal radius with dorsal displacement. This fracture disrupts the delicate degree of normal palmer tilt between the radius and the carpal bones: the scaphoid and lunate proximally and the capitate distally (Kauer, 1980). If left untreated, the mobility and dexterity of the hand may be lost as a result of immobility of the wrist joint. Depending on the type and degree of injury involved, the Colles fracture may be immobilized in a cast and/or external fixation anywhere from three to six weeks. The physician will determine the period of immobilization in a cast, splint, and/or external fixation. It is the responsibility of the occupational therapist to limit the potential for secondary complications, such as stiffness in the affected shoulder, elbow and forearm and digits, edema, and loss of active range of motion (AROM; Hunter, Mackin, & Callahan, 1995).

The Elbow

Orthopedic injuries that affect the elbow disrupt the fine motor coordination and dexterity of the hand in space as well as limit the flexibility and reach of the shoulder girdle. The elbow provides a solid weight bearing structure for the entire upper torso while providing the flexion, extension, and supination patterns that allow for discreet finger, hand, and wrist movements (Smith, Weiss, & Lehmkuhl, 1996). At the elbow, ligamentous flexibility coupled with bony stability allows the mobile radial head to rotate upon the fixed and rigid ulna. Without this efficient and unique design, most simple ADLs (especially feeding, grooming, and bathing activities) become almost impossible to perform (London, 1981).

Fractures to the olecranon and radial head are the most common sites of injury to the elbow. These conditions require management to maintain AROM and passive ROM (PROM) within the joint. Usually, the radial head will incur the majority of damage in a fracture involving the elbow.

A non-displaced fracture (Mason Type I) will usually require no immobilization, and quick return to mobilization is encouraged. In moderate fractures (Mason's Type II and III), an open reduction internal fixation (ORIF) operation is performed and protective motion is initiated as soon as possible. In all three of these fracture types, the goal is to maintain PROM and begin gentle AROM for flexion and extension motions only. By the third week, supination and pronation motions are initiated and focus is given to regain this motion.

The Shoulder

Orthopedic injuries that affect the shoulder girdle ultimately impact the function of the hand. The shoulder girdle (i.e., the clavicle, scapula, humerus, and thoracic spine and sternum) is multifunctional. The interplay of the humerus and scapula, commonly referred to as the scapulo-humeral rhythm, provides for increased range of motion in a number of different planes. This relationship is based upon an interplay comprised of muscular and ligamentous structures effectively suspending the humeral head within the glenoid fossa (Maitland, 1977).

In acute care, the occupational therapist may encounter the lack of AROM of the shoulder above 100 degrees of flexion, and lack of external rotation greater than 30 degrees. Simple explanations for this loss of motion, especially in the elderly population, can be attributed to a kyphotic position of the thoracic spine as well as common arthritic changes in the acromio-clavicular joint itself impacting the available ROM around the shoulder (France, 1991).

Hip Fractures

Hip fractures are common diagnoses treated in an acute care hospital setting. The prevalence is high in women: approximately 25% of women above age 65 experience hip fractures; 50% of whom return to independent ambulation (Melton, 1993). Most hip fractures are related to osteoporosis and result in 60,000 or more admissions to nursing homes annually (Melton, 1999). Three common surgical interventions an occupational therapist will encounter are total hip arthroplasty/replacement (THA/THR), open reduction and internal fixation (ORIF), and hemiarthroplasty (McGann, 1991).

Femoral Fractures

The primary site of hip fractures is at the femoral neck and intertrochantric region of the femur. If no displacement is noted in the fracture site, the physician will opt for ORIF or hip pinning (i.e., insertion of metal screws to stabilize the fracture). If the damage results in disunion of the bone in the femoral neck area, the physician may opt to perform a hemiarthroplasty or replacement of one part of the hip joint. If the damage is related to degenerative disease affecting the acetabulum as well as the femoral head and neck, then the physician may opt to replace the entire joint surface through a total hip replacement (Melton, 1995).

Total Hip Replacements

When other forms of intervention to decrease pain and improve mobility have failed, total joint replacement surgery is considered. There are three types of procedures: the anterolateral approach, the posterolateral approach, and the transtrochanteric approach. The age and health of the patient are considered in deciding on the surgical procedure (Pedretti & Early, 2001).

Target Areas for Intervention

Occupational therapy goals following fracture and joint replacement surgery include: (1) reduction of pain and edema in the affected joint after surgery, (2) maintenance of early active and passive range of motion (ROM) of the joint after surgery, (3) restoration of functional activities of daily living (ADL) skills independence, and (4) the return to pre-morbid occupational life roles.

Contextual Considerations

Clinical

The occupational therapist will usually encounter the patient one to three days postoperatively and will find the patient in a hospital gown, immobile, and in mild to moderate discomfort. The occupational therapist will complete a screening assessment to determine the need for adaptive devices and techniques, and degree of services that will be required at discharge to facilitate the person's resumption of life roles.

The early post-operative contact facilitates functional recovery and is cost effective. The initial evaluation is a brief summary of the patient's medical history, social history, presentation, sensory and perceptual assessment, cognitive evaluation, neurological, and muscular assessment. The evaluation should include ROM and manual muscle testing, functional assessment including performance in self-care and mobility, a problem list, a summary assessment of the findings, estimated length of stay, equipment needs, long-term goals and short-term objectives (made in collaboration with the patient), and discharge recommendations.

Information gathering is a team effort. The physiatrist or physician often makes first contact and assesses the rehabilitative prognosis for the patient including orthopedic and medical ongoing treatments, weight-bearing and ROM limitations, and the patient's pain and activity tolerance. Once the readiness for physical and occupational therapy is determined, the physiatrist's orders are placed and physical and occupational therapy is initiated. Alternatively, the orthopedic service may alert the rehabilitation service of pending or completed surgical procedures which require services. Information needs to be gathered on the social and physical environments to which the patient will return.

Family

Family involvement of persons with orthopedic diagnoses is critical to patients who may be discharged at a supervision or assistance level. Regular contact with family, including formal family training, can secure a safe discharge for the patient into his or her environment.

Practice Setting

The initial occupational therapy consult or referral for orthopedic diagnosis is most commonly encountered in the acute care hospital setting. The OT initiates and plans a continuum of care, initiates ROM as permitted by the surgeon, introduces and initiates self-care and functional transfers, and determines the follow-up need for inpatient rehabilitation, or a discharge to home with the necessary equipment and therapies. Areas that are addressed in the evaluation in acute care include ADLs, ROM, strength, functional mobility, skin integrity, cognitive perceptual skills, and the need for orthotics. In the acute care setting, the occupational therapist often works closely with the physical therapist to initiate bed mobility and transfers. In acute care, the time is limited and self-care training may include the introduction of assistive devices and their use.

The rehabilitation setting is typically the next step in the continuum of care from acute care for many patients with orthopedic problems. Typically, the therapist is given an hour and a half daily to work with the patient to return him or her to functional independence. In this high intensity setting, the focus of occupational therapy is to expand on the skills initiated in the acute care setting. Daily participation in self-care, bathing, grooming, upper extremity dressing, lower extremity dressing, and hygiene become routine for the patient until short-term and long-term goals are achieved. Transfer training expands to bathroom and kitchen mobility with an assistive device. Therapeutic exercise expands into light meal preparation and participation in home management tasks. Simple cognitive and perceptual activities expand into instrumental activities of daily living including money management, shopping, driving, etc. The occupational therapist, through ongoing re-evaluation and assessment of progress, will determine the possibility of the patient achieving functional independence and/or the necessity of family or caretaker involvement.

Sociopolitical

The primary sociopolitical issue facing persons with orthopedic injuries involves payment for services. Older persons who require hospitalization after a fall or fracture will typically have inpatient, outpatient, and home care costs covered by Medicare. Commercial insurance and workers' compensation may also cover hospitalization and related costs. The failure of both Medicare and commercial insurance to cover the cost of durable medical equipment and assistive devices for self-care may create a hardship for the patient who requires them to support ADL or instrumental ADL (IADL) during the healing process.

Lifespan/Lifestyle

The recovery from orthopedic injuries is, for most patients, a short-term process. With proper medical and therapeutic intervention, major changes to life style are not required.

Clinical Decision Making Process

Defining Focus for Intervention

The treatment focus for orthopedic patients is to improve ROM and strength, increase pain tolerance, activity tolerance, improve performance in activities of daily living, and return the patient to a normal routine with the aide of durable medical equipment, assistive devices, education in energy conservation, and adaptation of the home environment to facilitate functional independence.

The focus of treatment is related specifically to the injury or body part. Examination of the treatment approaches for Colles fracture, stiff shoulder, and total hip replacement will serve as examples for how the focus of treatment changes as the healing process progresses.

Colles Fracture

Early in treatment, the person with a Colles fracture should learn to "salute the ceiling." In order to reduce edema, lifting the affected extremity over the head and maintaining the arm on an elevated plane above the level of the heart will allow for good venous return and support the lymphatic system during the inflammatory phase of healing. Active motion is optimal, with movement at each joint (shoulder, elbow, forearm and digits) at least twice every waking hour. If the patient has difficulty moving any of the joints, the therapist should take each joint gently through its available ROM to prevent joint stiffness and aid in edema reduction. Elevation with a pillow or foam wedge is ideal for maintaining position above or at least level with the heart. Use of a sling to support the affected extremity is almost always contraindicated since it tends to foster the immobility of the extremity and can increase stiffness of the entire extremity. If the extremity is in a cast, care should be taken that the thumb motion is not restricted. Maximally, the cast should only reach the distal palmer crease, and should allow for full MCP extension and at least pinch to the third digit.

Tendon gliding exercises (TGE) are also important. TGEs allow for full excursion of the long digital flexor and extensor tendons, and prevent ligamentous shortening during the wrist immobilization phase. Additionally, these exercises help to stimulate circulation and reduce edema in the digits. Persistent digital edema can be reduced with the use of coban wrapping and retrograde massage. The coban is wrapped in a figure-8 style, beginning at the distal end of the digit and proceeding down to the level of the cast. The coban can be left in place for up to 24 hours but should be changed daily for hygiene and skin checks. Retrograde massage is performed by milking the digit, beginning at the distal end and moving back to the MCPs proximally. The use of lotion will aid in the movement over the digits as well as provide some lubrication to the skin.

Once the cast and/or external fixation are removed, therapy becomes more intense. The therapist's goal during this phase is to mobilize the wrist joint. The fabrication of a thermoplastic splint is utilized during this phase to support the weakened wrist extensors and provide stability to the digits as well. The splint can be made with either a dorsal or volar design with a bar that supports the distal palmer crease. It is imperative that the splint allows for full digital flexion and extension of the joints, as well as full mobility of the thumb with opposition available to the 5th digit. Out of the splint, the patient is guided through gentle active assistive ROM (AAROM) and PROM for wrist flexion and extension, as well as radial and ulnar deviation. It is also important to work on full supination. It is likely to initially be limited due to the pronation positioning in the cast. Initial movement will be very weak at first, so movement begins gently in gravity-eliminated planes to assist with good muscle recruitment throughout the wrist joint. The wrist joint will be stiff, so moist heat is often applied prior to mobilization. Gentle joint mobilization is also utilized, especially at the radiocarpal and midcarpal joints, to further enhance the motion.

From an occupational therapy perspective, utilization of light bimanual activities can be most rewarding to the patient and allow for increased mobility throughout the wrist joint. Weaving, knitting, kneading light dough or putty, buttoning, wringing out a rag, or threading nuts and bolts are just a few examples of exercises that require a variable amount of wrist and digital mobility that can be employed as part of a therapy regime at this stage of recovery. Another hallmark exercise is the "prayer position," which puts maximal stretch on the wrist and digital flexors and extensors and provides the patient with a simple reference guide for increasing joint mobility and AROM.

In the later phase (roughly by week 10), the most crucial motion that needs to be relearned is independent wrist extension. Due to the weakness of the wrist extensors (i.e., the extensor carpus radialis brevis [ECRB], the extensor carpus radialis longus [ECRL], and the extensor carpi ulnaris [ECU]), active wrist range of motion can be compensated utilizing the long axis of the digital extensors. (These are the extensor digiti communis [EDC] and to a lesser extent extensor indicis [EI] and extensor digiti minimi [EDM]). A fully closed, tightly packed fist during wrist extension eliminates the force arm of the digital wrist extensors and puts the load of wrist extension primarily on the extensor carpi radialis brevis, which gets assistance from the extensor carpus radialis longus (ECRL) and extensor carpi ulnaris (ECU). With the loss of independent wrist extension, the power grip and pinch of the hand is affected, as well as the power of the wrist joint itself. Without independent wrist stability, the mobility of the hand is significantly limited. As the stability of the wrist increases, the splint can be discontinued in favor of increasing the overall stability of the wrist joint. However, for individuals who will perform heavy and repetitive duty activities, the splint can provide increased stability until the muscular endurance around the joint is regained.

Stiff Shoulder

Conservative management of the stiff shoulder that is acute in origin, and has medically ruled out any other pathology, usually begins with a therapeutic modality such as moist heat. Placing the individual's shoulder in a lengthened position in which the joint is comfortable is usually optimal. Once the soft tissues have been heated, a gentle stretch can be applied. Placing the individual in a supine position allows the shoulder joint to become relaxed and helps to facilitate relaxation of the muscles, which, in turn, allows the therapist greater control of the joint. Gentle distractive forces can be applied to loosen the connection of the humeral head within the gleniod fossa. Additionally, gentle distractive and externally derived forces can be applied to unwind the humeral head within the gleniod. Usually, this external rotation force will be the most upsetting to the patient and care must be taken to allow the patient to relax and not recruit muscular forces to block PROM. Gently, passively guiding the joint through its available ROM and applying a gentle sustained stretch at the available end ROM will help to slowly increase shoulder joint mobility.

Utilization of overhead pulleys can further help to mobilize the shoulder by allowing the individual to aid his or her own muscular system to incrementally guide the shoulder through AAROM. This system also provides the individual with increased control over his or her mobility and allows participation in therapy at his or her own schedule. Additionally beneficial exercises are Codman or pendulum exercises that again provide stretch to the shoulder joint and allow for slow, gentle motion. Graded exercise should begin in supine to take further pressure off the joint, allow for gravity-minimized motion, and provide stability to the scapula throughout its ROM. Also, utilization of a dowel provides a visual and physiological feedback mechanism for comparison to the other shoulder for motion, and allows the unaffected upper extremity to assist the weaker shoulder through its ROM. Exercise should be provided not only for the shoulder itself but also for the scapula and upper back extensors to provide a stable base for shoulder mobilization.

Total Hip Replacement

The occupational therapist may begin treatment for a person with a total hip replacement on the first, second, and third day postoperatively. The physical therapist, often first on the case, may perform the initial bed mobility and transfer out of bed assessments, per the physician's orders. The occupational therapist frequently arrives at the bedside to find the patient in a hip chair (an elevated chair that promotes ease of transfers), in a hospital gown, often orthostatic, in mild to moderate discomfort, and possibly requesting to return to bed. The purpose of the therapist's visit and the frequency and the role of occupational therapy in the acute setting are explained to the patient. Vitals signs are taken and compared to the parameters set by physicians (usually, systolic blood pressure anywhere from 90 to 150 or 180, and diastolic blood pressure from 60 to 90; oxygen saturation between 92% and 100%; and pulse rate between 60bpm to 100bpm). Pain is assessed using the 0 to 10 pain scale.

Establishing Goals for Intervention

Physical limitations including ROM, strength, endurance, activity tolerance, balance, coordination, sensation, and overall ADL skill performance need to be addressed. Appropriate goals are set considering the patient's physical, social, and environmental factors.

When considering goal setting and treatment focus, the occupational therapist focuses on discharge planning. The question one should ask is: Where is this person going when he or she leaves the acute care environment? The options, although many, can include an acute rehabilitation setting where the person extends his or her hospital stay with emphasis on physical rehabilitation; a skilled nursing facility in which the person is transferred to a rehabilitative center where moderate intensity therapies are given; a nursing home in which the patient is given low intensity but daily physical and occupational therapies; a boarding home with few physical or occupational therapies; an independent living or assisted living center where therapies on a low intensity basis may be provided; and/or simply home with home therapies.

The next question to be addressed is: Who is at home with the patient? If the patient lives alone, it may be imperative that the patient be independent in ambulation and self-care upon discharge. Even though a person living alone may have neighbors, grown children, or grandchildren who can provide intermittent supervision, the patient must be independent and safe.

The person's spouse may be capable of providing assistance as needed, in which case the patient's goals can be independence with supervision. If the person lives with an elderly or disabled spouse with limited ability to help, the goals of the patient will reflect independence, or discharge planning will include continued home therapies and home-health services. In other cases, placement in a long-term care facility with physical and occupational therapies may be the option.

Another question is whether the patient's living space is conducive to the patient's recovery. Beyond the issue of supervision, is the patient safe? Falls resulting in orthopedic impairments are generally accidental in nature, such as tripping over an unsecured throw-rug, or slipping on an icy pavement. However, abuse and negligence (malnutrition, under-nutrition, history of previous burns, or multiple falls where no known neurological impairments exist) are also factors to be considered. Health professionals are required by law to report any and all cases of suspected abuse to authorities.

The next question is: Does the patient plan to return to his or her prior living space? The patient's family members may offer temporary or permanent living quarters until the patient is ready to return to their home. A person may have to consider moving to another location more conducive to his or her current situation.

Designing Theory-Based Intervention

The biomechanical and rehabilitation frames of reference are extremely useful for orthopedic patients in a hospital, rehabilitation, outpatient, or home-care setting.

The biomechanical frame of reference assumes that activity is used for the treatment of loss of ROM, strength, and endurance due to accident, injury, or surgery. As ROM, strength, and endurance improve, function is regained. Stress and rest need to be appropriately incorporated. This frame of reference is best suited for individuals who are cognitively intact. The biomechanical approach emphasizes structural stability, edema control, ROM, strength, and low-level and high-level endurance.

The rehabilitative frame of reference focuses on having the patient compensate for underlying deficits that cannot be remediated. The underlying assumptions for this frame of reference are: independence will be achieved through compensation, the person is motivated to be independent, the environmental context, the emotional and cognitive skills needed for independence are present, and adaptations and compensations are designed for the person to function in the discharge environment. The goal of rehabilitation is participation in activities of daily living, work, and leisure tasks in spite of physical limitations. Some of the tools used in rehabilitation are (1) adaptive equipment including adaptive devices and assistive technology, (2) upper extremity orthotics, (3) wheelchair modification, (4) ambulatory devices, (5) adaptive procedures, (6) environmental modification, and (7) safety education.

Evaluating Progress

As long as the patient continues to progress, occupational therapy intervention is warranted. Progress is continually evaluated via daily progress notes, weekly conferences if the patient is in a rehabilitation or a sub-acute nursing facility (SNF) setting, and monthly re-evaluations if the patient is in an outpatient or homecare environment. Goals are patient-centered, so that upon culmination of occupational therapy intervention, the patient has achieved functional independence and returns to former occupational roles.

Determining Change in or Termination of Treatment

Ultimately, change or termination of treatment is attained when the individual has achieved all of the goals, or when the patient has reached maximal therapeutic benefit. Usually, a team familiar with the case will meet with the individual and his or her family to recommend the best place to serve this person, and recommend equipment as needed.

Case Study

Upper Extremity Injury

KO is a 56-year-old female who suffered a fall on the ice while returning from lunch to a local bank where she works as a teller. She is married with three grown children. She is expecting her first grandchild in six months. She fell onto her right upper extremity and landed on her outstretched arm. She remembers hearing and audible "crack," and feeling intense pain in the dorsal and volar aspect of her wrist. She returned to the bank and immediately iced her wrist and finished her shift. The next day when she awoke her hand and wrist were severely swollen. Her husband took her to the emergency room. Her x-rays showed a distal radius fracture with an avulsion of the radial styloid. She was immediately taken to surgery. Her fracture was reduced, an external fixation system was applied, and her hand casted in plaster.

Following surgery, KO was sent to a bed in an acute care setting and occupational therapy received an order to evaluate and treat her for distal radius fracture, with stable fixation, digital mobilization, ROM exercises, and edema management. The acute care therapist assessed KO, instructed her in edema management, proper pin care and cast management, and issued a home program for KO to complete that included ROM exercises and tendon gliding exercises. KO was discharged to home.

KO's fracture has healed and her cast and pins have been removed. She is now being seen for more intense therapy in an outpatient setting. Her wrist, as expected, is stiff. She has been fitted with a volar wrist splint that immobilizes the wrist and supports the distal palmer crease. KO is spending more and more time in therapy without the splint. She moves her wrist in all positions. In addition, she is encouraged to supinate. Although her muscles and movement are weak, it is important for KO to move actively and recruit muscles throughout the areas of the wrist. Continuous movement and participation in activities that require graded increases in strength will assist her in achieving an optimum recovery.

Long- and Short-Term Goals

In the long-term, KO will demonstrate AROM, strength, coordination, and endurance in the right wrist and hand sufficient to support full independence in ADLs and IADLs.

In the short-term, KO will demonstrate AROM, strength, coordination, and endurance in the right wrist and hand sufficient to engage in a light bi-manual activity for three minutes.

Therapist Goals and Strategies

The therapist's goals include:

1. Reduce joint stiffness.
2. Increase ROM.
3. Increase muscle strength.
4. Improve coordination.
5. Increase endurance.

The therapist's strategies include:

1. Provide heat modality prior to activity.
2. Provide gentle joint mobilization prior to activity.
3. Provide a series of graded activities that facilitate range of motion, muscle strength, coordination and endurance.

Activity

Knitting a Small Baby Blanket

At this point in her recovery, KO will benefit from an activity that is bimanual and offers light resistance, requires movement throughout the wrist joint, and emphasizes wrist extension. Knitting is such an activity. It is easy to learn, it will offer light resistance, and it requires her to move her right wrist and fingers repetitively. Wrist flexion and extension are emphasized. KO can work on the project at home, and the baby blanket will allow her to focus her recovery on the impending happy occasion of the birth of her grandchild.

Treatment Objectives

The patient will demonstrate the AROM, strength, coordination, and endurance in the right hand and wrist to cast on fifty stitches and complete two rows of a knitting project.

Resources

The management of acute orthopedic injury is guided by treatment protocol. Since these are facility and physician specific, patients are encouraged to consult with their physician and treatment team for recommendations.

References

Cyriax, J. (1982). *Textbook of orthopedic medicine, volume I: Diagnosis of soft tissue lesions.* London: Bailliere Tindall.

France, M. (1991). Anatomy and biomechanics of the shoulder. In R. Donatelli (Ed.), *Physical Therapy of the Shoulder* (pp. 42–73). Edinburgh, Scotland: Churchill Livingstone.

Hunter, J., Mackin, E., & Callahan, A. (1995). *Rehabilitation of the hand: Surgery and therapy* (4th ed.). St. Louis, MO: Mosby.

Kauer, J. (1980). Functional anatomy of the wrist. *Clinical Orthopedics and Related Research, 149*(9), 92–106.

London, J. (1981). Kinematics of the elbow. *Journal of Bone and Joint Surgery, 63,* 529.

Maitland, G. (1977). *Peripheral manipulation.* London: Butterworth.

McGann, W. (1991). History and physical examination. In M. Steinberg (Ed.), *The hip and its disorders.* Philadelphia: Saunders.

Melton, L. (1993). Hip fractures: A worldwide problem today and tomorrow. *Bone, 14* (Suppl. 1), 1–8.

Melton, L. (1995). How many women have osteoporosis now? *Journal of Bone Mineral Research, 10,* 175–177.

Melton, L. (1999). Fracture incidence in Olmstead County, Minnesota: Comparison of urban and rural rates and changes in urban rates over time. *Osteoporosis International, 9,* 29–37.

Pedretti, L. & Early, M. (2001). *Occupational Therapy: Practice Skills for Physical Dysfunction,* (5th ed.). St Louis, MO: Mosby.

Rockwood, C. (1984). Subluxations and dislocations of the shoulder. In C. Rockwood & D. Green (Eds.), *Fractures in adults* (pp. 21–42). Philadelphia: Lippincott.

Smith, L., Weiss, E., & Lehmkuhl (1996). *Brunstrom's clinical kinesiology* (5th ed.). Philadelphia: FA Davis.

Burns

15

Josette Merkel, MBA, OTR/L
Jonathan Niszczak, MS, OTR/L

Synopsis of Clinical Condition

Prevalence and Etiology

In the United States, 1.4 to 2 million people are burned each year, and 75,000 of the victims require a hospitalization of at least two days. Of these hospitalized people, 85% have injuries to the hand or upper extremity. Approximately 5,000 deaths result from a burn injury or complications. The most common ages of injury are between 16 and 40. Burns are the primary cause of accidental death for children between the ages of 1 and 14, and the second most common cause of accidental death in the elderly. Burns are the second most common form of child abuse. Men have the highest incidence of being burned (Staley & Richard, 2001).

Burn injuries are classified into three major types: thermal, chemical, and electrical. Thermal injuries may include flame, scald, and contact. There are innumerable causes of injury, such as motor vehicle accidents, house fires, work-related accidents, or kitchen accidents. Children are often burned as a result of scalding (frequently, by the child pulling down a cup or pot full of hot water or beverage, or being put in a tub of hot water), playing with matches, and contact with a hot surface such as an iron.

Common Characteristics and Symptoms

The four major classifications of burn injury include:

- First degree (superficial) is usually characterized by red, dry, and edematous skin that is painful to touch and involves only the epidermal layer of the skin. It usually heals in three to five days, with possible slight discoloration and peeling but no scarring. The most common cause of first degree burn is sunburn.
- Second degree burns are divided into two categories: superficial partial thickness and deep partial thickness. Superficial partial thickness burns are characterized by red, blistering, weeping, and moist edematous skin that is very painful and sensitive to temperature. This burn involves the epidermis and some papillary dermis. It should heal in seven to 21 days without skin grafting. Minimal scarring and pigment change results. Deep partial thickness burns are pink, cherry red, or in the most severe cases, mottled white. There may also be small or large thick-walled blisters. This burn involves the entire epidermis, multiple layers of the dermis, and possibly the subcutaneous fat layer. It may heal in 21 to 35 days without skin grafting, however, significant pigment changes and scar contractures will develop.

- Third degree (full thickness) burned skin is dry, leathery, and non-pliable. No blisters appear, but the skin does have a mixed white or waxy white appearance. There is typically little to no pain. This burn involves the epidermis, the majority of the dermal and fat layers, and possibly the underlying fascial and muscular layers. This burn requires grafting, however small burns (<2% of the total body surface area) may heal without grafting after several months.
- Fourth degree (dermal injury) burned skin is white to dark charred in color and dry. It appears mummified and is anesthetic. This injury involves epidermis, dermis, fat, and commonly is associated with exposed bone and tendon. If the burned skin is not grafted, it will not heal. Amputations are often required, and in the absence of surgical wound closure, death may result.

There will often be a combination of burn classifications in the same person. For example, a person involved in a house fire may suffer first and second degree burns to his or her face and third degree burns to his or her hands as a result of crawling out to escape the burning house. The physician will estimate the total body surface area (TBSA) burned. The most commonly used methods are the Lund and Browder method and Berkow's percentages chart (Lund & Browder, 1955). First degree burns are not included in the estimation. An estimate of the total burned body surface area allows the physician to determine the resuscitation calculation and the severity of the injury. Generally, the higher the burn area percentage, the more critical the injury and more involved the rehabilitation will be. Specifically, burns of TBSA of 20% or greater in adults, 10% in children and older adults, and 5% or greater full thickness burn require hospitalization. Other people requiring hospital admission are those with chemical and electrical burns and suspected inhalation injury (Staley & Richard, 2001).

In addition to the obvious injury to the skin, the respiratory system can be injured as a result of inhaling toxic substances. This injury is referred to as a smoke inhalation injury. A severe inhalation injury alone or combined with a skin injury can indicate a poor morbidity and mortality prognosis. Mortality rates with inhalation injury are reported to be greater than 50%, with little change over the last 30 years. The incidence of inhalation injury is reported to be found in 3% to 21% of burn patients. The pulmonary injury is usually proportional to the depth and size of the cutaneous burn, (i.e., those with severe burn injuries commonly have an inhalation injury). As a result of severe inhalation injury, patients may need to be on mechanical ventilation and/or supplemental oxygen for a long period of time.

Target Areas for Intervention

Occupational therapy should begin as soon as the patient is medically stable. The occupational therapist focuses on maintaining range of motion (ROM), positioning, edema control and reduction, splinting, education, scar prevention and management, activity of daily living (ADL) adaptation and remediation, and return to occupation.

Contextual Considerations

Clinical

The clinical evaluation must incorporate information about the depth of the burn injury, the psychological status, and level of ADL independence. Data must be gathered regarding nature of the injury, any co-morbidity, and the leisure and occupational roles of the client. A thorough evaluation must be performed that assesses the patient's active and passive ROM, strength, sensation, coordination, ADL status, and functional mobility. Any joint involved in a burn should be measured and reassessed for changes on a daily basis.

Strength testing is particularly important to perform after an electrical injury. An electrical injury manifests in progressive weakness of effected muscles in the first days and weeks after the injury. Sensory testing helps to determine the classification of the burn injury and ascertain the level of risk for further injury due to diminished sensation. Self-care frequently begins with tasks at the bedside, including feeding and grooming tasks, toileting, and hygiene. Assessment regarding how the patient transfers and ambulates is also needed.

The *Functional Independence Measure*™ (Uniform Data Systems for Medical Rehabilitation, 1993) can provide information on many of these areas. Another widely used assessment for burns is the *Vancouver Scar Scale* (Baryza & Baryza, 1995). This instrument objectively assesses scar maturation across four distinct variables and provides a basis for the patient and therapist to chart progress. Pain is an inevitable consequence of burn injury and can be assessed in many formats. Most commonly used formats are the FLACC scale (Markel, 1997) and the Wong-Baker scale (Wong et. al., 1999). The FLACC scale can be used on unresponsive adults and children. The Wong-Baker scale may be used with children and with persons who speak a foreign language. Edema is measured with a tape measure over common joint areas and bony prominences (e.g., the wrist crease at the level of the styloids or at the level of the proximal interphalangeal [PIP] joint in the finger).

Family

Family support and encouragement is a critical component throughout the recovery process. Many patients require constant encouragement and persuasion to participate in the program. This is most critical when pain limits movement. Family members need to be encouraged and educated in the burn recovery process. It is important for them to understand that movement must ensue before healing has occurred. Family education in positioning, wound healing, scar management, home exercises, and participation in ADLs and instrumental ADLs (IADLs) is important. Family members may require emotional and psychological support to help the patient through episodes of depression, withdrawal secondary to disfigurement, and/or anxiety related to returning to school or work.

Practice Setting

Individuals are usually treated at a formalized burn center in a trauma hospital. Once the critical and surgical phase of recovery is complete, the patient can be transferred to an inpatient rehabilitation setting for further recovery and rehabilitation, if warranted.

Outpatient therapy can be performed at various settings including a hospital, hand center, and/or work hardening center.

Sociopolitical

Patients who are recovering from a severe burn injury will require services from an acute care hospital, rehabilitation inpatient services, and/or outpatient programming. Commercial insurance will be relied upon to cover acute care, rehabilitation, and outpatient services. For patients who sustain a work-related burn, workers compensation will provide funds for rehabilitation and the return to work. Patients who return to work will be covered under the Americans with Disabilities Act (ADA), which will provide a mechanism for reasonable workplace accommodations.

Lifestyle/Lifespan

Although most burn survivors can expect to return to roles and a level of independence close to premorbid levels, the process of complete recovery may be long and difficult. The acute care experience for inpatients is often fraught with fear of mortality, dependency, pain, stress, anxiety, and isolation. Further into the recovery process, the patient may experience depression, plus fear of and withdrawal from social situations, work, or school because of disfigurement and the need to wear pressure garments or splints. Patients will face a long process of rehabilitation, requiring compliance with a program of exercise, pressure garment use, and scar management until the burns are completely healed. Patients may experience prolonged periods of unemployment during recovery, and some may require a change in occupation and lifestyle.

Clinical Decision Making Process

Defining Focus for Intervention

The focus of occupational therapy depends on the location of the burn, the severity or depth of the burn, the TBSA, associated injuries (i.e., fractured leg as a result of jumping out a window), age, presence of an inhalation injury, past medical history, and occupation prior to admission. The therapist must also consider at which phase the patient is in the recovery process. The two phases in the recovery process are the acute phase and the rehabilitative phase. In the acute phase, from day 0 to approximately day 21, the critical factors that the therapist must address are edema management, positioning and splints, mobilization, maintaining active and passive ROM, patient education, self-care skill and adaptation, and skin and scar management.

In the rehabilitative phase, from approximately day 22 until full recovery (which may take six months to several years), the critical factors that the therapist must address are the same areas as in the acute phase, plus cardiovascular and strength training, psychosocial adaptation, and return to participation in life roles.

Psychosocial adaptation is a constant focus for occupational therapy in the acute and rehabilitative phases, and poses a lifelong challenge for the patient. Burn injuries create potential for pain, disfigurement, and the loss of independence. The challenge of therapy is to provide activity that fosters physical as well as psychosocial well being.

Establishing Goals for Intervention

The goals for intervention can be classified according to the phases or stages of recovery. In the acute phase, avoidance of deepening the burn injury and destroying the surrounding tissue is paramount. This translates into a treatment plan which will focus on reducing edema, preventing further loss of strength and endurance, preventing loss of mobility in the skin and joints, promoting independence in self-care, and providing education to the patient and family.

During the rehabilitative phase of recovery, the focus for occupational therapy intervention shifts toward providing patient and family education, promoting independence in self-care, controlling edema; scar management; teaching compensation techniques; fitting splints and pressure garments; restoring muscle strength, endurance and hand function, and restoring activity tolerance.

The development of discharge plans that facilitate the return to school or work forms the final phase of the rehabilitation process.

Designing Theory-Based Intervention

Successful long-term rehabilitation requires the combined application of the biomechanical and rehabilitation frames of reference. The biomechanical approach is used to address remedial issues such as edema control, scar management, strengthening and improvement of ROM, and hand and upper extremity function.

Several strategies address edema control; one of the most common is elevation of the extremities with pillows, bedside tables, or IV poles. Hand edema responds well to the muscle pumping of active ROM exercises and retrograde massage, Coban™, and Isotoner™ gloves. Patients should be encouraged to use and move their hands actively as much as possible through simple self-care tasks. Upper extremity and lower extremity edema may respond well to gradient pressure material such as Tubigrip™. In the rehabilitation frame of reference, issues of patient and family education and the use of adaptive equipment and strategies are the focus of intervention.

Upon admission, the patient needs to be positioned to minimize the potential for deformity and contracture. The ideal position is to stretch the burned skin. For example, if the burn is on the anterior surface of the elbow, the person should be positioned in elbow extension. If the burn is in the axilla, the person should alternate the positions of shoulder abduction and flexion to a least ninety degrees. If the patient is actively moving and performing self-care ADLs, this activity should be encouraged. But the person should resume positions of stretch during rest periods. A primary role of the occupational therapist is the fabrication of splints. Splints are used to prevent deformity, lengthen soft tissues, promote graft take, and prevent graft loss. A burn that will require grafting and crosses a joint surface must be splinted. The recommended position for upper and lower extremities is shoulder abduction 90 degrees to 100 degrees; elbow extension, neutral forearm, and wrist extension to 30 degrees; thumb abduction and extension, MP (metacarpal phalangeal) flexion 50 degrees to 70 degrees; and IP (interphalangeal) extension.

Splints are used to immobilize joints for the first three days post-graft. After the graft is stable, splints can continue to be used to stretch the healed skin and increase the motion in the joint and extremity.

In order to maximize pulmonary function and prevent weakness, the burn patient should begin to move around as soon as possible. Mobilization, depending on the patient's condition, may mean bed mobility, sitting upright in bed, sitting out of bed in a chair, or ambulating short or long distances. For a more involved patient, the therapist (in progressing the patient to get out of bed or at least move from supine) will need to consider many factors. The patient's medical status is imperative. Critical attention must be given to heart rate, oxygen saturation, respiration, and blood pressure initially and in response to position changes and movement. The patient may need to start slowly by having the head of the bed elevated to 30 degrees and progressed to 90 degrees. Mechanically ventilated patients may be medically stable enough to sit up in bed, at the edge of the bed, or even in a chair.

Date and location of skin grafts are very important. A skin graft less than three days old is at risk for shifting and loss. Generally, grafts more than three days old are not at great risk for loss and can withstand more aggressive movement.

The patient with a burn injury will most likely experience pain with mobility. Pain can be addressed with medication. Lower extremities can be wrapped with Ace™ bandages to prevent blood pooling.

A goal of occupational therapy is to maintain ROM of the involved joints. As skin heals, it will resist motion and contract. Second and third degree burns left in positions of comfort will develop limitations and contracture. Joints particularly at risk are the neck, axilla, shoulder girdle, elbow, wrist, thumb, and digits. ROM must be performed daily, unless contraindicated by a new graft. An optimal time to perform ROM is during dressing changes, when the occupational therapist can visualize the joint's motion and see how the joint reacts to stretch. Tightness and skin blanching indicate that the patient is at risk for scar bands and contracture. Accurate assessment of both active and passive ROM measurements must be used to determine gains and losses of joint range of motion.

The injury, skin grafting, recovery process, and rehabilitation will be a new experience for the patient. Education is vital. The more a patient understands the reason for therapeutic intervention, the more likely he or she will be an active and empowered participant in the process. For example, explaining to a patient that the purpose of a splint is to prevent contracture, and showing the patient a photograph of a person with a contracture, can illicit better compliance. Education should start in the hospital as soon as possible. During hospitalization, education focuses on the need for movement, the risk of contracture, ideal positioning, and splints.

In preparing the patient for discharge to home, education should include sun precautions, skin care needs, and follow-up instructions such as doctor visits and outpatient therapy appointments. Most patients need to learn an exercise program to perform at home as an adjunct to outpatient therapy visits. The ongoing care of healing skin is very important. Open, non-healed wounds need to be dressed with an anti-microbial topical dressing (typically SSD) and covered with bandages. This procedure will prevent infection and promote wound healing. Non-grafted skin and grafted skin are dressed with bandages until the wound has fully closed. Nurses usually perform dressing changes while the patient is hospitalized.

Once skin is closed and no longer needs dressing, the patient needs to be educated about skin and sun precautions. New skin is sensitive and fragile and it is at risk for scratches and cuts. Friction should be avoided, as it can cause blisters and reopening of the wound. Skin which has suffered a burn of any classification needs to be protected from the sun. The ultraviolet rays of the sun can damage the epidermis by increasing melanin production and therefore permanently darken the complexion of the burned skin. Protective clothing such as a hat with a wide brim, long sleeves, and socks should be worn to cover newly healed skin. Once skin has closed, the patient should apply a sunblock with an SPF of at least 30. Sunblock needs to be used even under clothes and in inclement weather days. A patient should avoid prolonged sun exposure during the first year after a burn injury.

Scars are an unfortunate consequence of burns. Burned skin that is not grafted and takes longer than 14 days to heal, and any grafted skin, is highly susceptible to scarring.

Scars result as an overproduction of collagen deposited in a disorganized fashion in the healing wound bed. The immature scar begins in the acute phase of recovery. The hallmark signs of the immature scar are red, raised and rigid skin, and most often limits to motion. Scar management is the employment of techniques to minimize scarring. Scars need to be managed immediately and continuously. It is never too early to begin scar management. Scars form quickly and will continue to grow until maturity.

In the acute phase, scar management includes active ROM, passive ROM, splinting, and positioning. Once the wound has closed, pressure therapy can begin. Pressure works to limit and organize the over-production of collagen bundles. In the acute phase, pressure can be applied with Tubigrip™, Coban™, custom-sewn Spandex™ gloves, and Isotoner™ gloves. The patient should wear the pressure garment 23 hours per day, and remove it for bathing and skin care.

Patients can begin self-care tasks in the burn unit. Depending on the patient's level and area of involvement, adaptations may need to be made for eating, grooming, dressing, bathing, and toileting. An effort should be made to encourage the patient to participate in self-care to promote his or her independence and recovery.

In the rehabilitative phase, approximately day 22 until full recovery, the critical factors that the therapist must address are the same areas as in the acute phase, plus cardiovascular and strength training, psychosocial adaptation, and return to occupational life roles. Edema may continue to be a problem in this phase. It will most likely have evolved from a pitting soft edema to a more brawny type. The same interventions used in the acute phase can apply. More aggressive techniques such as retrograde massage, contrast baths, or temporary fabricated garments may be required. Since hand edema is usually most prominent, the use of resistive active range of motion activities tends to be the most effective intervention. Whereas in the acute phase the goal was movement, now patients should do more resistive exercises and self-care tasks. At this time in recovery, the therapist will identify joints at risk for loss of ROM and contracture. This can be determined by decreasing and less than normal ROM measurements, scar bands and blanched skin with movement, and lack of active movement by the patient. Positioning techniques and splints are used to maintain a low load prolonged stretch (LLPS) on the healing skin. The patient should be positioned so that the stretch occurs against the direction in which the scar is pulling. For example, an anterior chest and neck burn will pull the patient into flexion as the scar contracts. To counteract the flexion force, the patient should be in extension and at times exercise into hyperextension. For example, the patient might be advised to sleep without a pillow, or wear a neck collar positioned in neutral.

If the patient is still in an inpatient hospital setting, every effort should be made to return the person to his or her former mode of ambulation. If no medical contraindications exist, efforts should be made to discontinue assistive devices and restore prior ambulatory status. Active and passive ROM exercises are an essential focus of therapy and recovery. The therapist, and most importantly the patient, needs to be aggressive in this area. Active ROM is performed against the pull of the burn scar. Every joint impacted by the burn must be stretched to its full available motion. This will usually be painful to the patient; however, joints not pushed to their limit will become contracted and non-functional. The burned hand needs to be stretched at every joint both in isolated passive ROM and active ROM, as well as total passive motion and active motion, to fully stretch the scar.

Scars form quickly and will continue to grow until maturity, usually one to one and a half years after a burn. Several techniques are used to decrease the chances for hypertrophic scars. Pressure modalities are paramount. The use of gradient pressure (i.e., Tubigrip™) and custom-fit pressure garments is a staple of burn treatment in this phase. For facial burns, a clear high-temperature plastic mask can be molded.

At this level, patients are expected to perform (or at least participate) in every aspect of the self-care activities of their daily routine. The movement and independence will be beneficial. Adaptive devices can be utilized when needed, but most importantly, the joint motion during daily skills will serve to increase overall ROM and decrease the chance for contracture. Loss of muscle mass and girth is common. Cardiovascular and strength training are employed as further adjuncts to active ROM. Stressing the cardiovascular system will help to challenge the skin and stretch the muscle tissue. Additionally, the skin's ability to respond to change in temperature, perspiration, and blood flow can be monitored.

Evaluating Progress

Periodic reassessments evaluate progress in areas such as edema and deformity control, scar mobilization, restoration of ROM, strength, endurance, and coordination. Demonstration of facility with adaptive equipment and techniques, and compliance with home programs, signal a positive outcome of patient and family education strategies. Improvement in these areas will be reflected in progressively higher levels of independence in ADLs and IADLs.

Determining Change in or Termination of Treatment

The wound healing process dictates treatment for the patient recovering from a burn injury. The status of the healing skin and related physical structures will be indicative of the course for therapy throughout all phases of recovery. Termination of treatment is indicated after the skin and structures are healed, the threat of scar or deformity formation is passed, and maximum function is restored.

Case Study

Description

J.J. is a 45-year-old male who has been referred to an outpatient clinic. He is employed in a warehouse stocking shelves and filling orders. J.J. lives with his wife and two small boys, ages eight and four years. His wife stays at home and cares for the children. J.J. is an active and involved father. He and his wife are restoring a historic home, and J.J. enjoys working on the house. In his spare time, he fly-fishes and coaches his son's soccer team. He is right hand dominant. Prior to his injury, he was employed full time and was independent in all ADLs and IADLs.

J.J. was involved in a chemical explosion when a coworker inadvertently combined two reactive chemicals. J.J. sustained second degree burns to the anterior chest on his right side and third degree burns to the right upper extremity (RUE) from the dorsal PIPs to the axillary fold. Immediately after the accident, J.J. was transported to the acute care hospital and admitted to the burn unit. He underwent a split thickness skin graft

(STSG) to the RUE. J.J. received occupational therapy in acute care for seven days. The focus of treatment was positioning, deformity, and edema control. The therapist provided J.J. with utensils that had built-up sponge handles and encouraged him to use his RUE. On post-burn day eight, J.J. was transferred to the rehabilitation unit. His progress was steady but slow. His graft sites and skin healed well, and strength and ROM improved throughout his RUE. His skin continued to heal and he was fitted with splints and pressure garments. Throughout his recovery, J.J.'s wife provided support and encouragement. J.J. is now at the point of sorting out vocational options. He would like to be able to return to work in the warehouse and looks forward to resuming work on the house.

Initial evaluation reveals that J.J. has resumed independence in all ADLs. He demonstrates some residual deficits in RUE function. Specifically, shoulder flexion is lacking 30 degrees, and elbow extension is lacking 25 degrees. Muscle strength, tested grossly throughout his RUE is 4 (good). Coordination, as measured by the nine-hole peg test, is below average. J.J. exhibits decreased endurance for completing upper extremity activities that require reaching while standing. He continues to wear pressure garments on his RUE.

The interview indicates that J.J. would like to return to the job that he held before his accident and his employer is willing to have him return if he is able to complete the job safely and efficiently. J.J.'s job consists of two distinct parts. Re-stocking shelves is a task that occurs early in his shift. There are no specific time limits or requirements for this task and J.J. is confident that he will be able to do this efficiently. A second component to his job requires that he read and fill orders on a conveyor belt. J.J. must read the order, obtain inventory from the shelf, and place it in a box before the conveyor moves the box out of his reach. In this job operation, timing is critical. J.J. is not as confident in his ability to complete this job task.

Long- and Short-Term Goals

The long-term goal of intervention for J.J. is to demonstrate the ability to fill orders by reading the request, securing products from a shelf behind him, and placing products in a shipping box at the rate of one order per minute (i.e., the industry standard).

The short-term goal of intervention for J.J. is to demonstrate the ability to fill a simulated order by reading the request, securing products from a low shelf, and placing them on a table in two minutes.

Therapist Goals and Strategies

The therapist's goals include:

1. Increase AROM in the right shoulder and elbow.
2. Increase strength throughout the RUE.
3. Increase endurance in the RUE.
4. Improve activity tolerance.
5. Improve skin tolerance to movement.
6. Educate J.J. about his body response to temperature during work.

The therapist's strategies include:

1. Have patient wear compressive garments during treatment.
2. Encourage attention to skin response and temperature.
3. Provide patient with opportunity to complete activities requiring combination movements of the shoulder, elbow, forearm, wrist and hand.
4. Provide graded activities that challenge ROM, strength, endurance, and activity tolerance.

Activity

Valpar Whole-Body Range of Motion

The *Valpar Whole Body Range of Motion* is a module in the Valpar series (Valpar International Corporation). It requires a patient to remove and reposition a variety of shapes on a frame, using screws to remove and reattach each piece. As the name implies, the *Valpar* requires the patient to demonstrate flexibility in the upper extremities, lower extremities, and trunk. It provides opportunities for the patient to produce combination movements of the shoulder, elbow, wrist, and hand. Removal and replacement of the shapes using screws requires sustained effort against gravity, which will help improve J.J.'s strength and endurance. Graded wrist weights could be used to increase the challenge for J.J. Performance on the *Valpar Whole Body Range of Motion* may be timed and related to industry standards. Throughout completion of the activity, J.J. will be able to judge the impact of such movement on the shearing forces between his compression garments and skin.

J.J. has come to this clinic with the goal of returning to work. He has been through ongoing rehabilitation since his injury and has received occupational therapy in both acute care and rehabilitation. It is important that the activities in which he engages now are clearly work related. The job to which J.J will be returning requires him to stand and use both upper extremities (BUEs) to place and retrieve objects of varied weights and sizes on shelves. J.J. will complete all activities with his compression garments on. It may take up to 18 months for scar tissue to mature. J.J. will return to work with pressure garments in place.

Treatment Objectives

J.J. will remove and reposition all shapes of the *Valpar Whole Body Range of Motion*, taking rest breaks as required.

Resources

Baryza, M.J., & Baryza, G.A. (1995). The Vancouver Scar Scale: an administration tool and its interrater reliability. *Journal of Burn Care and Rehab,16*(5), 535–538.

Merkel, S., et.al. (1999). The FLACC Scale: a behavioral scale for scoring postoperative plan in young children. *Pediatric Nursing, 23*(3), 293–297.

Uniform Data Systems for Medical Rehabilitation™. (1993). *Functional independence measure (FIM).* Buffalo, NY: The State University of New York University at Buffalo.

References

Burn Survivors Online. (2003). www.burnsurvivorsonline.com

Lund, C.C. & Browder, N.C. (1955). The estimation of areas of burns. *Surgery, Gynecology, and Obstetics, 79,* 352–358.

Staley, M.J. & Richard, R. (2001). Burns. In S.B. O'Sullivan & T.J. Schmitz (Eds.), *Physical rehabilitation assessment and treatment.* Philadelphia: FA Davis. p 845–873.

Uniform Data Systems for Medical Rehabilitation™. (1993). *Functional independence measure (FIM).* Buffalo, NY: The State University of New York University at Buffalo.

Wong, D.L., et.al. (1999). *Wong-Baker scale. Whaley and Wong's nursing care of infants and children.* (6th ed.). St. Louis: Mosby.

Spinal Cord Injuries

16

Kendall Daly, OTR/L
Ellen Rosenberg Pitonyak, MS, OTR/L

Synopsis of Clinical Condition

Prevalence and Etiology

An understanding of spinal cord injury requires a basic knowledge of anatomy of the spinal cord, the vertebral column, spinal nerves, and the cord's vascular supply.

The spinal cord makes up part of the central nervous system. It is responsible for sending messages from the brain to the muscles, to produce voluntary movement. The spinal cord also controls involuntary functions not associated with the autonomic nervous system, including skin sensation and respiration. The spinal cord is $\frac{1}{2}$-inch wide and 18-inches long extending from the medulla oblongata to the level of the L1 or L2 vertebrae. The spinal column consists of 7 cervical, 12 thoracic, 5 lumbar, 5 sacral, and 4 coccygeal vertebrae. A typical vertebra consists of a body, located anteriorly, and an arch. The spinal cord is encased in the spinal canal formed and protected by the vertebral bodies and arches. The cervical, thoracic, and lumbar vertebrae are separated by intervertebral discs and are connected and stabilized by ligaments. The sacral and coccygeal vertebrae are fused (Smith, Weiss, & Lehmkuhl, 1996).

A cross section of the spinal cord reveals an H-shaped area in the center referred to as the gray matter, and a surrounding area called the white matter. The dorsal horn of the gray matter contains cell bodies that are predominantly sensory, and the ventral horn contains cell bodies that innervate the skeletal muscles that control motor function. The white matter contains various motor and sensory tracts. The nerves that lie within the spinal cord are called upper motor neurons (UMNs), and their function is to carry messages back and forth from the brain to the spinal nerves along the spinal tract. There are also spinal nerves called lower motor neurons (LMNs) that branch out from the spinal cord to specific areas of the body. There are motor and sensory portions of LMNs. The motor portions send messages from the brain to various body parts to initiate movement. For example, the C7 spinal nerve controls the biceps. The sensory portions carry messages about sensations from the skin and other organs to the brain.

There are 8 cervical, 12 thoracic, 5 lumbar, 5 sacral, and 1 coccygeal pairs of spinal nerves. The C1–C7 spinal nerves exit the vertebral canal above the corresponding numbered vertebrae. The C8 spinal nerve exits the canal below the C7 vertebrae, because there is no C8 vertebra. Because the spinal cord is shorter than the vertebral column, the spinal nerves need to travel caudally to exit the column forming the cauda equina. The spinal cord receives its blood supply from a single anterior artery and from two posterior spinal arteries.

Spinal cord injury (SCI) is damage to the spinal cord that results in loss of motor function and sensation. Spinal cord injury is catastrophic and impacts almost all aspects of the injured person's life. It is estimated that every year in the United Sates 7,500 individuals are injured (National Spinal Cord Injury Statistical Center, 2001). The recovery is often long and frustrating for the person with the injury as well his or her family and friends. It is estimated that 250,000–400,000 persons in the United States are living with spinal cord injury (National Spinal Cord Injury Statistical Center, 2001). The etiology of the condition may be either traumatic or non-traumatic. There are many causes of SCI including motor vehicle accidents (38.5%), violence (24.5%), falls (21.8%), sports (7.2%), and others (7.9%) (National Spinal Cord Injury Statistical Center, 2001). Sixty percent of persons with spinal cord injury are 30 years old or younger. Most injuries occur between 16 and 30 years of age. The majority of persons with SCI are men with a 4 to 1 male to female ratio.

Fracture dislocation is the most common injury to the cervical spine at C5–C6. Gunshots and stab wounds may damage the cord either by direct penetration or by bone fragments causing laceration of the cord. This type of injury can occur at any level. Hemorrhage, aneurysm, thrombosis, or emboli can disrupt the blood supply to the cord resulting in a spinal cord injury. Compression due to tumors may also cause permanent damage.

A spinal cord injury may be either complete or incomplete. The designation of the level of SCI is determined by the most caudal normally functioning segment. A complete injury involves the loss of all motor and sensory function in the dermatomal distribution below the level of the lesion. In incomplete lesions, some combinations of neurologic function are retained below the level of the injury. Residual muscle function depends on which spinal fibers remain intact. With incomplete lesions, sensation may be intact, impaired, or absent below the level of the lesion. Incomplete spinal cord injuries are often described as syndromes.

Central cord syndrome and Brown-Sequard syndrome are the most common types of incomplete spinal cord injuries. In central cord syndrome, the middle of the cord is more damaged than the outer areas, causing more upper extremity involvement than lower extremity. This syndrome occurs most often in older people who fall and experience neck hyperextension. It can also occur at any age following a flexion injury. Brown-Sequard syndrome is characterized by one side of the spinal cord being damaged, causing motor and proprioceptive loss on one side of the body and loss of pain and temperature on the other side of the body. This is the most common spinal cord injury following a ruptured disc, burst fracture, or penetrating trauma. Almost all people with this syndrome ambulate and regain a large part of their independence (Atrice, Morrison, McDowell, & Shandalov, 2001).

Anterior cord syndrome results from trauma to the anterior cord or the anterior spinal artery or both. This is caused by flexion injuries and/or pressure to the anterior cord from a ruptured disc or fracture. Loss of pain and temperature and motor function is noted, while proprioception remains intact (Atrice, Morrison, McDowell, & Shandalov, 2001).

Posterior cord syndrome describes damage to the dorsal columns, causing loss of proprioception with other sensory and motor function remaining intact. Cauda Equina is usually due to massive disc herniation at the lowest discs on the spinal column. It can also stem from vertebral collapse resulting from tumor, infection, or trauma and results in bowel and bladder dysfunction and lower limb involvement. Conus Medullaris describes injury to the sacral cord above the cauda equina and also results in bowel, bladder, and lower limb dysfunction.

Spinal cord injuries may be grossly divided into two categories: tetraplegia and paraplegia. Tetraplegia, which consists of injury to one of the high cervical segments, is characterized by a pattern of motor and sensory deficits in all four extremities. Paraplegia, which involves injury to the thoracic, lumbar, or sacral regions, is characterized by a pattern of sensory and motor deficit in the lower extremities. Since 1990, the most frequent distribution of spinal cord injuries is incomplete tetraplegia (29.5%), complete paraplegia (27.3%), incomplete paraplegia (21.3%), and complete tetraplegia (18.5%) (National Spinal Cord Injury Statistical Center, 2001).

Common Characteristics and Symptoms

The most obvious symptom of spinal cord injury is the loss of voluntary muscle control in the trunk and extremities. Impaired sitting posture and balance is also evident with the loss of muscle control. This affects control over the body and the ability to manipulate the environment resulting in loss of independence. In the months and years following, most people with spinal cord injury experience some recovery in the musculature that is innervated by cord segments one to two levels below the lesion.

Sensory impairment is evident in most spinal cord injuries. A loss of sensation can lead to incoordination of body movements, decreased body awareness, and vulnerability to trauma. Initially, after the injury, there is a period of spinal shock lasting one day to eight weeks. Spinal shock refers to a state of decreased excitability of the spinal cord secondary to withdrawal of the excitatory influences from higher centers.

During spinal shock, muscles are flaccid. As spinal shock resolves, muscle reflexes below the level of the lesion return causing spasticity. Spasticity is characterized by flexor or extensor tone, or by myoclonus. This increase in tone can be uncomfortable or painful and can limit function or lead to contractures. Contractures can also result from disuse, overuse, or poor positioning.

A person with a complete spinal cord injury experiences loss of body temperature regulation. Sweating is not evident below the level of the lesion, and an inability to sweat can lead to overheating. Individuals also experience frequent intolerance to either hot or cold.

Respiratory dysfunction is another symptom of spinal cord injury. Because the muscles involved in respiration are not functioning, persons with high tetraplegia may require a ventilator. Some individuals can be weaned off the ventilator eventually, but individuals with an injury at C1, C2, or even C3 most likely will not be. Respiratory difficulties, including difficulty coughing and clearing the lungs of secretions can lead to pneumonia and other respiratory complications, which are the most common cause of death following spinal cord injury. Decreased endurance can also result from respiratory insufficiency.

Cardiovascular function can also be altered following spinal cord injury. Common problems are slowed heart rate, hypotension (low blood pressure), and orthostatic hypotension, which is a decrease in blood pressure that occurs with movement into an upright position. An abdominal binder and compression stockings are indicated in order to reduce orthostatic hypotension.

Most spinal cord injuries result in an inability to voluntarily control bowel and bladder function. Voluntary control requires an intact sacral cord, and most injuries occur above this level. Bowel and bladder dysfunction varies with incomplete injuries. Incontinence must be managed carefully, as it can cause a variety of physical and psychological problems.

Spinal cord injury can also result in a loss of sexual functioning. The genitals receive their innervations from the thoracolumbar and sacral regions of the spinal cord. With a spinal cord injury, messages from the genitals to the brain are disrupted, and men may experience difficulty with erection. Female fertility remains unchanged. Many people also have problems related to body image and feelings of unattractiveness.

Feelings of loss, depression, anger, and anxiety are common psychological symptoms following spinal cord injury. Changes in individual's roles as well as social functioning and interests can be very challenging. Adjusting to disability requires patience, education, and communication.

The medical complications that can occur as a result of spinal cord injury include autonomic dysreflexia, deep vein thrombosis, osteoporosis, heterotopic ossification, as well as gastrointestinal (GI) tract and urinary tract dysfunction. Autonomic dysreflexia can occur in people who sustain a spinal cord injury at T6 level or above. Complete and incomplete injuries are vulnerable to this condition. Autonomic dysreflexia is a "hyperreflexia" caused by an irritation or other noxious stimulus, such as a full bladder or bowel, a plugged catheter, a skin ulcer, pain, muscle spasm, sexual activity, etc. Signals from the affected area cannot reach the brain, so the body continues to send the message, and the reflex becomes "hyper." Symptoms of autonomic dysreflexia include a sudden increase in blood pressure, pounding headache, flushed face, goose bumps, sweating above the level of lesion, slowed pulse, and anxiety. Treatment requires sitting the person up and looking for the stimulus to relieve the irritation. An untreated autonomic dysreflexia can result in a serious medical condition with risk of stroke or seizure.

Persons with spinal cord injury are also at risk for deep vein thrombosis (DVT). A DVT is a blood clot that can occur in the lower extremities as a result of decreased circulation and inactivity. Pulmonary embolism is one of the leading causes of death in persons with spinal cord injury and it usually occurs within three months post injury. Anticoagulants and compression stockings are indicated.

Following spinal cord injury, bones lose both calcium and collagen. Osteoporosis progresses gradually and increases the likelihood of fractures. Heterotopic ossification (HO) is the formation of new bone, which occurs below the level of injury. This usually occurs in the first four months after the injury, and treatment includes aggressive range of motion (ROM) and radiation. Surgery is indicated if changes in function and positioning problems arise.

Pressure sores are caused by loss of blood supply to an area, secondary to prolonged pressure over a bony prominence. In patients with spinal cord injury, muscle atrophy and sensory loss complicates the process. Skin abrasion during movement is also a problem. Symptoms of pressure sores include a red or discolored area, blistering or an opening in the skin.

Gastrointestinal complications following spinal cord injury include stomach ulcers, GI bleeds, paralytic ileus, gastric dilation, fecal impaction, and bowel obstruction. Proper medical management can prevent these complications. Bladder dysfunction following spinal cord injury can lead to multiple medical issues including urinary retention, bladder infection, and reflux of urine into the ureters, kidney stones, and kidney failure. Before urologic advances in the late 1980s and early 1990s bladder complications were a leading cause of death for persons with spinal cord injury.

Life after spinal cord injury can be enjoyable and productive. In 1999, the average length of stay in the hospital was 16 days in acute care and 44 days of rehabilitation (National Spinal Cord Injury Statistical Center, 2001). Eighty-eight percent of those with spinal cord injuries return to their homes; the remainder find residence in group homes or other lodging. Approximately 40% of persons with paraplegia and 30% with tetraplegia eventually return to work (Krause, Newman, DeVino, Maynard, Roach, & Ducharme, 1999).

Target Areas for Intervention

Occupational therapy intervention provides unique opportunities for people with spinal cord injury to return to their prior life roles. Through purposeful functional activity, education, and support, occupational therapists facilitate increased independence. A thorough initial interview is conducted with the patient and family in order to determine the patient's prior level of function as well as interests and hobbies. It is also important to understand the occupational roles, such as those of parent, spouse, worker, homemaker, etc. in which the patient engaged prior to the injury. Areas that are initially addressed are feeding, self-care, skin care, bed mobility, and transfers. Instruction in the appropriate weight shift is an immediate concern due to the high risk of pressure ulcers. Often, self-care skills need to be performed at the bedside until the patient can progress to a seated level. Once the patient progresses, more complex skills such as bowel and bladder management, home management, and meal preparation are addressed. Further progression leads to participation in community activities such as shopping, driving, using public transportation, and working. Occupational therapists provide the necessary resources in order to help people achieve future goals and to plan for future needs. Accessibility is a major concern for people with spinal cord injury. Occupational therapy plays a major role in evaluating the home environment and in making the appropriate recommendations for home set-up, equipment, and strategies to increase independence, safety, and accessibility. Since not all people with spinal cord injury ambulate, wheelchair level skills and wheelchair accessibility is a major focus of intervention. Occupational therapists also involve the family to a great extent in the form of education and training in order to prepare everyone for discharge.

Contextual Considerations

Clinical

The clinical evaluation incorporates biographical information, sensorimotor components, cognitive components, psychological components, activities of daily living (ADL) performance, and functional mobility performance.

Biographical information is obtained by an interview with the patient and includes information about prior living situation, prior level of function, activities and interests, occupational role performance, and individual goals. This information is important when choosing activities and treatment planning.

Sensorimotor components include information about sensation and sensory awareness, neuromusculoskeletal skills, and motor skills. Using the ASIA scale, key sensory areas are tested to identify the neurologic level of injury. The sensory evaluation should also include light touch, stereognosis, kinesthesia, pain and temperature, and joint proprioception. In order to prevent ulcers and irritations, it is imperative that patients with spinal cord injury understand that the insensate parts of the body are extremely vulnerable to pressure and trauma.

The neuromusculoskeletal evaluation of the upper and lower extremities and the trunk includes range of motion, muscle tone, strength, endurance, and postural control.

Strength is tested using the Manual Muscle Test (MMT), and the dynanometer for grip. Muscle tone is tested using the Ashworth Scale. Gross motor coordination and fine motor coordination/dexterity are also identifiers of arm and hand function. Fine motor coordination is tested using the 9-hole peg test. The information gathered from these evaluations is important, because it will affect performance on mobility skills, ADLs, skin care, and bowel and bladder care. It will also indicate a patient's need for adaptive equipment, a universal cuff, positioning devices, upper extremity splints, and lower extremity bracing. It is important to communicate with the physical therapist regarding the status of the lower extremities and the ambulation devices that he or she recommends.

Due to the traumatic events that cause spinal cord injury, it is not uncommon for people to suffer a head injury at the same time. It is important to evaluate cognition with assistance from the neuropsychologist. This provides important information about memory and problem solving, which are skills that contribute to a patient's ability to learn new information, to adapt to new strategies, and to direct care. The psychologist also assists with the evaluation of psychosocial skills, which contribute to a patient's ability to cope with disability and to participate in therapeutic activities.

Activities of daily living are evaluated using the *Functional Independence Measure*™ (Uniform Data System for Medical Rehabilitation, 1993). This provides information about feeding, grooming, bathing, dressing, homemaking, community skills, bowel and bladder function, bed mobility, and transfers. Once baseline status is formulated, a treatment plan and goals can be established with the patient and family.

Family

An important task of rehabilitation that begins immediately is to prepare the patient and family for discharge to home. In addition to an interview with the patient, it is important to conduct an interview with the family to determine a primary caregiver and family priorities. It is also necessary to consider family values, cultural and religious practices, and family goals when establishing the treatment plan. It is important to know where and with whom the patient is going to live, and what resources the family has. The social worker can assist with gathering financial information, contacting appropriate community resources, and supporting counseling. Since the length of stay for inpatient hospitalizations has decreased over the years, a bigger burden of care falls on the family of the spinal cord injured patient. A family meeting, including the patient and all treatment team members, is useful in educating the family about the present functional status as well as future needs. This is also a good time to schedule a home visit with the family in order to evaluate home accessibility and the presence of architectural barriers. Further family training sessions are scheduled to assure that all caregivers are competent and safe with equipment and with assisting the patient.

Practice Setting

The occupational therapist provides treatment at many stages of recovery for the patient with spinal cord injury. Following stabilization and/or surgery, therapy in the acute care setting occurs. Positioning, splinting, and range of motion are the focus of treatment to maintain range of motion and to prevent contractures and pressure ulcers. Once the patient is medically stable, therapy continues in a more intensive inpatient rehabilitative setting. Following inpatient therapy, treatment continues in homecare, outpatient, or work-site settings. It is very important for therapists to communicate along the continuum of care to ease the transition to the new environment.

Sociopolitical

Persons with disabilities may be devalued in society and may be subject to discrimination in a variety of ways. Architectural and transportation barriers may make it difficult for people with mobility impairments to access home, work, and community settings. A disabled person is likely to experience discriminatory behavior related to returning to prior housing situation, work, and school. Lack of adequate medical coverage and funding sources provide another challenge for people with disabilities. The Americans with Disabilities Act of 1990 (ADA) promotes the inclusion of people with disabilities into mainstream society. This act ensures that people with spinal cord injury have equal opportunity for employment as well as equal access to public facilities, institutions, and transportation. Modifications may need to be made to the workplace to make it more accessible, and by law employers are required to make the necessary changes to accommodate a person with a disability. The ADA empowers individuals with disabilities to advocate for their rights and to take the necessary actions against institutions or facilities that deny equal opportunity or access.

Financial assistance may be needed to meet the needs of the spinal cord patient in returning to home and to the community. The social worker at the hospital helps identify available resources at the federal, state, and local levels. The Social Security Administration determines eligibility for financial assistance based on disability. There are Veterans Administration offices located regionally to assist veterans with needed services. State vocational rehabilitation offices assist with the purchase of equipment, job placement, counseling, and other forms of financial assistance. The Crime Victims Association as well as other voluntary and charitable organizations on the national, state, and local levels exist that can provide information about services to which the disabled individual is entitled.

Lifestyle/Lifespan

Persons with spinal cord injury have the same hopes, desires, and interests as people without a disability. The spinal cord injured person can return to a satisfactory lifestyle. Due to the extent of losses a person faces following spinal cord injury, a number of issues will be faced throughout the lifespan. The patient and family should be made aware of social, medical, accessibility, and financial concerns.

The extensive physical, functional, and personal losses that a person with spinal cord injury faces can lead to feelings of grief. Each patient progresses through stages of grief in a variable way and time. It may take years for a person to adjust to a disability from spinal cord injury. The function of relationships changes, and it is not uncommon to lose friends and sexual partners as a result. It is the function of the rehabilitative team to educate and support the patient and family as they cope with these social changes. Due to changes in body image and feelings of worthlessness, it is important to access social supports in the community including psychology and peer support.

Primary medical issues that remain during the life of the spinal cord injured patient include respiratory, skin, bowel and bladder, and autonomic dysreflexia. For higher-level cord injuries, respiratory complications are a threat whether or not mechanical ventilation is needed. Respiratory rehabilitation includes measures to manage secretions and to enhance breathing ability. The patient and family need to be provided the knowledge and skills necessary to prevent respiratory complications that result from the inability to effectively clear secretions and decreased vital capacity. The threat of skin breakdown in the spinal cord injured person is continuous, especially as aging decreases skin elasticity. A rigid pressure relief system and skin care routine is essential to the prevention of decubitus ulcers. Bowel and bladder dysfunction can lead to urinary tract dysfunction and gastrointestinal problems. Autonomic dysreflexia, an exaggerated, sympathetic response to a noxious stimulus below the level of the spinal cord lesion, can be life threatening. There are many causes, signs and symptoms, and treatment for dysreflexia that should be reiterated to the patient and family in order to prevent a serious medical emergency.

The extensive set of issues that the person living with SCI will face throughout his or her lifetime is summarized below.

Table 16.1
SCI–Related Issues

Accessibility	Financial	Medical	Family	Social
Home	Daily medical supplies	Skin care: prevention of decubiti	Support for daily care	Interaction with peers
School/Work	Cost of attendant care	Orthostatic hypertension	Role interruption	Role resumption
Community	Home modification	Heterotropic bone	Potential role reversal	Role reconfiguration
Driving/transportation	Work site modification	Bowel and bladder control	Adjustment to disability	Adaptive leisure
	Vehicle adaptation	Respiration		
	Planning for future living arrangements			
	DME			

During rehabilitation, the spinal cord injured patient and family must be taught the knowledge and skills necessary to remain healthy. If the patient is unable to be independent in certain skills, then communication and assertiveness skills are required to facilitate the patient's ability to manage his or her care.

Clinical Decision Making Process

Defining Focus for Intervention

In defining a focus of treatment for the patient with a spinal cord injury, the five most important factors are:

1. Level and pattern of injury.
2. Degree of head and upper extremity control.
3. Degree of wrist and hand function.
4. Trunk control.
5. Psychosocial adjustment to the disability (Hill, 1986).

The occupational therapist is most interested in which muscles and sensory systems are intact and functional.

For patients with high-level injuries (C1–C5), head control and/or proximal upper extremity control will need to be captured and utilized to access environmental control systems and adaptive equipment. The degree of residual wrist and hand function present will determine the need for training alternative grasp patterns (i.e., tenodesis grasp at C6) versus the development and strengthening of more traditional grasp patterns (at C7 and below). The degree of residual trunk control will impact decisions regarding seating and positioning, wheelchair selection, and functional mobility training. Finally, the degree of adjustment to disability will impact the patient's motivation to learn adaptive strategies and participate in redesigning a productive life.

Establishing Goals for Intervention

Goals for intervention reflect the patient's motivation, energy level, and expected level of independence. Targeted levels of independence for persons with spinal cord injury are summarized below:

Table 16.2
Target Levels of Independence

Level of Injury	Level of Independence
C1	Respirator dependency. Motorized wheelchair dependency. Computer and environmental control system powered by sip/puff; tongue switch, eye gaze, or voice activation. Dependent in all self-care but able to direct caregiver.
C2–C3	Motorized wheelchair dependency. Computer and environmental control system powered by head switch or voice activation. Dependent in all self-care but able to direct caregiver.
C4–C5	Motorized wheelchair or light manual wheelchair with quad spokes. Mobile arm support and quad cuff for self-feeding. Computer and environmental control system powered adapted upper extremity switches. Self dressing with dressing loops. Maximum assistance required for all self-care. Able to direct caregiver.
C6	Tenodesis function in upper extremity may limit need for assistive devices for self-care. Tenodesis splint to support hand function. Manual wheelchair with quad spokes and wheelchair gloves. Sliding board transfers with supervision. Can access standard controls for computer systems and environmental controls.
C7–C8	Same as above with increased strength and endurance noted in distal musculature of wrist and hand.
T1–lower	Independent manual wheelchair use. Combination of braces and crutches for ambulation in home environment. Independent in all transfers. Independent in self-care.

Close examination of the expected levels of independence above illuminates the difficulty that patients with SCI may experience. Specifically, lower extremity dressing for patients at C4–C6 takes practice and even the most accomplished patients finds it time and energy consuming. Such patients may choose to have an attendant assist with that activity during the day. This allows them to conserve time and energy for more valued work or leisure activities.

Designing Theory-Based Intervention

The biomechanical frame of reference guides the components of the treatment plan designed to maintain range of motion, prevent deformity, and increase residual muscle strength. The rehabilitation frame of reference guides the selection of adaptive devices such as a quad cuff and compensatory techniques such as the use of tenodesis grasp.

Evaluating Progress

From the biomechanical perspective, progress is noted if increased strength is achieved in innervated muscles and splinting, serial casting, and positioning have decreased or prevented deformity. From the rehabilitation perspective, progress is noted if the patient no longer relies on the therapist for verbal cues, correction, or assistance in carrying out daily living activities.

Determining Change in or Termination of Treatment

Because recovery and rehabilitation of spinal cord injury is such a long process, termination of treatment is rarely a concern. More commonly, goals are adjusted to fit the energy patterns of the life the patient is constructing. As noted earlier, lower extremity dressing may be difficult and/or time consuming for the patient. Although it may have been set as a goal in combination with other self-care tasks, that activity may be abandoned for direct care in this area so that more energy can be given to work or leisure activity. Prioritization of goals continues throughout the rehabilitation process.

Case Study

Description

HR is a 21-year-old male injured in a diving accident at a family reunion. Prior to his injury, HR was living with a roommate in a third floor apartment in a large city. He worked full time at an auto detail shop and was studying to be a pharmacy technician at a local community college and planned to pursue a pharmacy degree in the future. HR and his roommate share simple meal preparation and homemaking. To HR, "basketball is life." He plays in a local league and is an avid fan of local NBA teams—he attends every game. HR is a member of a large, supportive family that lives in a nearby suburb. He is the oldest sibling in a family of three brothers and sisters. He has a girlfriend who attends college in a nearby state.

Immediately after the accident, HR was admitted to the acute care hospital that was designated as a component of regional spinal cord injury care system. He remained in the acute care hospital for 10 days. During that time, his spine was stabilized. It was determined that HR's level of injury was at C6. In acute care, HR was evaluated by an occupational therapist. The occupational therapy program included the design of bilateral resting splints to maintain HR's hand position and prevent deformity, skin care and breath control education, sitting practice to diminish dizziness when upright, and transfer training. HR has made good progress and is now in the rehabilitation hospital. Assessment in rehabilitation confirms the C6 level of injury. HR's head control, upper extremity function, and trunk control are consistent with a C6 injury. Goals and care plan are outlined for HR in the areas of self-feeding, communication, oral/facial hygiene, dressing, bowel and bladder management, splinting, and deformity control.

In the area of self-feeding, it is anticipated that HR will be independent with equipment for drinking, utensil feeding, finger feeding, and cutting food. The equipment that he will use is a cup holder, bicycle water bottle, utensil cuff, sandwich holder, and adapted knife. In the area of communication, it is anticipated that HR will be independent with equipment for writing, typing, page turning, telephone, and computer use. The presence of tenodesis action in HR's wrists and hands will be valuable in this area. Equipment that he may use includes a writing splint, tenodesis training splint, typing stick, and phone holder with shoulder rest. For oral/facial hygiene, HR is expected to be independent in washing his face, brushing and flossing teeth, shaving, nail care, combing, brushing, washing and drying hair, and applying deodorant. Equipment that HR will use to support oral/facial hygiene includes a tooth paste stabilizer, dental floss holder, electric razor with adapted handle, adapted shaving cream can, adapted brush and comb, and adapted shampoo dispenser. In dressing, HR is expected to be independent for upper and lower extremity dressing with equipment. He will use a dressing stick or dressing loop, Velcro™ shoe closures, loops on socks, zipper pull, and sock donner. For bowel and bladder management, HR is expected to empty a catheter bag, and apply an external male catheter. He may use a suppository inserter or digital stimulator for bowel management. HR is interested in becoming as independent as possible. He is motivated to build a future for himself.

Long- and Short-Term Goals

The long-term goal of intervention for HR is to be independent with equipment for communication skills including writing, typing, page turning, and telephone and computer use.

The short-term goal of intervention for HR is to demonstrate tenodesis action bilaterally sufficient to manipulate one-inch objects.

Therapist Goals and Strategies

The therapist's goals include improving tenodesis function in HR's right upper extremity to reduce reliance on adaptive devices and techniques.

The therapist's strategies include:

1. Fabricate a tenodesis training splint for the right hand to encourage development of a strong and functional tenodesis pattern.
2. Design and implement activities to develop more precise tenodesis control allowing for the manipulation of progressively smaller and heavier objects.

Activity

Velcro and Standard Checkers

Prior to beginning the session, the therapist collects a standard checker board with $1\frac{1}{2}$ inch checkers and an adapted checker game constructed of $1\frac{1}{2}$ inch blocks with hook Velcro on the bottom of each checker. Each checker is fitted on top with a plastic loop. Loop Velcro is attached to each block square of the checker board. The Velcro surfaces provide resistance when the checkers are lifted from the board. HR is seated at the table and fitted with the tenodesis training splint. The therapist sits by his side. The checker game starts with the standard checker set. The therapist provides a demonstration and verbal cues regarding how to approach and grasp the checkers using a tenodesis grasp. The therapist describes the role of the splint in training the movement. The game is completed. As HR's tenodesis becomes more habitual, the therapist upgrades the activity by moving to the adapted set. The small plastic top loop represents a smaller target then the standard sized checkers. This requires finer application and placement with the tenodesis grasp. A stronger tenodesis is required to remove and place the Velcro checker than a standard checker. By challenging HR to manipulate finer and heavier or more resistive objects, the therapist helps HR to develop the most functional tenodesis possible.

It is critical for HR to focus on an activity that will systematically allow for the development of a strong and functional tenodesis in the right upper extremity. He will need to learn coordinate wrist flexion, finger extension, wrist extension, and finger flexion patterns. This movement can be reinforced by the use of a tenodesis training splint. A functional tenodesis will reduce HR's reliance on adaptive equipment for self-care.

Treatment Objectives

HR will complete a competitive game of checkers using a standard checker game and a tenodesis training splint for support.

Resources

National Spinal Cord Injury Association:
www.spinalcord.org

Spinal Cord Injury Network International:
www.sonic.net/~spinal

Christopher Reeve Paralysis Association:
500 Morris Avenue
Springfield, NJ 07081

References

Atrice, M., Morrison, S., McDowell, S., & Shandalov, B. (2001) in Umphred, D. (Ed.), *Neurological rehabilitation* (4th ed.). St. Louis, MO: Mosby.

Hill, J. (1986). *Spinal cord injury: A guide to functional outcomes in occupational therapy.* Rockville, MD: Aspen.

National Spinal Cord Injury Statistical Center (2001). Facts and figures at a glance. http://www.spinalcord.uab.udu.

Nobunago, A., Go, B., & Karunas, R. (1999). Recent demographics and injury trends in people served by the model spinal cord injury care system. *Archives of Physical Medicine and Rehabilitation, 80,* 372–382.

Smith, L., Weiss, E., & Lehmkuhl (1996). *Brunstrom's clinical kinesiology* (5th ed.). Philadelphia: FA Davis.

Uniform Data System for Medical Rehabilitation (WDSMR). (1993). *Guide for the uniform data set for medical rehabilitation (Adult FIM), versions 4.0.* Buffalo, NY: WB Foundation Activities.

Repetitive Trauma Disorders: Carpal Tunnel Syndrome

17

Marlene J. Morgan, Ed.D., OTR/L

Synopsis of Clinical Condition

Prevalence and Etiology

Repetitive trauma disorders is a term that is used to describe a number of conditions that involve soft tissue structures such as nerves, tendons, tendon sheaths, muscles, and blood vessels. Repetitive trauma disorders occur from repeated physical movements. Symptoms associated with repetitive trauma disorders include:

- Tightness, discomfort, burning or soreness in the elbows, forearms, wrists, hands, or fingers
- Coldness, tingling, or numbness in the hands
- Lack of strength and coordination in the hands
- Pain that wakes a person up at night
- Feeling the need to massage the hands or wrists (Fast, 1995)

In addition to the symptoms outlined above, repetitive trauma disorders share a number of common characteristics. Repetitive trauma disorders are affected by both the intensity and duration of work or activity and symptoms, are poorly localized, episodic, and non-specific. Close examination of the activity patterns of the patient may reveal a work cycle that is short and repetitive, a stressful work environment, or prolonged periods of working with poor posture in a static position. The development of symptoms is slow and insidious. It may take months or years for the condition to develop and subsequent recovery may also take months or years (Fast, 1995). Repetitive trauma disorders may occur throughout the upper extremity. Fast (1995) includes the following in a list of conditions commonly treated by occupational therapists:

- Bicipital tendonitis
- Thoracic outlet syndrome
- Lateral epicondylitis
- Carpal tunnel syndrome
- de Quervain's syndrome
- Trigger digit

Common Characteristics and Symptoms

In this chapter, carpal tunnel syndrome is the term used to illustrate the clinical reasoning and problem solving approach that an occupational therapist would use to treat a patient who presents with symptoms of repetitive trauma disorder. Carpal tunnel syndrome results from the impingement of the median nerve as it passes through the carpal tunnel at the wrist. Eight flexor tendons of the fingers, one flexor tendon of the thumb, and the median nerve all pass through the carpal tunnel. Carpal tunnel syndrome is accepted as the most frequent entrapment neuropathy (Vender, Truppa, Ruder, & Pomerance, 1998). It is the diagnosis most frequently seen by occupational therapists working in outpatient orthopedic practices. Common symptoms of carpal tunnel syndrome include tingling, numbness, and pain in the hand especially in the thumb, index and middle fingers. Numbness and pain may also radiate into the forearm or shoulder. Many patients experience increased pain and tingling at night, and may also experience weakness and atrophy of the thenar muscles. A pattern of weakness in the muscles innervated by the median nerve may result in weak grip and limited ability to make a fist, and decreased fine motor coordination may also be apparent.

Median nerve compression and the resulting symptoms usually occur in stages. In the early compression stage, the patient typically complains of intermittent symptoms. In the moderate compression stage, the patient complains of ongoing abnormal sensation. Thenar weakness is also evident at this stage. Sensory changes are persistent in the severe compression stage. Some degree of atrophy in the thenar muscles is observed and electromyographic examination (EMG) by a physician shows denervation of the muscles supplied by the median nerve. Although there is no universally accepted treatment for carpal tunnel syndrome, surgical treatment is usually preferred to nonsurgical or conservative treatment (Verdugo, Salinas, Castillo & Cea, 2002).

Target Areas for Intervention

Carpal tunnel syndrome is more common in men than women. Patients usually begin to experience symptoms between 30 and 50 years of age, but it can occur at any age. The development of symptoms of carpal tunnel syndrome may be related to work or other activities. Repetitive activities and, most specifically, activities that require forceful wrist flexion, are thought to contribute to the development of the condition. Activities such as computer use, assembly line work, knitting, needlework, and woodworking are examples of those that may contribute to the exacerbation of the symptoms of carpal tunnel syndrome. A major contributing factor to the condition is the patient's lifestyle. After treatment, many patients need to alter the way they do tasks. Carpal tunnel syndrome may also be seen in patients with seemingly unrelated medical conditions such as diabetes, rheumatoid arthritis, and obesity. Additionally, carpal tunnel syndrome may be associated with pregnancy and use of an oral contraceptive.

Carpal tunnel syndrome is difficult to cure. Although this condition is disabling to some persons, it can usually be managed effectively through a plan of coordinated care involving the physician, the therapist, and the patient.

Contextual Considerations

Clinical

A combination of pathological, histological, and clinical findings is used to decide the course of treatment for a patient with carpal tunnel syndrome. The physician may complete a nerve conduction study to assess the status and conduction capacity of the median nerve. Additionally, the physician may use an EMG to test for the integrity of the muscles innervated by the median nerve. The components of the clinical occupational therapy evaluation for the patient with carpal tunnel syndrome must incorporate information about the musculoskeletal status, activities of daily living (ADL), instrumental activities of daily living (IADL), and work history (Lisak, Personal communication, December 15, 2002; Headley & Singer, 1998). The OT assessment includes:

- Musculoskeletal status which is assessed by completing ROM, manual muscle test (MMT), assessment of the wound site, sensory testing, coordination testing, grip, and pinch strength.
- Patient interview to determine the effect that carpal tunnel syndrome is having on the patient's abilities in the areas of ADL and IADL.
- Detailed work history and information about the person's job tasks and the physical requirements of the tasks.

The components and frequency of the data collected in the musculoskeletal component of the clinical data varies with the treatment plan for the patient—surgical or nonsurgical (conservative) treatment.

For patients receiving nonsurgical (conservative) treatment, the initial musculoskeletal assessment consists of:

- Sensory evaluation
- Active range of motion (AROM) and passive range of motion (PROM)
- Manual muscle test (MMT) with special emphasis on those muscles innervated by the median nerve

The complete series of assessments is repeated monthly, and data is compared to detect positive or negative changes in median nerve function (Lisak, personal communication, December 15, 2002). For patients who are seen after surgical intervention, assessment is phased in consistent with the healing of the postsurgical wound:

- First Postsurgical Visit: ROM and wound assessment
- Three Weeks Post Surgery: MMT
- Four Weeks Post Surgery: sensory evaluation

Family

Family support and encouragement are critical throughout recovery from carpal tunnel syndrome. Changes in lifestyle and activity patterns required to prevent the reoccurrence of this repetitive trauma will need to be reinforced and rewarded on an ongoing basis. Patients may struggle with the interruption of their work role during recovery and may fear that their vocation is in jeopardy. Family education regarding the etiology of carpal tunnel syndrome and subsequent prevention measures is also critical.

Practice Setting

Patients with carpal tunnel syndrome typically receive occupational therapy services in an outpatient clinic. This is true for patients whose carpal tunnel syndrome is being treated post-surgically or without surgical intervention.

Sociopolitical

Patients with carpal tunnel syndrome that is work related may have services paid through worker's compensation funds. A gradual and graded plan for returning to work will be required to insure that the worker is able to return to work. Work site modifications and/or job restructuring may be required to insure that the symptoms of carpal tunnel syndrome are not exacerbated upon the return to work. Both the occupational therapist and the physician use an ongoing assessment of the patient's progress to determine both the steps and the pace of a return to work strategy. Return to work for patients with carpal tunnel syndrome is guided in the legal arena by the employment title of the Americans with Disabilities Act (ADA).

Lifestyle/Lifespan

A major contributing factor to carpal tunnel syndrome is the patient's lifestyle. Patients with carpal tunnel syndrome may experience problems with ADLs (such as buttoning and fastening garments), IADLs (such as driving and using the phone), work related tasks (such as computer use and assembly line work), and leisure activities (such as digging in a garden or knitting). Activities that require repetitive wrist flexion, extension and circumduction, and those requiring forceful wrist flexion are problematic and often exacerbate the symptoms of carpal tunnel syndrome.

In addition to the physical symptoms and problems associated with carpal tunnel syndrome, patients may have psychosocial concerns. Some patients may fear that carpal tunnel syndrome will result in a permanent disability. Others may eliminate desired activities from their routine because of associated pain. Still others may fear losing a job if they are not able to return to work or require a modified workstation or schedule.

After treatment, many persons need to alter the way they do tasks or use specially designed or adapted tools. Tools that have larger or built up handles, tools with padded handles, and commercially available tools that are ergonomically designed are recommended. Additionally, patients may need to be educated to change the way they approach tasks. During task performance, patients should be encouraged to keep their wrist as straight (neutral) as possible. In this position the carpal tunnel is at its widest and alleviates pressure on the median nerve. Patients should be reminded not to repeat the same movement over a period of time and to take frequent rest breaks during activity. Sustained grip and pinch should be avoided if possible and patients should be encouraged to substitute their whole hand when grasping and carrying objects rather than relying on the thumb, index, and middle fingers. Patients should be encouraged to ask for help when engaging in activities that make the symptoms worse (AOTA, 2002).

Clinical Decision Making Process

Defining Focus for Intervention

The clinical findings are the primary determinant of the focus of OT treatment for patients with carpal tunnel syndrome. To reduce the compressive forces on the median nerve as it passes through the carpal tunnel, the physician may choose to use either a surgical or non-surgical (conservative) approach. Non-surgical or conservative methods rely on reducing the symptoms of carpal tunnel syndrome by modifying the patient's work station and activity pattern and splinting the wrist in a neutral position (Lisak, Personal communication, December 15, 2002). These OT strategies are complimented by anti-inflammatory medications that are prescribed by the physician. Surgical intervention is directed at the etiology of the condition. The carpal tunnel is opened by releasing the transverse carpal ligament, allowing more space for the median nerve. Following the surgical release of the carpal tunnel, the patient participates in an OT program that focuses on supporting the wrist and a systematic program to increase strength, coordination, and function in the areas of the hand supplied by the median nerve (Lisak, Personal communication, December 15, 2002).

Establishing Goals for Intervention

The goals for successful rehabilitation of patients with carpal tunnel syndrome are consistent whether they are receiving nonsurgical (conservative) treatment or surgical intervention. The overarching goals for intervention are:

- Reduce pain and paresthesias.
- Maintain or increase muscle strength.
- Maintain or improve hand function.
- Educate the patient.

Designing Theory-Based Intervention

Patients with carpal tunnel syndrome benefit from a program designed to use a combination of the biomechanical and the rehabilitation frames of reference. The biomechanical frame of reference is the driving force behind the components of a treatment plan designed to restore function in the hand by promoting wound healing, controlling edema, increasing strength and range of motion, and improving sensation and coordination. The rehabilitation frame of reference is instrumental in guiding the selection and design of the compensation techniques, adaptive equipment, work site modifications, and lifestyle changes that will be required to promote a symptom-free life for the patient.

Routine treatment for patients with carpal tunnel syndrome is protocol driven. It is important to note that treatment protocols for patients of this type are facility- as well as physician-specific. It is important to consult with the physician (most especially post-surgically) to inquire as to how the patient should be managed. A surgeon generally has a preferred method for the postsurgical care of a patient. For a patient being treated in a nonsurgical (conservative) way, the protocol may include all or a selection of the following:

- Fabrication of a wrist splint with the wrist positioned in a neutral position (Burke, Burke, Stewart, & Cambre, 1994). The splint remains in place and is removed only for hygiene and cleaning. Splint is worn for 3–4 weeks.
- The full time splinting regime described above is replaced after 3–4 weeks with a splint regime that requires the patient to wear the splint only at night for 3–4 weeks.
- The physician injects the carpal tunnel with steroids.
- Cryotherapy (cold compress) is applied to the wrist and hand by OT and by the patient as part of a home program.
- Iontophoresis
- The physician prescribes non-steroidal anti-inflammatory agents.

Evaluating Progress

For patients who present with mild symptoms, a conservative approach is tried first. The goal of this strategy is to see if the symptoms of carpal tunnel syndrome can be relieved without surgical intervention. The conservative approach, as described above, is deemed ineffective if the patient experiences persistent pain and parasthesias, the development or increase in atrophy of the thenar muscles, and continued loss of function. When conservative treatment is not found to be effective, the surgical approach is recommended. A surgical approach is also the first treatment of choice when a patient presents initially with moderate to severe symptoms. For a patient being treated post-surgery, the following offers a general protocol:

Table 17.1
Postsurgical Protocol

Days 1–14	Day 15	Day 24	Day 28
Wrist stabilization–neutral position	Sutures removed	Begin strengthening	Sensory evaluation and retraining
	Wrist AROM		Work hardening may begin
AROM to all digits	AROM to all digits		
	Scar management techniques		
	Edema control		
	Desensitization, if needed		

Determining Change in or Termination of Treatment

The surgical intervention is deemed to be successful if the symptoms of carpal tunnel syndrome (pain and parasthesias) are decreased, and hand function (including muscle strength, sensory status and coordination) are improved or restored.

Case Study

Description

RCM is a 45-year-old woman who is employed as a medical biller. A primary task of her job involves entering patient information and records into a computer billing system. She is a single woman who lives alone in a one-story ranch house. She was independent in all ALDs and IADLs. Additionally, she takes care of her home including mowing the lawn and completing minor home repairs. She is a gourmet cook and enjoys taking classes and cooking for her friends and family. About three months ago, she presented with symptoms of pain and tingling in her right (dominant) wrist and hand. An interview revealed that RCM had been experiencing these symptoms for several months. Pain in her wrist was waking her up at night, and she experienced pain, tingling, and numbness during the day as she entered data at work.

The doctor decided to treat her conservatively at first. After two months of a regime of splinting and medication, RCM continued to have symptoms. The physician then chose to do surgery and RCM had her carpal tunnel released. She has seen OT since that time following a postsurgical protocol. She has had a splint fabricated for her that places her wrist in a neutral position. She knows how to clean and apply it. She wears the splint to support her wrist when she is engaging in activities that require wrist flexion, extension, or circumduction. She has been educated in edema control techniques and scar massage. Her surgical site is healing well. On the 15th day after surgery, following protocol, RCM was instructed in tendon gliding and nerve gliding exercise and encouraged to do gentle AROM at the wrist (with no resistance) (Rozmaryn, Dovell, Rothman, Gorman, Olvey, & Bartko, 1998). In anticipation of returning to work, the OT has been discussing with RCM some of the things that she will need to consider and modifications that may need to be made to her work station to protect against reinjury. Some of the recommendations that RCM feels will be most helpful include:

- Adjusting the height of her chair to a position where her elbows are at her side with her forearms parallel to the floor.
- Using her whole arm and shoulder to control the computer mouse rather than relying on her wrist.
- Replacing her existing standard keyboard with one that is ergonomically designed to fit her hand.
- Remembering to rest her wrists on a padded surface when she is not actively entering data.
- Taking frequent breaks to rest her wrists and hands.
- Taking her splint to work for those times that she feels the need for extra support.

RCM has expressed that it will be "hard" to remember to take rest breaks during her busy day.

Long- and Short-Term Goals

The long-term goals of the postoperative phase of treatment for RCM are to exhibit hand function (strength, sensation, endurance, coordination) sufficient to complete ADLs and IADLs independently; incorporate proper wrist positioning into all self-care, work, and leisure activities; incorporate frequent rest breaks into all self-care, work, and leisure activities; utilize a wrist splint for support as needed during activities that require forceful wrist flexion; and continue to monitor her wrist for symptoms of reoccurring carpal tunnel syndrome.

RCM will reach these goals in part through successfully achieving the following short-term goals:

1. Exhibit full AROM in the wrist and fingers.
2. Demonstrate and describe the proper neutral position for the wrist.
3. Describe the list of symptoms related to carpal tunnel syndrome.
4. Identify times during her work day when she will be able to rest.
5. Demonstrate the ability to properly position her chair, incorporate her elbow and shoulder into mouse use, and select an ergonomically designed keyboard.
6. Demonstrate proper technique for tendon gliding exercises.
7. Demonstrate proper technique for nerve gliding exercises.
8. Demonstrate proper use of splint for wrist support.

Therapist Goals and Strategies

The therapist's goals include:

1. Provide support to healing surgical site.
2. Reduce or prevent edema.
3. Manage scar formation.
4. Increase strength and restore hand function.
5. Teach compensation techniques and adaptive strategies to reduce stress and compression of the carpal tunnel.
6. Assess patient for adaptive devices that will provide proper wrist support and promote function.
7. Complete work station evaluation and make recommendations for work site modification.

The therapist's strategies include:

1. Construct splint that supports the wrist in a neutral position.
2. Teach patient edema control techniques to be incorporated into a home program.
3. Teach scar management techniques.
4. Provide a graded exercise program designed to increase muscle strength and restore hand function.
5. Teach patient tendon and nerve gliding exercises to be incorporated into a home program.
6. Teach patient proper positions and approaches to activity for both home and work.
7. Complete work site assessment and recommendations.
8. Provide patient education.

Activity

Cream Cheese Mints

RCM needs to increase strength and maintain the mobility that has been gained through the tendon gliding, nerve gliding, and active exercises. Activities that include flexion and extension of the wrist against light resistance, circumduction of the wrist, opening and closing of the hand, extending the thumb and opposing the thumb and middle finger are appropriate choices during this time. The procedure for making cream cheese mints fits these criteria. As RCM kneads the mixture of powdered sugar, cream cheese, and mint flavoring mixed in a zip lock bag, the therapist observes for wrist position, reinforces rest breaks, and recommends the application of the splint as appropriate. The fact that the cream cheese mint mixture is in a zip lock bag allows for the kneading to be stopped and started at any time. The mixture may be stored for up to a week before molding, therefore this activity provides an appropriate context for educating the patient on wrist position, rest breaks, and splint application. For RCM, making cream cheese mints is also consistent with her interest in cooking and may provide the opportunity for her to identify other cooking tasks that may be modified or adapted in the future.

Treatment Objectives

The objective for this session is to engage the patient in an activity that provides gentle exercise to the wrist, thumb, and fingers while at the same time providing the opportunity to reinforce important patient education concepts regarding wrist position, splint application, and activity pacing.

Resources

The following resources can be helpful for gathering clinical data:

- MMT
- Sensory test
- ROM
- Coordination test

The following are common practice settings:

- Outpatient rehabilitation services

The following resources can be helpful for gathering sociopolitical data:

- Workers compensation offices
- ADA

The following can be helpful in managing and understanding lifestyle/lifespan issues:

- Work site
- Job responsibilities
- Activity patterns

Internet and Published Resources

American Occupational Therapy Association:
www.aota.org

Carpal Tunnel Syndrome: A Guide to Daily Activities, American Occupational Therapy Association

References

American Occupational Therapy Association (2002). *Carpal tunnel syndrome: A guide to daily activities.* Upper Marlboro, MD: AOTA Press.

Burke, D. T., Burke, M. M., Stewart, G. W., & Cambre, A. (1994). Splinting for carpal tunnel syndrome: In search of the optimal angle. *Archives of Physical Medicine and Rehabilitation, 75*(11), 1241–1244.

Derbery, V. J., & Howard, L. L. (1998). Management of the painful arm: Cumulative trauma revised. *Physical Medicine and Rehabilitation: State of the Art Reviews, 12*(2), 215–224.

Fast, C. (1995). Repetitive strain injury: An overview of the condition and its implications for occupational therapy practice. *Canadian Journal of Occupational Therapy, 62*(3), 119–126.

Headley, B., & Singer, G. (1998). Carpal tunnel syndrome: Making the right diagnosis. *Advance for Occupational Therapy, 4*(14), 18–30.

Rozmaryn, L.M., Dovell, S., Rothman, E. F., Gorman, K., Olvey, K. M. & BArtko, J. J. (1998). Nerve and tendon gliding exercises and the conservative management of carpal tunnel syndrome. *Journal of Hand Therapy, 11*(3), 171–179.

Vender, M. I., Truppa, K. L., Ruder, J. R., & Pomerance, J. (1998). Upper extremity compressive neuropathies. *Physical Medicine and Rehabilitation: State of the Art Reviews, 12*(2), 243–262.

Verdugo, R. J., Salinas, R. S. & Cea, J. (2002). Surgical versus non-surgical treatment for carpal tunnel syndrome (Cochrane Review). *The Cochrane Library, 4*. Chichester, UK: John Wiley & Sons, Ltd.

Substance Abuse 18

Nancy Beck, MA, OTR/L
C. Thomas North, Ph.D., OTR/L

Synopsis of Clinical Condition

Prevalence and Etiology

Substance abuse is a complex problem with physiological and psychological ramifications. Physiological dependency means that the body requires repeated use of the substance to maintain physiological homeostasis. The structuring of behavior around the habitual use of the substance constitutes psychological dependency. Alcohol, barbiturates benzodiazepines, cocaine, opiates, amphetamines, methamphetamines, cannabis, and hallucinogens are substances that are frequently abused. The number of persons at risk for alcohol abuse is greater than other substances because alcohol is a legal substance and readily available. Illegal substances or street drugs pose additional risks in that they may have additives such as arsenic or other lethal agents.

Metabolic processes and the structural integrity of the central nervous system are frequently compromised as a result of long-term substance abuse (Sadock & Sadock, 2003).

Common Characteristics and Symptoms

Alcohol intoxication is characterized by animation and elevation of mood followed by reduced reaction time, impaired coordination, slurred speech, depressed affect, and, eventually, unconsciousness. Withdrawal may be characterized by dehydration, nausea, hypersensitivity to sound or light, and psychomotor impairment. There is a 20% fatality rate associated with untreated alcoholism (Sadock & Sadock, 2003).

Sedatives, hypnotics, and anxiolytics include barbiturates (secobarbital, phenobarbital) and benzodiazepines (Ativan™, Halcion™, Valium™, Xanax™). Barbiturate abuse occurs in two forms. The first is considered chronic and frequently the result of dependency upon a prescription. The second form is episodic and usually related to recreational use. These substances are usually taken orally, but they also can be taken intravenously. With injection, there is an added risk of HIV, hepatitis, or other infections from the use of contaminated needles. Barbiturate abuse is associated with increased risk for lethal overdose resulting from respiratory depression. It is also associated with suicide related to the progressively severe dyphoric episodes associated with reduced drug levels between dosages. As therapeutic use of benzodiazepines replaces barbiturates, the risk of lethal overdose is greatly decreased as the user will most likely doze off before he or she has ingested enough to have lethal effects. However, dependency with benzodiazepines is similar to that of barbiturates. If the patient has been treated with a moderate to high dose of a benzodiazepine, medical staff will attempt to gradually reduce the dosage. Immediate cessation should be avoided (Sadock & Sadock, 2003).

Opiates (morphine, heroin, codeine, methadone) are central nervous system depressants that precipitate dysphoria on the first use and euphoria on subsequent uses. Additional reactions are psycho-motor retardation, drowsiness, impaired memory, and decreased attention. Signs of overdose include coma, pinpoint pupils, and decreased respiration. Withdrawal is characterized by elevated blood pressure, tachycardia, fluctuations in temperature, cramps, aching, and fluid loss through diarrhea, lacrimation, and rhinorrhea. Medical intervention includes administration of another opiate, such as methadone, to facilitate withdrawal. The patient under treatment for withdrawal experiences flu-like symptoms and depression (Sadock & Sadock, 2003).

Cocaine is classed with opiates even though it is a stimulant. Its use is associated with a quick, euphoric high that is often followed by depression and suicidal ideation. It is highly addictive, and death from overdose is usually due to heart attack. This drug can be ingested, inhaled, or injected. Crack is a freebase form of cocaine; it is extremely potent, and persons have been known to become addicted after one or two uses (Sadock & Sadock, 2003). Ten separate diagnoses have been developed to label conditions that result from cocaine abuse: Cocaine Withdrawal, Cocaine Intoxication Delirium, Cocaine-induced Psychotic Disorder with Delusions, Cocaine-induced Psychotic Disorder with Hallucinations, Cocaine-induced Mood Disorder, Cocaine-induced Anxiety Disorder, Cocaine-induced Sexual Dysfunction, Cocaine-induced Sleep Disorder, and Cocaine Induced Disorder Not Otherwise Specified (*DSM–IV–TR*, 2000). Intoxication is characterized by euphoria, increased perception of self, and increased endurance. Withdrawal from crack/cocaine is characterized by agitation and irritability. Recovery is usually within 48 hours, with depression continuing for several weeks (Sadock & Sadock, 2003).

In the U.S., amphetamines (Dexedrine™, Desoxyn™, Adderall™, Ritalin™) are the third most widely used drugs after cannabis and cocaine. Drugs containing amphetamines have been used as stimulants, weight loss aids, cold remedies, and as treatment for attention deficit/hyperactivity disorder and narcolepsy. Amphetamines are contraindicated for those with hypertension and are habit forming. They have been known to induce a toxic psychosis, and can be fatal (Sadock & Sadock, 2003). Amphetamine intoxication resembles that of cocaine. The typical dependency picture is one of weight loss and paranoid ideation. Withdrawal symptoms include anxiety, tremors, dysphoric mood, lethargy, fatigue, nightmares, headache, excess perspiration, stomach cramps, muscle cramps, and ravenous appetite. Depression can be a reaction to long-term, high dose use and can lead to suicide (Sadock & Sadock, 2003).

Cannabis (marijuana, hashish, hemp, ganga, bhang), is the most frequently used illicit substance (Sadock & Sadock, 2003). Although the evidence for physiological addiction is weak, a high potential for psychological addiction exists. As tolerance is developed, a withdrawal syndrome, including irritability, restlessness, insomnia, and anorexia will be experienced once the drug is stopped (Zickler, 2000).

Hallucinogens (natural: psilocybin from mushrooms, mescaline from peyote cactus; synthetic: lysergic acid diethylamide—LSD) are sometimes called psychedelics or psychotomimetics because they mimic psychosis (Sadock & Sadock, 2003). Hallucinogenic intoxication includes paranoia, anxiety or depression, fear of loss of control, impaired judgement, distorted perceptions, depersonalization, derealization, and hallucinations. Physiological changes may include: pupillary dilation, tachycardia profuse perspiration, palpitations, blurred vision, tremors, and/or incoordination. Approximately 10% of the American public have used a hallucinogen at least once, and more than 50% were less than 20 years of age. Relative to other illicit substances, hallucinogens are related to less morbidity and less mortality (*DSM–IV–TR*, 2000).

Target Areas for Intervention

Over the long-term, behaviors related to substance dependency take precedence over those associated with more productive life roles (Sadock & Sadock, 2003). The focus of occupational therapy intervention is on the facilitation of the patient's ability to chose more adaptive, substance-free methods of dealing with the stressors of daily life.

Contextual Considerations

Clinical

The context of the dependency and the type of substance used will affect the tenacity of the condition and its long-term ramifications. For instance, the patients with a physical or emotional condition who inadvertently become dependent upon substances because of "self-medication" will be more likely to have the insight and motivation to become independent of the substances than those who have a life style and life history of consistent substance abuse. For the latter, a self-concept of being sober is foreign and may be sufficiently uncomfortable to discourage investment in recovery. A history of the client's substance use can help to alert the practitioner to the existence of substance dependence.

Alcoholics and most drug abusers present with somewhat different symptoms. Alcoholics and clients who abuse other depressants often present with a quiet and compliant demeanor when not actively using. They often have difficulty expressing their feelings and seek alcohol as an outlet.

Clients who abuse amphetamines are often highly distractible, demanding, talkative, impulsive, and moody. The drive to use and abuse substances is a powerful force that continually lures them back into active use even as they pursue recovery. Many long-term users may go through detoxification programs and participate in rehabilitation programs in order to support their drug dependency. By lowering their drug tolerance, they can achieve a "high" on smaller doses, thereby lowering the cost of the habit.

A study by Volkow (Zickler, 2002) found that, compared with participants who never used the drug, methamphetamine abusers had reduced control of movement, attention, and motivation. This loss of judgement may explain the tendency of substance abusers to engage in risky behaviors related to their addictions without regard for the dangers that may befall themselves or others.

Long-term substance abuse can result in permanent changes to neurological structures causing conditions such as dementia and related short-term memory deficits and/or permanent damage to respiratory, gastrointestinal, liver, or cardiac systems.

The Mini-Mental Status Exam (MMSE) (Folstein, Folstein, & McHugh, 1975) uses short-term memory function as an indicator of degree of dementia. Two things should be noted: 1) patients who may be agitated or depressed, as may be seen in intoxication or withdrawal, can produce a score that is lower than their actual capacities; 2) short-term memory may provide an indicator of capacity for learning, but does not provide information about the patient's ability to function.

The Routine Task Inventory (RTI) (Allen, Earhart, & Blue, 1992) and The Allen Cognitive Levels Test (Allen, 1990) are practical performance measures. The Allen Cognitive Levels Test (Allen, 1990) assesses cognitive capacity, or an ability to learn, and it uses such landmark phenomena as error recognition, use of three dimensional concepts, and ability to problem solve. Again, agitation and depression may produce a lower score than the patient's capacity. Also, it does not provide information about how the patient may have adapted. Low scores, especially those below 5.0, indicate that the patient is limited in understanding cause and effect, and is therefore at risk for safety. The Kohlman Evaluation of Living Skills (KELS) (Kohlman, 1992) is a tool used to assess the patient's instrumental activities of daily living (IADL). It is not unusual for someone with a low score on the ACL to perform moderately well on the KELS. However, it is fairly consistent that a low ACL will accompany a poor performance on the safety measures on the KELS.

The Occupational Case Assessment and Inventory Rating Scale (OCAIRS)(Kaplan & Kielhofner, 1989), is a useful tool to get a view of the patient's perception of his or her role within the household, as well as how the substance dependence has effected others.

Because of the complexities listed above, assessment is less straightforward than in many other conditions. Because of the feelings of inadequacy that may have encouraged the person to use drugs, or the feelings of guilt from being dependent, a Role Checklist (Oakley, Kielhofner, & Barris, 1986) may be helpful in determining the patient's perception of self. Something like the OCAIRS (Kaplan & Kielhofner, 1989) may provide some insight into the patient's perception of how others see him or her, and how this impacts his or her behavior.

If a client has a long history of substance abuse, dementia should always be considered. An MMSE (Folstein, Folstein, and McHugh, 1975) will help to identify possible dementia, but it focuses primarily on short-term memory function as an indicator. A score on the MMSE below 26 is a strong indicator of possible dementia. The ACL (Allen, 1990) is a good performance assessment. If the person performs poorly (below 5.0), it may be useful to follow up with a KELS (Kohlman, 1992) or an RTI (Allen, Earhart, & Blue, 1992). If the patient does well on these performance tests, then he or she may be able to use old skills effectively but have difficulty with learning new skills. However, a low ACL score or low MMSE reflect an impaired capacity for learning, which creates a safety risk as he or she cannot adequately grasp cause and effect.

Family

A comprehensive assessment of the social support systems available to the patient and the patient's insight regarding the family impact of substance abuse yields important information regarding the scope of intervention. The support systems available to the patient can either represent a strong barrier to rehabilitation or provide a strong impetus for recovery. If others in the household tolerate or condone the substance abuse, the enabling behaviors and codependent relationships that are engendered by these attitudes may complicate the rehabilitation effort. Conversely, recovery is facilitated by family and friends who are actively engaged in reinforcing a substance-free lifestyle.

There is a considerable amount of literature on the effects of substances upon children whose mothers used substances while pregnant. Learning disabilities, Attention Deficit

Disorder (ADD), and Attention Deficit Hyperactivity Disorder (ADHD) have all been shown to be related to substance abuse during pregnancy.

Family members may not be willing to trust and support substance abusers through repeated attempts at recovery. Although the clients may be demanding, they are frequently masking a sense of being undeserving of care. They often have difficulty recognizing success, don't trust success, and often unconsciously sabotage the successes they make in the recovery process. Habitual behaviors have led the clients to hide their feelings and hurt others before the others hurt them, hence they have few nonabusing friends. They often blame others for their problems and see life as devoid of meaning.

Family education increases the understanding of the addiction phenomenon. Alcoholics Anonymous (AA), Narcotics Anonymous (NA), Alateen, and Al-Anon are examples of support groups.

Practice Setting

An occupational therapy practitioner can expect to work with clients who are abusing or dependent on substances in any setting (schools, hospitals, community programs, assisted living centers, etc.) and in any age group (children through geriatrics).

The problem of substance abuse can occur due to or in addition to other problems. Persons with substance abuse problems may be encountered in homeless shelters, the prison population, and physical medicine and rehabilitation facilities. Any hospital facility may provide detoxification services for those undergoing withdrawal. Drug rehabilitation can be provided only in a designated facility which may be freestanding and often will neither provide nor allow medications.

Sociopolitical

The practice setting for those suffering from substance abuse is determined by reimbursement regulations. The coverage available for treatment of substance dependence is variable. Private insurance will often pay for detoxification programs and may provide for rehabilitation. Those who are gainfully employed by a moderate to large organization will have access to employee assistance programs (EAP). These programs will provide counseling and may also pay for treatment. The allotment will depend upon the company. Often, the coverage for rehabilitation is predetermined by days per year, or lifetime days. Comorbidity units are available and funded by some third party payors. Comorbidity is a label to describe persons with substance dependence as well as a psychiatric disorder.

Government funding for substance abuse programs began to diminish in the late 1990's and early 2000's as public and political trends became more punitive. In response to the increase of drug related crimes, the government started to allocate more funds for building prisons and detention centers than supporting rehabilitation programs for substance abusers. This changing attitude with its lack of sympathy for the frightening and enduring struggle which recovering substance abusers face, is leading to fewer programs, harsher laws governing illegal acts committed while under the influence of substances, and a reliance on free self-help programs like Alcoholics Anonymous (AA). The change in public attitude also leads to a limited number of private funding sources to support the recovery process.

Lifestyle/Lifespan

Dependence upon a substance can be a life-changing event. Because it is an expensive habit that becomes more expensive as the patient becomes more dependent, financial resources are soon exhausted. When abusing drugs, the patient is not as functional, and may have trouble keeping a job. Persons who are recovering from opiate addiction may require a lifelong dependence upon methadone. Dementia and physical deterioration limit the ability to adapt to the demands and stresses of everyday life. Physical and psychological isolation is a common outcome.

Clinical Decision Making Process

Defining Focus for Intervention

In the early stages of recovery, the focus of OT intervention is education about the recovery process and engagement in activity that rekindles a sense of self-efficacy and hope for the future. As treatment continues, the emphasis shifts to self-expression, the development of coping strategies, and exploration of aftercare plans. Clients need to experience feelings and activities that are related to their recovery and identify healthy ways to get support, express their feelings, have fun, find excitement in living, cope with stress, and find peace within themselves.

Ongoing treatment in the community focuses on many of the above issues as well as practical issues like finding or continuing employment, relationship building skills, recreational and stress reduction skills, and building healthy support systems.

Prisons and other correctional or forensic facilities are sites where OT practitioners may work with substance abusers. The goals and expectations of treatment are not always geared toward discharge, but paced in accordance with the stressors present in the facility and the lengths of the sentences of the clients. A goal may be to help the prisoner find ways to function safely and effectively without substances within the correctional facility.

Establishing Goals for Intervention

The goals for treatment need to be practical and understandable to the client. When the clients are part of the goal planning, they feel a stronger sense of control in their treatment. The treatment becomes meaningful to them and can increase their level of participation. Common issues around which goals are developed are: anger management, stress management and outlets for feelings, effective self-expression and communication, building support systems, awareness of self and values, spirituality, relational skills, education on symptoms of relapse, relapse prevention, wellness, and self-care. Each of these issues becomes a meaningful goal when it is coupled with particular events or personal stressors.

Designing Theory-Based Intervention

Theoretical frameworks with a basis in learning theories such as a developmental model or one that address roles and values like the Model of Human Occupation, effectively guide the OT practitioner in developing interventions for treatment of substance abusers. The habituated process of developing a dependence on substances and the associated roles and distorted values developed through an addiction require a major life change as the client works toward recovery. Each of these theoretical models guide the OT in understanding the development of the aberrant behaviors and the enduring process of changing the ingrained habits the substance dependent client has developed. As with goal planning, the clients need to be involved in understanding their actions. Feedback from the assessments the OT does with the clients is the basis for their self-discovery. The feedback needs to be direct, honest, and supportive even when the information is difficult to hear.

In a psychiatric hospital or psychiatric unit in a general hospital, the patients will have co-occurring disorders, a combination of substance abuse and a mental illness like schizoaffective disorder or depression. Allen Cognitive Level Theory (Allen, Earhart, and Blue, 1992) is helpful in determining the functional level of the client and impacting the course of treatment in a meaningful way.

Evaluating Progress

The move from one phase of recovery to the next and finally to discharge is determined by the client's progressive and consistent application of adaptive coping strategies. Engagement in community-based support groups may aid in the transition to after care. Termination occurs when the client has abstained from substances for a specified period of time, has realistic plans for post-discharge, and has arranged to follow up with a supporting organization.

Determining Change in or Termination of Treatment

Long-term effects of treatment are difficult to evaluate due to the high incidence of recidivism among substance abusers. The occupational therapist assesses the clients' progress in treatment by listening to what they say and observing their approach to tasks and activities. In concert with other members of the rehabilitation team, the occupational therapist ascertains the congruency and consistency of the clients' words and actions.

Case Study

Description

Sabina is a 33-year-old woman who has been addicted to cocaine for four years. She quit work as a lawyer to raise her three children who are four, six, and nine years old. Her husband works quite a distance from the home and stays near the office three nights per week. She doesn't think she has any friends or other supports. Her brother also abuses cocaine, using her money to pay for the cocaine that he buys for her. She frequently supplements her cocaine use with alcohol to increase the high or when she runs out of cocaine. She thinks she has hidden her addiction from her family by only using when the children are at school and her husband is at work. Her children and husband have noticed a change in her (she appeared slovenly and seemed distant and secretive), but didn't question it until a neighbor told Sabina's husband that Sabina had not been picking up the four-year-old from daycare. Sabina tried outpatient treatment, but didn't like it. She tried Cocaine Anonymous, but thought she was better than the people there and could just quit anytime on her own. She continued using saying, "I don't really have a problem. Everyone is making too big a deal out of a little recreational cocaine." Her husband found her unconscious on the kitchen floor when he came home for a weekend. After having her stomach pumped at a local hospital, she was diagnosed with Major Depressive Disorder and Substance Abuse Disorder and admitted to a psychiatric hospital co-occurring disorder unit. Denying her problem, she angrily blames her brother "for getting me into this." Trying to rationalize her addiction, she complains of being "bored and lonely at home." Recognizing the effect of her addiction on her family, she expresses feelings of shame for hurting the people she loves, saying, "I don't deserve their love." A Role Checklist (Oakley, Kielhofner, & Barris, 1986) assessment shows she highly values her family, home, being productive at work and hobbies, spiritual life, and being a friend. Due to her depression, she sees no hope for the future, as she is unable to identify roles she has in the present or future. She has doubts that she will ever be able to live without using.

Long- and Short-Term Goals

The long-term goal of intervention for Sabina is to identify and pursue meaningfully satisfying activities that are healthy and practical alternatives to using cocaine while in an intensive outpatient program.

This goal will be reached in part through successfully achieving the short-term goal of identifying meaningful activities she can do with her family.

Therapist Goals and Strategies

The therapist's goals include:

1. Stimulate Sabina to think about her role in the family.
2. Rekindle Sabina's interests in doing activities without using cocaine.
3. Facilitate Sabina's recognition of her self-worth.

The therapist's strategies include:

1. Provide concrete evidence of Sabina's interests and roles in the family through activity.
2. Facilitate Sabina's self-reflection through group process and direct, honest feedback.

Activity

Spiritual Daisy

In a group setting, each member will use construction paper, magic markers, and glue to create a large daisy-like flower with a center circle identifying his/her primary support person, whom they value. Sabina picked her husband. The group members are asked to write an activity that each enjoys doing with this support person on each of the 6 petals of the daisy, and glue the petals to the daisy. When the daisies are complete, each member, in turn, will display his or her daisy and explain what each has created. The facilitated discussion will support the group members in helping each other clarify what they have written, discuss ways to overcome obstacles that prevent them from doing the activities, and make suggestions for other ways they can connect to their support person.

Sabina feels worthless and is doubtful that she can gain a sense of control over her addiction and relationships with her family. Sabina's habituated lifestyle does not include a feeling of productivity in any area, although being productive is very important to her. Her addiction has consumed her leisure and reduced her ability to relate effectively to her family and friends. She has become neglectful of herself and her responsibilities. She has a history of successful functioning and a caring and potentially supportive family. The addiction coupled with the depression has distorted her self-concept and ability to recognize and address problems effectively. She is bright, well educated and able to engage in logical, sequential thought process if given a rational basis for processing.

Sabina, like many addicts, denies or rationalizes the extent of her habit and the hypnotic lure of the cocaine. The change in lifestyle that recovery demands is overwhelming and frightening for Sabina. Her impulsive actions and thoughts make it difficult for her to accept that there are no quick cures for the addiction. The lack of spiritual energy in her life makes the ordinariness of everyday living seem boring. She will need to make strong connections with her healthy values and roles while in treatment in order to embrace a future without cocaine that seems worth living to her.

Treatment Objective

Sabina will identify six activities she can do without using cocaine and accept feedback from her peers about her choices.

Resources

The following resources can be helpful for gathering clinical data:

History of abuse, related conditions including:

- What substance(s)
- Length of time
- Intoxication, dependent, or withdrawal
- Neurological or organ tissue involvement
- Comorbidity

Assessments:

- ACL
- RTI
- KELS
- OCAIRS
- MMSE

The following resources can be helpful for gathering family data:

- Family interview
- Family history

The following resources are common practice settings:

- Acute care general for detox or withdrawal
- D & A rehabilitation
- Prisons
- Shelters
- PM&R settings
- Support groups
- Dual diagnosis (Comorbidity) units

The following resources can be helpful for gathering sociopolitical data:

- Employee assistance programs
- Private insurance

The following issues can be helpful in understanding and managing lifestyle/lifespan issues:

Financial needs:

- Resources lost supporting habit
- Problems with keeping a job

Medical needs:

- Comorbidity
- Possible dementia
- Possible organ damage

Personal adaptation

Support system

Family, friends, support groups such as AA, NA, Alateen, Al-Anon.

Internet Resources

Al-Anon/Alateen:
www.al-anon.alateen.org

Alcoholics Anonymous (AA):
www.alcoholics-anonymous.org

Narcotics Anonymous (NA):
www.na.org

National Institute on Alcohol Abuse and Alcoholism
www.niaaa.nih.gov

The National Institute for Drug Abuse (NIDA):
www.drugabuse.gov/NIDA_Notes

References

Allen, C.K. (1990). *Allen cognitive level test.* Colchester, CN: S&S Worldwide.

Allen, C. K., Earhart, C. A., & Blue, T. (1992). *Occupational therapy treatment goals for the physically and cognitively disabled.* Rockville, MD: The American Occupational Therapy Association.

American Psychiatric Association. (2000). *Diagnostic and statistical manual of mental disorders* (4th ed., text revision). Washington, DC: Author.

Folstein, M. F., Folstein, S, & McHugh, P. R. (1975). Mini-mental state: A practical method for grading the cognitive state of patients for the clinician. *Journal of Psychiatric Research, 12,* 189.

Kaplan, K. & Kielhofner, G. (1989). *Occupational case analysis, interview, and rating scale.* Thorofare, NJ: Slack Incorporated.

Kohlman, L. T. (1992). *Kohlman evaluation of living skills.* Rockville, MD: American Occupational Therapy Association.

Mathias, R. (2003). New approaches seek to expand Naltrexone use in heroin treatment. *NIDA Notes, 17*(6) March. http://165.112.78.61/MDA_notes/NNVol17N6/Approaches.html

Oakley, F., Kielhofner, G. & Barris, R. (1986). The role checklist. *Occupational Therapy Journal of Research, 6,* 157–170.

Sadock, B. J., & Sadock, V.A. (2003). *Kaplan and Sadock's synopsis of psychiatry: Behavioral sciences/ clinical psychiatry* (9th ed.). Baltimore: Williams & Wilkins.

Waxman, S. G., & DeGroot, J. (2000). *Correlative neuroanatomy* (24th ed.). Norwalk, CT: Appleton and Lange.

World Health Organization. (1992). *International statistical classification of diseases and related health problems.* Geneva, Switzerland: Author.

Zickler, P. (2000). Evidence accumulates that long-term marijuana users experience withdrawal. *NIDA Notes, 15*(1), March. http://165.112.78.61/NIDA_notes/NNV0l15Nl/Evidence.html

Zickler, P. (2001). Cues for cocaine and normal pleasures activate common brain sites. *NIDA Notes, 16*(2), May. http://165.112.78.61/NIDA_notes/NNVol16N2/cues.html

Zickler, P. (2002). Methamphetamine abuse linked to impaired cognitive and motor skills despite recovery of dopamine transporters. *NIDA Notes, 17*(1), April. http://165.112.78.61/NIDA_notes/NNVol17Nl/Methamphetamine.html

Schizophrenia and Related Disorders

19

C. Thomas North, Ph.D., OTR/L
Nancy Beck, MA, OTR/L

Synopsis of Clinical Condition

Prevalence and Etiology

Thought disorders (psychoses) represent some of the most serious mental disorders. They include Schizophrenia and the other psychoses. Typically, they develop early in life and are chronic. The disorders in this grouping are characterized by a predominance of psychotic symptoms. Psychotic symptoms may be present in other disorders such as the mood disorders and the dementias, but as secondary features. The disorders to be discussed in this chapter are:

- Schizophrenia
- Schizophreniform Disorder
- Schizoaffective Disorders
- Delusional Disorder

Diagnosis is dependent upon psychiatric history and the mental status exam. No single characteristic is definitive. *DSM–IV–TR* (American Psychiatric Association, 2000) lists five primary symptoms of Schizophrenia. Of these symptoms, the patient must experience at least two, and they must be present in some combination for more than six months. Employment, social interaction, or self-care must be impaired significantly as a result of the symptoms. All other disorders must be ruled out.

Common Characteristics and Symptoms

The five primary or positive symptoms are delusions, hallucinations, disorganized speech, and grossly disorganized or catatonic behavior. Negative symptoms may also be present and include flattened or dulled affect, poverty of speech, apathy, anhedonia, withdrawal, and inattentiveness. If delusions are bizarre, no other symptoms are necessary for the diagnosis of Schizophrenia (*DSM–IV–TR*, 2000). Similarly, if the hallucinations are auditory and consist of a running commentary of the patient's thoughts or behaviors, or are a conversation of two or more voices, no other symptoms are necessary. Sadock & Sadock (2003) states that auditory hallucinations are by far the most frequent of hallucinatory symptoms. They strongly suggest that if the patient experiences gustatory, olfactory, or tactile hallucinations that the clinician should suspect a neurological (dementia or delirium) or physical cause before diagnosing Schizophrenia.

There are five subtypes of Schizophrenia. Paranoid Type is characterized by a predominance of delusions and possibly hallucinations, but with a minimum of disturbance of speech, thought, disorganized or catatonic behavior, or affect.

If the patient's predominant symptoms are disorganized speech, disorganized behavior, and disturbed affect, the appropriate diagnosis would be Schizophrenia Disorganized Type. A third subtype is Schizophrenia Catatonic type. A patient with this diagnosis can exhibit:

- motoric immobility or stupor,
- excessive or purposeless activity,
- extreme negativism or muteness,
- peculiar posturing, stereotyped movements, peculiar mannerisms, or grimacing, or
- echolalia or echopraxia.

At least two symptoms from this list are necessary to make the diagnosis. The most typical manifestation of Schizophrenia is the Undifferentiated Type. This label is applied if most of the criteria for Schizophrenia apply, and none are sufficiently prominent to be labeled as Catatonic Type, Paranoid Type, or Disorganized Type. Schizophrenia Residual Type differs from the others in that there is a preponderance of negative symptoms, while positive symptoms are virtually absent (*DSM–IV–TR*, 2000).

The major differences between Schizophreniform Disorder and Schizophrenia are the duration of symptoms and the level of impairment. In Schizophreniform Disorder, the duration exceeds a month, but is less than six months and does not usually precipitate a significant change in social, occupational, or self-care function. (*DSM–IV–TR*, 2000). Between 60% and 80% of persons diagnosed with Schizophreniform Disorder will progress to Schizophrenia (Sadock & Sadock, 2003).

The diagnosis of Schizoaffective Disorder is somewhat complex. The patient must carry the symptoms that would diagnose him or her with Schizophrenia, and at some point concurrently experience Depressive Episode, Manic Episode, or Mixed Episode (see chapter 20, Depressive Disorders). Although delusions or hallucinations must be present, they must be in the absence of the mood symptoms. Delusional Disorder is a condition that is also known as Paranoia, Paranoid Psychosis, or Paranoid State. The *DSM–IV–TR* (2000) criteria are: presence of non-bizarre delusions for at least a month, possible presence of delusion-congruent tactile or olfactory hallucinations (other schizophrenic symptoms are absent), minimal impairment of functioning, and mood episodes (if present) are brief relative to delusional periods. In both instances, substance use and medical causes must be ruled out (*DSM–IV–TR*, 2000).

Worldwide, the prevalence of Schizophrenia is between 0.5% and 1.5% of the population. The age of onset in men occurs in the late teens or early twenties, and onset in women is more commonly a decade later. Onset may be insidious or abrupt. There is typically a prodromal phase, which is characterized by a decrease in hygiene, social withdrawal, and loss of interest in school or work. Some individuals may remain chronically ill, while others may experience remissions and exacerbations. Full recovery is uncommon.

Among those factors associated with a better prognosis are: good premorbid adjustment, acute onset, later onset, retention of insight, precipitating events, presence of mood disorder symptoms, good family support, education beyond high school, and marriage. Factors associated with poor prognosis include: early onset, no precipitating factors, insidious onset, poor premorbid adjustment, history of negative symptoms prior to diagnosis, lack of meaningful social relationships, family history of Schizophrenia, poor support systems, no remissions within three years, numerous relapses, and limited education. The risk of violent outbursts accompanying hallucinatory or delusional behavior is greater if there is a history of violent behavior and persecutory delusions. It is estimated that about 50% of persons with Schizophrenia attempt suicide, and 20% to 30% of that number are successful. The causes of suicide in this group may include an underlying depression, a sense of emptiness, auditory hallucinations and/or a belief that suicide is an escape from painful hallucinations or delusions (Sadock & Sadock, 2003).

The causes of Schizophrenia are unknown. Recent research suggests that Schizophrenia is not one disease, but possibly several different diseases with different causes that manifest as similar disorders. It has been speculated that factors such as dopamine processing, seratonin imbalance, and viral infection may be linked to schizophrenia.

Schizophrenia is a complex disorder and a result of biochemical and psycho-social factors (Sadock & Sadock, 2003). The occupational therapist should be aware of the side effects of the pharmacological treatments used with this population. Antipsychotic medications fall into two major groups: the Dopamine Receptor Agonists, and the Serotonin-dopamine Antagonists. The Dopamine Receptor Agonists (DRAs) (Thorazine™, Stelazine™, Prolixin™, Mellaril™, Serentil™, Navane™, Loxitane™, Moban™, Haldol™) were formulated to control the positive symptoms of psychosis such as delusions and hallucinations. These medications have unpleasant side effects such as akathisia (increased muscular tension resulting in restlessness) and Parkinson-like tremors and rigidity (extra pyramidal signs). Possible serious side effects include tardive dyskinesia (involuntary movement disorder involving puckering of lips and tongue and writhing of extremities) (Merck Research Laboratories, 1999) and neuroleptic malignant syndrome (rigidity, fever, autonomic instability, potentially fatal) (Merck Research Laboratories, 1999).

The Serotonin-Dopamine Antagonists (SDAs; Clozaril™ [clozapine], Risperdal™ [risperidone], Zyprexa™ [olanzapine]) treat the positive and negative symptoms of psychosis. Patients on SDAs have fewer relapses and less hospitalizations than patients who are not. (Sadock & Sadock, 2003). The adverse effects of clozapine include: dizziness, sedation, tachycardia, hypotension, EKG changes, nausea, sialorrhea (excessive salivation), anticholinergic effects, and muscle weakness. At high doses, there is a 4% risk of seizures. Blood disorders (leukopenia, granulocytopenia, agranulocytosis) occur in less than 1% of the patients, but are potentially lethal (Sadock & Sadock, 2003).

Target Areas for Intervention

Foci for occupational therapy intervention include the development of functional interactive and self-care skills, reality orientation, and task modification to compensate for disorders in judgment and organization.

Contextual Considerations

Clinical

Persons with Schizophrenia have difficulty with social interaction, new learning, and comprehending causality. The *Allen Cognitive Level Test* (ACL) (Allen, 1990) provides information regarding the patient's capacity for learning unfamiliar tasks. The *Routine Task Inventory* (RTI, Allen, Earhart, & Blue, 1992) and the *Kohlman Evaluation of Living Skills* (KELS) (Kohlman, 1992) are performance-based tests that employ familiar IADL tasks. Typically, the person who does poorly on the ACL will not do well on the safety tasks in the KELS because the latter require an understanding of cause and effect. The *Occupational Case Interview and Rating Scale* (OCAIRS; Kaplan & Kielhofner, 1989) is useful in that it provides an indication of the patient's insight into the personal and family impact of his or her illness. In addition to assessments of function and insight, the occupational therapist should conduct an interest inventory and a leisure assessment to inform the design of an occupational therapy program that is motivating and engaging for the patient.

Family

The severity and chronic nature of Schizophrenia often precludes full time employment and limits access to health insurance. The emotional and financial cost of caring for the patient with schizophrenia can be burdensome to the family. These factors, in combination with the disordered social and communication patterns of the patient, can be very challenging to family interactions, and the patient may become alienated. As a result, a primary support system may be comprised of fellow residents of a group home or Community Rehabilitative Residences (CRRs). Education regarding the maintenance of a structured, supportive environment that fosters independence is important for the patient and the members of his or her support system.

Practice Setting

Although individuals who are severely involved remain in state hospitals, the trend has been to treat these patients in the least possible restrictive setting. When patients are admitted for inpatient treatment, the plan is to return them to the community as quickly as possible, thereby reducing a potential dependence on institutional living. In these settings, occupational therapy treatment focuses on symptom recognition and management.

Partial hospital programs allow the patient to live in the community while he or she attends a daily treatment program. Partial programs emphasize the development of social skills, communication skills, stress management, symptom recognition, and disease management. Although occupational therapy is indicated in this aspect of treatment, reimbursement for this type of intervention is limited.

The "clubhouse" format is an example of a community-based day program. Although few professional staff members are present, this venue provides the patient with the opportunity to develop a social community and engage in productive activity. Locally funded drop-in centers that provide chronic mental patients with a safe haven are other examples of community programs and provide the patient with an opportunity to engage in productive activity and to practice social skills.

Sociopolitical

State legislation mandates that the purpose of an inpatient hospital stay be documented. Voluntary admissions require a document signed by the patient and involuntary admissions require a commitment by the civil court. If the patient is committed by the civil court, his or her cost of treatment is paid with public funds.

In general, most health insurance plans are limited for inpatient psychiatry. This is particularly troublesome for disorders such as Schizophrenia which may require extended hospital stays. Most plans have an annual limit of hospital days, as well as a lifetime limit. Because psychotic disorders often prevent the patient from gainful employment, the possibility of employer-subsidized health insurance may be out of reach.

Lifestyle/Lifespan

Delusions may result in the patient not taking prescribed medication. The dosages, timing, and number of different medications may confuse the patient who is cognitively involved. Inconsistent management or cessation of a medication regimen may cause repeated hospitalizations. The maladaptive behaviors associated with this condition, if not mitigated, may put the patient at risk for lifelong social isolation.

The devastating and enduring effects of the illness create a lifelong need for support for clients and their caregivers. Local chapters of organizations like NAMI (National Association for the Mentally Ill) provide ongoing support for persons and families who live with Schizophrenia and other psychotic disorders.

Clinical Decision Making Process

Defining Focus for Intervention

Utilizing data gathered from referral documentation, the medical history, patient and caregiver interviews, and assessment tools such as the *Occupational Case Interview and Rating Scale* (OCAIRS) (Kaplan & Keilhofner, 1989), and the *Kohlman Evalauation of Living Skills* (KELS) (Kohlman, 1992), the occupational therapist assesses the client's habits, roles, and capabilities. A history and description of the client's routines give an indication of the client's goals and aspirations, the barriers to those goals, and the potential for productive participation in the client's chosen life tasks.

The focus for occupational therapy intervention is usually the reduction of the barriers to the client's active participation in life tasks. For instance, if diminished cognitive abilities and/or distracting hallucinations impair the client's ability to consistently manage his or her medication routine, then reality orientation and task simplification may become the focus for occupational therapy. If maladaptive communication skills hinder the client's social interaction, then activities that provide practice in differentiating passive, assertive, and aggressive communication patterns may be the focus for intervention.

Establishing Goals for Intervention

In an inpatient setting, the primary goal is reduction of symptoms so they do not interfere with function and safety of the client and others. Specific goals may include the mitigation of delusional thoughts, the reduction of impulsive behaviors, and the improvement of concentration and attention through the use of activity. In a community setting, intervention will be focused on public demeanor, family and peer relationships, self-care, and employment. Both the patient and the family should be educated in the nature of the disease and symptom recognition. As clients and caregivers become more skillful in recognizing the signs of impending exacerbations, they will be able to seek professional assistance before a crisis results.

Designing Theory-Based Intervention

The Model of Human Occupation and occupational behavior theory are key sources for the development of intervention strategies. By using an occupation-based perspective, the therapist can frame interventions that will facilitate successful engagement in the life tasks which define personal identity. Assessments like the *Role Checklist* (Oakley, Kielhofner, & Barris, 1986) and OCAIRS (Kaplan & Kielhofner, 1989) provide a method by which therapist and client can prioritize life tasks and occupations, identify barriers to successful engagement in these occupations, and design strategies for overcoming these barriers. Activities that are designed to elicit coping behaviors form the core of occupational therapy intervention while educational sessions and group discussion are employed to relate the activity experience to daily life and stimulate internalization of newly learned coping skills. In addition to engagement in structured therapy activities and discussion groups, occupational therapists may encourage client interest in leisure and/or exercise activities that can foster self-reliance and self-efficacy and be continued post discharge. For example, the patient, though limited in some areas, may need to identify and assume a role (parent, child, sibling, student, worker). The occupational therapist can assist in the process through analysis of the patient's skills and the skills necessary for the successful execution of the life tasks that are inherent to the roles that have been identified. The focus of intervention may be on the identification, modification, and/or adaptation of the tasks or environment in which they are performed.

The Cognitive Disabilities framework (Allen, Earhart and Blue, 1992) helps to define the client's cognitive abilities and limitations based on observation of performance on a series of unfamiliar tasks. The cognitive disabilities that often accompany Schizophrenia are frequently manifested in an inability to manage medication routines. Occupational therapists may often simplify tasks by reducing the number of decisions or steps required for successful task completion. For instance, in order to simplify the management of many daily medications, the therapist might construct a partitioned pillbox and place a picture of each pill in each of the partitions. This strategy would provide the patient with visual and physical cues as he or she fills the pillbox on a daily basis. The Recapitulation of Ontogenesis frame of reference (Mosey, 1986) focuses on the developmental nature of interaction. A patient who suffers from irritability, agitation, and withdrawal due to paranoid ideation may be treated in a series of activity sessions that require progressive levels of interaction (solitary, parallel, dyadic, group) in order to increase social interaction skills.

Evaluating Progress

Functional activity is evidence of mastery for the client and an essential ongoing evaluation tool for the practitioner. A client easily dismisses words of encouragement, but a completed task (craft, picture, written exercise) provides tangible evidence of functionality. The manner in which the client approaches a task, the level of support the client requires for successful completion of a task, and the reaction of the client to task completion are all indicators of progress. Through the analysis of the client's performance on the activity, the practitioner can measure improvement and assess to what extent the client is progressing toward the goals of treatment.

Determining Change in or Termination of Treatment

Clinical observation helps the practitioner assess the client's reality orientation, attention span, social interaction, safety awareness, and other skills that will be required in the discharge environment. At times it may be necessary to terminate a client from a group or session because behavior, peer interaction, verbal outbursts, or sudden paranoid response may compromise the safety of the patient or others.

Case Study

Description

James is a 55-year-old man who was diagnosed with Schizophrenia when he was 21 years old. James has been in and out of hospitals for most of his adult life. Before the onset of his illness, he graduated from high school and successfully held a series of clerical positions of which he was very proud. After the onset of his illness, which included auditory hallucinations, he attempted to work but was fired from several jobs. He applied for state funded medical assistance. He now lives with his four brothers and his mother who are supportive caregivers. They are a little confused about how to handle his periodic irrational thoughts and outbursts, but are basically good supports for him. He is ambulatory and in good physical health. James frequently engages in long, boisterous harangues and vehemently denies that he has any problems. When he started attending occupational therapy groups in a partial hospitalization program, he would loudly proclaim, "Hi, I'm fine. I don't have any problems. Let me help you. How are you?" James has a good memory of working and takes pride in the service he provided through work. He is clean and well dressed and eager to help his peers and the staff. He enjoys doing many of the activities provided in the program. He follows through with responsibilities he is given, but needs direction to get started.

James takes pride in working with and helping others. He has a boisterous voice and friendly helpful demeanor. He needs to do concrete tasks and be in a supportive atmosphere with reduced stimuli in order to be an effective worker and he no longer requires the partial hospitalization environment. He is anxious about leaving the partial program with which he has become familiar and comfortable. He doesn't want to change and asks, "Why can't I just be picked up by the van, come to partial, and work in ceramics instead of attending groups?" Although he is resistant to taking public transportation, he is capable of independently negotiating the bus routes. He is capable of caring for himself with guidance and support from his family. Although he is not a self-starter, he is reliable in independently completing tasks that are given to him. He requires regular, supportive, and encouraging feedback to gain a sense of satisfaction in his work, and feels whole and "normal" when he is able to help others.

His family makes sure that he is clean and dressed. He has been attending the partial hospitalization program five days per week, and is transported to and from the program by city-funded transportation for individuals with handicapping conditions who cannot negotiate public transportation. He has expressed interest in ceramics.

Long- and Short-Term Goals

The long-term goal of intervention for James is to independently use public transportation to commute to volunteer activities.

This goal will be reached in part through successfully achieving the short-term goal of negotiating bus travel with the assistance of his brother.

Therapist Goals and Strategies

The therapist's goals include:

1. Increase organizational skills.
2. Increase self-confidence.
3. Increase independence.

The therapist's strategies include:

1. Gradually reduce partial program days and use of supportive transportation.
2. Provide maps that clearly delineate the bus route and walking route from the bus stop to the hospital. Include significant landmarks.
3. Practice walking from bus stop to hospital. Note significant landmarks.
4. Enlist James' brother to accompany James as he learns and practices the bus route to and from the hospital.
5. Gradually withdraw assistance and accompany each independently achieved milestone with praise.

Activity

Assisted Travel on Public Transportation

The therapist will enlist James's brother to help James learn the bus schedule and bus route and plan the trip from home to the hospital. The first trip will be on a weekend when the number of travelers is light. James will be encouraged to talk about his experience and the family and therapist will use praise to encourage his continued use of public transportation.

James wants to help others, but is not interested in a full time job. He has expressed some curiosity and interest in ceramics. In order for James to begin his journey toward independence, it is decided that he will transition from his status in the partial program to a volunteer program in the ceramics room; however, his resistance to change results in anxiety. Making the transition from partial hospitalization to volunteerism needs to be gradual to avoid a stress induced exacerbation of his illness. The gradual change gives James a chance to gain mastery over his responsibilities as a volunteer and an independent commuter. The continued support of the treatment program helps him process the feelings that arise as he makes the transition. The involvement of his family helps them learn what James is doing and understand the problems he might face using public transportation. They help him address safety issues and learn the route.

Resources

The following resources can be helpful for gathering clinical data:

Family history of mental illness

Patient report

Observation of behaviors and adaptive skill

Reports from other treating professionals

Assessments:

- ACL
- OCAIRS
- KELS

Interest inventory

Leisure assessment

The following resources can be helpful for gathering family data:

Support system:

- Family
- Friends
- Neighbors

Workplace history

Family education

The following are common practice settings:

Acute inpatient psychiatric program

Partial hospital program

Community-based programs:

- Drop-in center
- Clubhouse

The following resources can be helpful for gathering sociopolitical data:

Mental health legislation

Health insurance coverage

The following can be helpful in understanding and managing lifestyle/lifespan issues:

Employment and other opportunities for participation in life roles

Medication regimen and related side effects

Availability of caregivers

Internet Resources

American Occupational Therapy Association:
www.aota.org

National Alliance for the Mentally Ill:
www.nami.org/illness/

National Institute of Mental Health:
www.nimh.nih.gov

World Fellowship for Schizophrenia and Allied Disorders:
www.world-schizophrenia.org

References

American Psychiatric Association. (2000). *Diagnostic and statistical manual of mental disorders* (4th ed., text revision). Washington, DC: Author.

Allen, C. K. (1990). *Allen cognitive level.* Colchester, CN: S&S Worldwide.

Allen, C. K., Earhart, C. A., & Blue, T. (1992) *Occupational therapy treatment goals for the physically and cognitively disabled.* Rockville, MD: The American Occupational Therapy Association.

Kaplan, K., & Kielhofner, G. (1989). *Occupational case analysis, interview, and rating scale.* Thorofare, NJ: Slack Incorporated.

King, L. J. (1974). A sensory integrative approach to schizophrenia. *The American Journal of Occupational Therapy, 28*(9), 529–536.

Kohlman, L. T. (1992) *Kohlman evaluation of living skills.* Rockville, MD: American Occupational Therapy Association.

Korb-Khalsa, K., Azok, S. D., & Leutenberg, E. (1991). *Life management skills.* Beachwood, OH: Wellness Productions.

Mental Health Procedures Act of July 9, 1976, PA (P.L. 817) §§ 50-7201-7304.

Merck Research Laboratories. (1999). *The Merck manual* (17th ed.). Whitehouse Station, NJ: Author.

Mosey, A. C. (1986). *Psychosocial components of occupational therapy.* New York: Raven Press.

Sadock, B. J., & Sadock, V. A. (2003). *Synopsis of psychiatry: Behavioral sciences/clinical psychiatry* (9th ed.). Philadelphia: Lippincott Williams & Wilkins.

Depressive Disorders 20

C. Thomas North, Ph.D., OTR/L
Nancy L. Beck, MA, OTR/L

Synopsis of Clinical Condition

Prevalence and Etiology

Depression is often used to describe a sad mood, a lack of motivation, or a lack of interest. In clinical depression, these symptoms may exist, but a broad array of other symptoms is also possible. Depressed individuals may have low energy and appear disengaged from the environment, or they may also appear agitated and have difficulty concentrating. Weight loss or weight gain and insomnia or prolonged sleepiness may also be present. Depression is a factor in all Mood Disorders (Diagnostic and Statistical Manual of Mental Disorders, 4th ed. Text Revision [*DSM–IV–TR*; American Psychiatric Association, 2000]).

The Diagnostic and Statistical Manual of Mental Disorders, 4th edition, Text Revision (American Psychiatric Association, 2000) details several disorders under the heading of Mood Disorders, including those that impact function and some that do not. All are chronic, but manageable with medication (Kaplan & Sadock, 2003).

The list of conditions includes:

- Major Depression
- Dysthymic Disorder
- Depressive Disorder Not Otherwise Specified
- Bipolar I Disorder
- Bipolar II Disorder
- Cylcothymic Disorder
- Bipolar Disorder Not Otherwise Specified.
- Mood Disorder Due to General Medical Condition
- Substance Induced Mood Disorder
- Mood Disorder Not Otherwise Specified

The designation of major Depression is further classified into two subheadings: Major Depression, Single Episode, and Major Depression, Recurrent. Single Episode is specified further by 16 subtypes while the additional specifiers describe the nature of the current or most recent phase of the Recurrent classification (American Psychiatric Association, 2000). Classification depends upon the number, duration and severity of symptoms, the duration of symptom-free periods, and the degree to which daily function is disrupted. (Kaplan & Sadock, 2003) Mood Disorder Due to General Medical Condition and Substance Induced Mood Disorder require evidence that the symptoms can be explained by physiologic disturbances or the use of medications or other substances, respectively (American Psychiatric Association 2000). When the patient is clearly mood disordered, but none of the symptoms meet the definitions provided in *DSM–TR* (2000), the most appropriate label is Mood Disorder Not Otherwise Specified.

Major Depressive Disorder is most prevalent in the population at about 5% to 12% for men and twice that for women and typically develops in adolescence or early adulthood. A later onset is usually attributable to a medical condition and would be labeled Mood Disorder Due to General Medical Condition. Dysthymic (6%), Bipolar I (.4%–1.6%), Bipolar II (.05%) and Cyclothymic (.4%–1%) disorders are relatively rare. Immediate relatives of individuals with these disorders are at a higher risk for developing these disorders as well as alcohol dependence and anxiety disorders. Men tend to have more Manic Episodes, while women tend to have more Depressive Episodes. (*DSM–IV–TR*, 2000). *DSM–IV–TR* (2000) notes that up to 15% of persons diagnosed with Major Depressive Disorder die of suicide. It also cites death the rate among those over 55 years of age with Major Depressive Disorder is four times that of the general population.

Common Characteristics and Symptoms

Most mood disorders are cyclical, but individuals with mood disorders tend to lead normal and productive lives between clinical episodes. Four phases/episodes are associated with mood disorders: major depressive episode, manic episode, mixed episode, and hypomanic episode. In order to be diagnosed with a mood disorder, the patient must have a history of two episodes with at least one depressive episode. To meet the criteria for a major depressive episode, the patient must experience symptoms for a period exceeding two weeks and the symptoms must significantly impact daily functioning. At least five of the following symptoms must accompany a depressed mood: diminished interest or pleasure in most activities, significant weight loss or gain, decrease or increase in appetite, loss of sleep or increased sleeping, irritability or psychomotor retardation, fatigue, feelings of worthlessness or unfounded guilt, poor concentration, and/or thoughts of death or suicidal ideation. It is also possible that the patient may experience mood congruent hallucinations or delusions. It should be noted that depressive symptoms as a result of bereavement should not be considered as a clinical issue unless the symptoms exceed two months (American Psychiatric Association 2000).

In contrast, the manic episode is characterized by a period of elevated, expansive, or irritable mood that lasts at least one week, significantly impairs function, and is accompanied by at least three of the following symptoms: inflated self-esteem or grandiosity, decreased need for sleep, pressure of speech, flight of ideas or racing thoughts, distractibility, agitation, and/or excessive involvement in activities that could produce long-term negative results (sexual indiscretion, overspending, etc.). The mixed episode, sometimes referred to as "rapid cycling," is comprised of symptoms of both depressive and manic episodes on a daily basis. Symptoms must be present or cycling for a period exceeding one week. Again, the symptoms must be adequately severe to significantly impair day to day functioning. The hypomanic episode differs from the manic episode only in that there is not a significant impact upon day to day functioning. In all cases, other causes for the symptomatic behavior, such as medical conditions or substance abuse must be ruled out (*DSM–IV–TR*, 2000).

Occupational therapists should be aware of the side effects of the medical treatments that are frequently used in this population. The current medications of choice are all in the Selective Serotonin Reuptake Inhibitor (SSRI) family. Familiar brand names of SSRIs include: Prozac™, Paxil™, Zoloft™, Luvox™, and Celexa™. Side effects can be strong enough to discourage drug compliance and include: gastrointestinal effects (diarrhea, nausea, anorexia), headache, CNS (anxiety, insomnia, EPS, seizures), anticholinergic effects, hematologic effects, and galactorrhea. All of these tend to be temporary or reversible. One side effect, sexual dysfunction, tends to remain throughout the drug regimen, and may affect as many as 80% of the patients, but can be treated with supplemental medication (Kapllan & Sadock, 2003).

Lithium has been the traditional drug of choice for Bipolar disorders. Side effects include thirst, polyuria, gastric distress, weight gain, tremor, fatigue, and mild cognitive impairment (Kaplan & Sadock, 2003). Many anticonvulsants such as Depakote™, Neurontin™, and Topamax have been shown to be effective in treating Bipolar disorders (Physician's Desk Reference, 2000) (PDR). Also effective have been some antipsychotics such as Zyprexa, Risperdal, and Clozaril (Kaplan & Sadock, 2003). Tricyclics and tetracyclics (TCAs) are traditionally used to treat some mood disorders but they are not used to treat Bipolar I disorder because they may trigger manic episodes. Initial side effects are dry mouth, constipation, blurred vision, and urinary retention. Patients should be made aware of all side effects and instructed that these effects fade as the medication is tolerated. Patients with narrow angle glaucoma are particularly at risk. Medications with known negative interactions include: antihypertensives, antipsychotics, CNS depressants, sympathomimetics, and oral contraceptives (Kaplan & Saddock, 2003).

Electroshock therapy (ECT) is very effective in treating Mood Disorders and is not painful. The regimen for ECT therapy is an induced convulsion every second day for a period of two to four weeks. The typical series is at least six treatments. Before each treatment, patients are premedicated to reduce the risk of respiratory failure, cardiac arrest, and bone fractures. Because of the medications, the patient may be groggy and confused following treatment. The greatest side effect is temporary memory loss, lasting approximately four weeks (Kaplan & Saddock, 2003).

Target Areas for Intervention

The profound sadness and sense of hopelessness that is experienced by individuals who are diagnosed with Major Depressive Disorder or other Mood Disorders leads to isolation, helplessness, and disengagement from all the activity that supports self-efficacy and gives meaning to life. Occupational therapy focuses on the re-establishment of self-efficacy through engagement in structured activity that is designed to develop a broad repertoire of strategies for coping with the stressors of daily life and an ability to resume engagement in life roles.

Contextual Considerations

Clinical

The clients experience a feeling of hopelessness and helplessness to which suicide or homicide may seem the only way out. They have lost their ability to cope with the stresses in their lives, have become disconnected from their support systems, and have no energy and/or ability to concentrate on engaging in daily activities. Posture, gait, level of alertness, and affect are frequently good indicators of mood. Most mood disorders are cyclical and characterized by manic, hypomanic, and/or depressive cycles punctuated by remission periods in which the patient is fully functional. Persons are more likely to carry out a suicide attempt during the manic phase of the illness.

Mood disorders are not usually accompanied by cognitive disorders; therefore, clients who do not have cognitive limitations are capable of logical sequential thought process and are capable of synthesizing information and integrating it into their lives. During periods of remission, clients will often have insight into the life impact of the illness. The Role Checklist (Oakley, Keilhofner, & Barris, 1986) and the Occupational Case Analysis Interview Rating Scale (OCAIRS) (Kaplan & Kielhofner, 1989) provide data regarding the impact of the illness on the patient as well as the patient's perception of others' understanding of the illness. The Kohlman Evalaution of Living Skills (KELS) (Kohlmnan, 1992), is an instrument designed to assess skill in handling daily living activity.

Family

A family history of mood disorders, maladaptive behaviors, or depressive episodes is usually present in persons with mood disorders. Family education and training can facilitate the development of insight into the nature of the illness and strategies for coping with the patient. Both patient and family should be trained to recognize the signs of impending manic or depressive episodes.

Practice Settings

Patients with mood disorders are seen in acute psychiatric hospitals if they are to receive electro-convulsive therapy (ECT), if they are so debilitated that survival without supervision is unlikely, or if they pose a suicide risk. In this setting, the goals for occupational therapy are:

1. Reduce stress and increase receptiveness to treatment.
2. Identify and practice functional coping strategies.
3. Gain insight into problem solving life issues (Rehabilitative Services Department Manual 2001, Belmont Center for Comprehensive Treatment, Philadelphia, PA).

Patients are discharged as soon as the risks are mitigated. However, one does not come out of a depressive phase precipitously. Often, there is a need for group and individual therapy in a partial setting until the patient is able to return to work.

In an Intensive Outpatient Program or Rehabilitation Partial Hospitalization Program, the goals focus on gaining independence and consistency in the identification and practice of coping skills and life management. In outpatient settings, goals may focus on coping with work problems, relational problems, parenting, pain management, and depression due to medical problems.

In all settings, the goals of treatment need to be practical and understandable to the client. Goal attainment is very dependent on the clients' commitment to and participation in their own recovery. For many clients, using coping skills to address problems is a process of rethinking how they approach living. They have begun to think that suicide or homicide is the only solution to problems. At one time, most clients have used more positive coping skills. Treatment can be a process of the clients rekindling or relearning coping strategies that they have used in the past and expanding their repertoire of skills to be able to manage their daily stressors in a more satisfying and productive way.

Community-based programs include support groups and self-help groups. These approaches work best for those who fully understand their illness, and benefit from offering and accepting support from others with similar experiences. These patients are usually veterans of hospitalization or outpatient treatment.

Sociopolitical

Virtually all states in the United States have a mental health code that requires a legal document stating the purpose of hospitalization be included in each patient's chart. If the admission is voluntary, the document also provides for withdrawal from treatment and is signed by the patient. If the patient has been committed to treatment by the mental health court, commitment time is limited and requires a case review by the court with input from treating staff.

Patients may receive treatment based upon insurance coverage rather than treatment need. A broad range of coverage is available since psychiatry, unlike most other services, is not reimbursed under the Diagnosis Related Group (DRG) system that is used by Medicare. Therefore, no normative data addresses costs or length of treatment. If the commitment for treatment has been court mandated, treatment is provided at county government expense. Most government and private third party payers allow for a few days with frequent reviews, and other insurers have a days-per-year coverage for inpatient services, with an upper limit determined by lifetime days. Unlike Medicare and many private third party insurers, Medicaid does not provide for partial hospital programs. Employers may be willing to provide coverage for mood disorders since recovery is likely.

The social stigma of mental illness has ramifications in treatment and recovery. Although legal protection for persons with mental illness has been assured by civil rights legislation, lack of public understanding and acceptance of the mentally ill may provide barriers for community integration.

Lifestyle/Lifespan

Any disorder that impairs function will have a negative impact upon financial resources. Medications are a costly, lifelong need. The cyclical nature of mood disorders allows the patient to be productive in periods of remission. The successful patient will learn to recognize the cycles as natural phenomena and can learn to use coping skills and the support of family and friends.

Clinical Decision Making Process

Defining Focus for Intervention

An initial interview that includes a perspective on family relationships, support systems, interests, work/school issues, pain and medical issues, psychiatric history, living arrangements, precipitating factors leading to treatment, anticipated length of stay in the practice setting, and discharge options helps to inform the development of occupational therapy intervention.

Establishing Goals for Intervention

The first step in the treatment process is to assist the client in identifying how the illness has impacted the roles, routines, and habits inherent to functional daily living. Once the therapist, in concert with the client, has established the life tasks that are most meaningful to the client, the general goals for intervention are focused on increased awareness of more adaptive coping strategies, assisted engagement in structured activities that require the repeated employment of these strategies, and the progressively independent deployment of these strategies for use in every day life.

Designing Theory-Based Intervention

The Model of Human Occupation and occupational behavior theory are key sources for the development of intervention strategies. By using an occupation-based perspective, the therapist can frame interventions that will facilitate successful engagement in the life tasks which define personal identity.

Assessments, like the Role Checklist (Oakley, Kielhofner, & Barris, 1986) and OCAIRS (Kaplan & Kielhofner, 1989) provide a method by which therapist and client can prioritize life tasks and occupations, identify barriers to successful engagement in these occupations, and design strategies for overcoming these barriers.

Activities that are designed to elicit coping behaviors form the core of occupational therapy intervention, and educational sessions and group discussion are employed to relate the activity experience to daily life and stimulate internalization of newly learned coping skills.

In addition to engagement in structured therapy activities and discussion groups, occupational therapists may encourage client interest in leisure and/or exercise activities that can foster self-reliance and self-efficacy and be continued post discharge.

Numerous sources are available that can be used to promote and educate clients on a wide variety of coping skills. Life Management Skills (Korb-Khalsa, Azok, & Leutenberg, 1991) are excellent resources to begin building a repertoire of materials to use during group sessions. Therapy board games, paper and pencil exercises, (available in catalogues like *Wellness Production, Inc* and *Child's Work, Child's Play, Inc.*), role playing, relaxation exercises, discussion, and sports or physical activity are examples of approaches that can be taken to address most coping skills.

Evaluating Progress

Diminished lability, reduction of suicidal ideation, increased initiative, increased reflectivity, active engagement in activity, and planning for the future are all indications of progress.

Determining Change in or Termination of Treatment

If a client shows either no signs or diminished signs of progress after 1–2 weeks, it is important to assess the course of treatment. A history of treatment resistance (noncompliance with medications, prolonged depressive episodes, personality disorder with chronic suicidal ideation, chronically dependent personality traits, chronically obsessive or racing thoughts) may indicate that more time in treatment is needed. It also may indicate that the client has a baseline of diminished function that will not change substantially before discharge. The safety of the client is most important. Discharge plans should include an intensive "step down" from hospitalization like a Partial Hospitalization Program or a rigorous outpatient regime.

Support systems become very important when considering discharge and are an ongoing issue addressed in almost all treatment interventions. Depression does not suddenly appear and it does not suddenly go away. The recovery process continues after discharge from all settings. The clients' support network can strengthen the process adding increased stability for the transition from discharge to quality lifestyle. Prior to discharge, it is helpful to meet with the family or other support network to provide education about the illness or facilitate communication between the client and the supports.

Discharge readiness occurs when the client is stable enough to safely move on to the next level of care or able to resume daily functions using the support of outpatient services, medication, family, or significant others.

Case Study

Description

Brian is a 28-year-old, second year medical student who attends school in the Northeast. He admitted himself to the hospital for the second time in a year, after taking an overdose of his psychiatric medication. He lives alone and has minimal contact with his family who live in the West. He has casual friends from class, but no close friends or relatives in the area. In the initial assessment interview, he was quiet and somewhat reluctant to talk, but admitted that he had stopped going to classes for about two weeks, had stopped eating, and was sleeping a lot. He was having difficulty concentrating and had been refusing to answer the phone. His limited interests included studying, running by himself, and occasionally going to the park to watch the boat races. He admitted spending a lot of time alone in his apartment. His psychiatric history revealed that he had been seeing a psychiatrist at school for the past year. He appeared in OT group for the first time with sad affect, quiet demeanor, clean, conservatively dressed, and sitting somewhat stiffly by himself not talking to his peers.

Upon further assessment via interview, Brian talked about his family life saying abruptly with a slight edge in his tone, "My parents aren't affectionate. They only tell me what I do wrong. Sometimes my mom encourages me, but not too often. We live in a small town where everyone knows about me going to school in the Northeast and don't think that I'll make it." The *Role Checklist* revealed that of his roles in life, he valued being a family member and student with some interest in friendship although it was not a role he defined for himself in the present. He also did not define family member as a role in the present. He pictured his future as being a student. He indicated that he used to like going places and doing things with his friends and wanted his family to be more supportive.

The results of the assessments indicated that he is a shy person who has difficulty expressing his feelings effectively. He also seems to have difficulty expressing anger in a satisfying way, turning his anger inward toward himself. His view of the future is sparse and limited to the immediate future with student being the only role he envisions. He may be feeling an overwhelming fear and pressure to prove to his hometown that he can succeed. He has marginal confidence in his psychiatrist, and is fearful of changing to a new psychiatrist. Brian has a limited repertoire of activity and seems unable to expand his interests. His supports are limited to his psychiatrist and a casual female friend whom he only sees in class. He has pervasive hopelessness about the future and is unable to or helpless in coping with his relational and school stressors. His goal is to return to school and not be so lonely.

Long- and Short-Term Goals

The long-term goal of intervention for Brian is to resume his classroom studies, communicate his needs to others, and continue seeing a psychiatrist for aftercare support.

This goal will be reached in part through successfully achieving the short-term goal of identifying ways to express anger and other feelings through healthy outlets.

Therapist Goals and Strategies

The therapist's goals include:

1. Provide activities to express feelings.
2. Facilitate integration of experience and knowledge.

The therapist's strategies include:

1. Education about how to express feelings.
2. Provide experiences to practice expressing feelings through activity participation.
3. Process the activity through facilitated discussion to help client relate the experience to his life.

Activity

Balloon Volleyball

The group will begin by brainstorming a list of feelings. Each member will pick a feeling from the list and identify one outlet for that feeling. This exercise helps to get the group focused on the topic or goal of the group.

The group will then participate in an activity that requires communication from all the members. The activity is a cooperative challenge activity or noncompetitive sport activity. The group is asked to stand in a circle and keep a balloon in the air by hitting it in the air to various group members. After the group gets the first balloon successfully bouncing from person to person, a second balloon and third balloon are introduced. The group is reminded to talk to each other to help keep all of the balloons in the air. The activity ends when the balloons begin to fall, break, or the group looks tired and frustrated, or when they begin to laugh so much they begin to miss the balloons (about 5 to 10 minutes). The activity usually produces stress relief and laughter.

The activity is followed by a discussion about the activity and its relevance to the topic of expression of feelings. The therapist encourages clients to talk about their roles in the activity, the things they said to encourage each other, and the feelings they experienced during the activity. Clients are also encouraged to discuss how they can use what they learned in this activity in their home or work environment.

This activity was chosen based on the following information:

1. Brian is an adult interested in going to school with secondary interests in running, sports, and relating to peers.
2. Brian is focused on his work (going to school). He has difficulty seeing the relevance of leisure outlets and has extreme difficulty expressing his feelings. He seems to lack role models and methods for feeling expression, hence his thoughts are internalized without benefit of others' perspectives. As his feelings of anger and stress build, he has no regular outlet for them except running. He is lonely, but lacks the skills or confidence to reach out to his peers unless it concerns schoolwork. He has no friends or social life.
3. Brian is a bright, pleasant young man who feels powerless over his life and views suicide as the only way out. He is not confident in his outpatient psychiatrist, but does not have the energy nor assertiveness to change psychiatrists. At this point it would probably provide more stability for him to continue with the same psychiatrist upon discharge. The fear of the change or unknown may be greater than his lack of confidence in the caretaker and only confidante.
4. Brian does not seem to have a history of using activities to provide outlets for feelings. Meeting goals in this area will require education, practice, and reflective discussion. He needs to build support systems in his new environment. Through treatment, he can learn to communicate his thoughts and feelings in a productive way that helps him relate to peers, develop friendships, and release anger/feelings in ways that are comfortable for him and help him achieve his social and career goals.

Treatment Objectives

1. Brian will experience stress relief during the activity.
2. Brian will identify three outlets for feelings.
3. Brian will identify one person with whom he can do activities.

Resources

The following resources can be helpful for gathering clinical data:

Family history of mental illness and Depression

Patient report about illness experience (new or seasoned patient)

Risk of suicide

Observation of behaviors and adaptations

Reports from team and other treating professionals

Assessments:

- Role Checklist
- OCAIRS
- KELS
- Interest Inventory leisure assessment

The following resources can be helpful for gathering family data:

Support systems (family, life partners, significant others, children, friends)

Workplace history

The following are common practice settings:

Acute inpatient psychiatric programs

Partial hospital program

Private pay outpatient programs

Community-based programs, e.g. self-help, support group, etc.

The following resources can be helpful for gathering sociopolitical data:

Health insurance companies

Mental health code

The following resources can be helpful in understanding and managing lifestyle/lifespan issues:

Financial:

- Loss of income
- Cost of medication
- Insurance costs

Medical:

- Chronic pain
- Illness related to depression
- Depression related to medical treatment

Personal Adaptation:

- Cycling
- Agitation
- Low energy
- Loss of self-esteem
- Withdrawal
- Medication precautions

Internet Resources

American Occupational Therapy Association:
www.aota.org

Depression, Bipolar Support Alliance (formerly: Depression, Manic Depression Alliance):
www.dbsalliance.org

National Alliance for the Mentally Ill:
www.nami.org/illness/

National Institute of Mental Health:
www.nimh.nih.gov

References

American Psychiatric Association. (2000). *Diagnostic and statistical manual of mental disorders* (4th ed., text revision). Washington, DC: Author.

Kaplan, B. J., & Sadock, V. A. (2003). *Synopsis of psychiatry: Behavioral sciences/clinical psychiatry* (9th ed.). Philadelphia: Lippincott Williams & Wilkins.

Kaplan, K., & Kielhofner, G. (1989). *Occupational case analysis, interview, and rating scale.* Thorofare, NJ: Slack Incorporated.

Korb-Khalsa, K., Azok, S.D., & Leutenberg, E. (1991). *Life management skills.* Beachwood, OH: Wellness Productions.

Medical Economics Co, Inc. (2000). *Physician's desk reference* (54th ed.). Mountvale, NJ: Author.

Oakley, F., Kielhofner, G., & Barris, R. (1986). The role checklist. *Occupational Therapy Journal of Research, 6,* 157–170.

Rehabilitative services department manual. Albert Einstein Health Network, Belmont Center for Comprehensive Treatment (2001). Philadelphia: Author.

Osteoarthritis and Rheumatoid Arthritis

21

Rosalyn Lipsitt, MHL, OTR/L

Synopsis of Clinical Condition

Prevalence and Etiology

Osteoarthritis and rheumatoid arthritis are chronic conditions characterized by painful joints. Osteoarthritis develops due to a breakdown of cartilage between joints, and is a diagnosis commonly associated with adults and older adults. Rheumatoid arthritis, on the other hand, is a systemic disease caused by an autoimmune response which attacks the synovium, the thin membrane which lines and lubricates the joint, ultimately causing a breakdown of the joints' supporting structures. In addition, rheumatoid arthritis may involve an individual's internal organs, eyes, skin, and may be diagnosed in children (as juvenile rheumatoid arthritis) as well as adults. Both types of arthritis result in joint pain and decreased physical functioning.

Persons with arthritis are challenged to come to terms with issues relating to mobility, vocation, occupational satisfaction, competence in activities of daily living, body image, and ability to cope. Although this challenge may result in anxiety and depression for many people with arthritis, it is not universal. Significant predictors of psychosocial adaptation are, "perceptions of social and emotional support, perceptions of disease control, self-efficacy, favorable comparisons of disease activity, and favorable social comparisons of valued abilities and activities" (Livneh & Antonek, 1997, p. 247). It is important for occupational therapists to understand the condition and its repercussions, treat each person as an individual, and take a holistic approach by including psychosocial issues in practice.

According to the U.S. Centers for Disease Control and Prevention, arthritis and related diseases affect approximately 43 million Americans, 50% of whom are aged 65 and older. It is estimated that by the year 2020, the number of individuals with arthritis will increase to sixty million. Over 100 different forms of arthritis have been identified, and are divided into eight categories (Hansen & Atchison, 2000). Some form of arthritis is evident in most individuals over the age of 50. As the population ages, more cases are expected to be diagnosed. According to Hunter, et al (1990), forms of arthritis are one of the leading causes of work disabilities, second only to cardiac conditions.

Most Common Types of Arthritis

Ankylosing Spondylitis
Bursitis

Cervical Arthritis
Gout
Infectious Arthritis
Juvenile Rheumatoid Arthritis
Osteoarthritis
Osteonecrosis
Psoriatic Arthritis
Reactive Arthritis (formerly Reiter's)
Fibromyalgia
Rheumatoid Arthritis
Lumbosacral Arthritis
Rheumatoid Foot and Ankle
Tendonitis

Autoimmune Diseases That Can Cause Arthritis

All of the following are connective tissue diseases:

Lupus Erythematosus
Systemic Lupus Erythematosus
Scleroderma
Polymyositis
Dermatomyositis

Osteoarthritis is the primary example of degenerative arthritis. It is primarily an adult condition and, in the older age groups, is more prevalent among women than men. It affects the weight-bearing joints (knees, hips, and spine), and the distal interphalangeal (DIP) joints of the hands or metatarsophalangeal joints of the feet (Hunter, et al., 1990). It is believed to be related to age and genetics. In osteoarthritis, also referred to as degenerative joint disease (DJD), the thinning or other damage to cartilage creates a rough or eroded surface. As opposing bones attempt to glide in the absence of "cushioning," inflammation develops, contributing to the formation of bony ridges and spurs. These bony malformations, and the inability of the opposing bones to meet uniformly, cause deformity and pain during activity or at rest.

Some etiologies of osteoarthritis are less common than the process described above. Because cartilage naturally breaks down with age, due to wear and tear of the joint, it is believed that in some cases, arthritis may develop as a result of, or secondary to, other physiological conditions such as congenital defects and obesity. Some of the other risk factors associated with arthritis are bowed legs, dislocated hips, genetic defects, overuse or injury to a joint as a result of an accident, diabetes, and certain hormonal disorders such as gout and poor posture.

Early in the disease process, an individual will experience morning stiffness in the joints, which subsides during the course of the day, and possibly a crackling sound (crepitus) with movement of the joint. As the disease progresses, movement will be accompanied by increasing pain as well as swelling, caused by synovitis, increased amounts of synovial fluid, or changes in bone or cartilage, such as the formation of marginal osteophytes protruding into the joint space (Hunter, et al., 1990). These are observable on the DIPs and are referred to as Heberden's nodes, and, those at the proximal interphalangeal joints (PIPs), are known as Bouchard's nodes. Ulnar deviation of the wrists, also known as a "zig-zag" deformity, is also a common manifestation of rheumatoid as well as osteoarthritis.

Rheumatoid arthritis (RA) is a chronic and systemic (vs. localized) disease and is the most common form of inflammatory arthritis. There are actually over 100 different types of RA. In this form of the disease, an unknown event triggers the immune system to produce chemicals which stimulate an inflammatory reaction. This reaction causes inflammation of the synovium (the thin membrane which lines and lubricates the joint), which then proliferates, creating pannus (an overgrowth of synovial tissue), resulting in swelling. Eventually, the pannus, a rough, grainy tissue, invades the joint cavity and destroys the components of the joint, namely, the capsule, ligaments, and tendons. Unlike osteoarthritis which is localized, RA may involve body systems other than joints alone, such as the blood, lungs, and heart.

The symptomology of RA differs somewhat from osteoarthritis. RA usually affects joints bilaterally. Symptoms may be constant, or present with intermittent "flares" and remissions. Pain may be present, as well as other symptoms such as fatigue, low-grade fever, weight loss, dryness of the eyes and mouth, color changes in fingers and toes, inflammation of the eyes, heart, lungs, skin and nerves, and the appearance of rheumatoid nodules, most often seen near a joint. Other manifestations of RA as well as their descriptions are as follows:

1. Fusiform swelling: Digits become spindle-shaped due to swelling in the PIP joints.
2. Boutonniere deformity: The PIP is flexed due to a detached central slip. This causes the DIP to hyperextend.
3. Swan neck deformity: MCP joint exhibits a flexion contracture, which in turn creates hyperextension of the PIP, and flexion of the DIP. The processes which result in these abnormal positions of the IPs, are set into motion as a result of contractures of the interosseus and flexor muscles and tendons.
4. Thumb deformities:
   - boutonniere-type deformity,
   - volar subluxation of the thumb,
   - exaggerated adduction of the thumb, flexion of the MCP joint, and hyperextension of the DIP (Nalebuff, 1990).

Target Areas for Intervention

Occupational therapy intervention focuses patient education in the following areas: coping skills, joint protection, energy conservation, pain management, safe exercise, adaptive strategies, assistive devices, and self-empowerment in seeking information and social support in the community.

Contextual Considerations

Clinical

Several assessments are usually employed by the occupational therapist in order to evaluate the physical manifestations of the condition, the psychosocial aspects, and the functional challenges. Many assessments are available today which address each of the above aspects of diagnosis and treatment, however, for the purposes of this text, an example of each type has been chosen.

The types of assessments which will prove most helpful in determining goals and interventions for this diagnosis are: an interview, a physical examination of all joints and systems of the hand, a functional assessment, and a semi-structured, client-centered interview to help prioritize focus for treatment.

The initial interview provides key data when determining priorities for goals and intervention. It is during the interview that the therapist gains rapport with the patient, learns about his or her physical and social environment, his or her cognition, affect, experience of the illness, and priorities for treatment.

The hands and wrists are evaluated by observation, palpation, goniometry, and manual muscle testing. Each hand is inspected for trophic changes (condition of skin, degree of warmth and redness). Palpation is used to determine structural abnormalities of the joints and crepitus. Active range of motion will reveal any limitations due to stiffness, pain, tenderness, or locking of the tendon (trigger finger). Active and passive range of motion is measured with the goniometer, respecting any pain that may be present. Manual muscle testing may also be performed, unless the patient is in an acute stage and in pain. If the patient complains of nerve pain, or if the examination suggests deficits, sensory testing is also performed. Some patients with RA experience neuropathies or carpal tunnel syndrome, due to tenosynovitis of the digital flexors. Functional evaluations are also important. A self-care assessment is very valuable in determining the degree of function, and will reveal compensatory techniques used by the patient. The Occupational Performance History Interview (Henry & Kielhofner, 1989) is a semistructured interview allows for a more in-depth observation of the individual and an occupational history.

The Canadian Occupational Performance Measure (COPM) (Law, et al., 1994) is another interview-based instrument that allows the patient to report personal perceptions of self-care and leisure function and productivity. The patient is able to rate the degree of difficulty for each type of task, and how important each of those tasks are to him or her. This assessment assists with collaborative goal setting.

Family

The diagnosis of arthritis impacts the lives of individuals and their families in different ways. Some individuals may experience anxiety, depression, or anger if they are faced with increasing dependency on others and limitations in their ability to carry out the tasks that are associated with roles such as spouse, parent, worker, or student.

Practice Settings

Individuals with a diagnosis of arthritis may be encountered in long-term care facilities, assisted living, rehabilitation hospitals, adult day care, community programs, outpatient facilities, and home care settings.

Sociopolitical

Most managed care systems require arthritis patients to be managed by a primary care physician (PCP) who may not possess the specialized knowledge of a rheumatologist and may not be aware of the special needs of the patient with arthritis and the benefits that occupational and physical therapy may provide. The capitation system imposed by some managed care systems may actually discourage PCPs from referring patients to rheumatologists. Therapists will need to stress patient education to empower individuals to become active participants in developing a healthy and productive lifestyle and managing their health care needs.

The development of measurable, functional goals for occupational therapy is of paramount importance since current cost containment strategies call for shorter medical treatment sessions and evidence of the value of services prior to reimbursement (Melvin & Jensen, 1998).

Lifestyle/Lifespan

According to Livneh & Antonak (1997), there is extensive variability in psychological responses related to adaptation to arthritis. Fatigue, pain, limited flexibility, and neuropathies will influence the level of participation in many life tasks. Some common responses to a diagnosis of rheumatoid arthritis are: initial disbelief, denial, anxiety, and depression. Some people experience anger, which may be internalized or externalized. These emotions are in response to the patient's changing lifestyle in which many adaptations may need to be made due to loss of function.

Home, community and workplace accessibility, and medical costs are a few of the challenges persons with arthritis must face over the course of their lifetime.

Many individuals will benefit from having special devices such as a raised toilet seat, grab bars, special scissors, cooking, kitchen, and eating equipment; some of which may not be covered under insurance and will add to living expenses. Depending on severity of symptoms, some individuals may need environmental adaptations to the workplace to reduce overuse of joints, such as waist-level filing drawers, built-up writing implements and other tools, and an ergonomically correct chair. For others, an adjusted work schedule or vocational change may be required.

Clinical Decision Making Process

Defining Focus for Intervention

In defining the focus for intervention, the therapist is guided by the type of arthritis with which patient presents, the results of the physical assessment (range of motion, sensation, deformities, functional abilities), how they impact the patient's life roles (Occupational Performance History Interview), and their perception of the impact of the condition their independence (COPM). Comorbidities, such as cardiac conditions, and medications which may affect cognition or motor functioning are taken into consideration, to assure that the interventions will be appropriate and safe for the patient. Most commonly, occupational therapists intervene with this diagnosis, in any or all of the following focus areas.

1. Preparatory or enabling activities to prepare the patient for treatment (e.g. paraffin baths, active and passive range of motion, heat).
2. Patient education regarding work simplification, joint protection, energy conservation, exercise programs, use of assistive devices, resources for support in the community.

3. Activities of daily living (ADL) training, and instrumental activities of daily living (IADL) (e.g. use of assistive devices for cooking).
4. Exploration of leisure activities. This would include adapting an existing activity if needed or learning a new activity.
5. Work or productive activities. This would include instruction in how to perform the required tasks using joint protection and energy conservation and adapting the environment, if needed.
6. Splinting to rest painful joints or to slow the process of deformities.
7. Coping strategies. Occupational therapists will address patients' concerns and anxieties regarding the progressive nature of the condition. Intervention each of the areas mentioned above assists with increasing a sense of self-efficacy and serves to decrease anxiety and depression in the patient.

Establishing Goals for Intervention

Occupational therapy goals for persons who present with arthritis are determined by several factors including the physician's referral, the setting, the results of the initial evaluations, and the insurance coverage defining the length of treatment. Informed by these factors, the occupational therapist analyzes data collected from interview and assessments and collaborates with the patient in the establishment and prioritization of long- and short-term goals for treatment.

Designing Theory-Based Intervention

The complex nature of arthritis warrants the employment of more than one frame of reference. For example, issues of joint deformity and weakness may be addressed by the biomechanical and the rehabilitation frames of reference. Splinting to prevent further deformity, the institution of an exercise program to maintain and increase muscle strength, and the employment of modalities such as paraffin for pain relief represent the biomechanical frame of reference. Training in the use of adaptive devices, and the incorporation of energy conservation techniques and work simplification strategies represent the rehabilitation frame of reference. Additionally, the Model of Human Occupation provides the therapist with a holistic view of the patient that incorporates the physical ramifications of the conditions within the context of the patient's personal values, needs, and life roles (Kielhofner, 1997).

Precautions that should be taken during assessment and intervention are as follows:

1. During acute exacerbation, when patients present with joint swelling, redness, and pain, manual muscle testing and passive range of motion should be avoided.
2. Patients using heat at home to relieve pain and stiffness should be advised to use the heat for no more than 20 or 30 minute intervals and to avoid the use of heating pads overnight.
3. Care should be taken with patients on blood thinners, not to offer activities or tasks which require sharp objects (e.g. sewing needles, handling flowers with thorns).
4. Sharp objects should also be avoided with patients who have peripheral neuropathy in the hands.

5. Activities requiring excessive pinching and gripping should be avoided. Tools and implements should be built-up with padding whenever possible.

Evaluating Progress

Progress is demonstrated by an increase or stabilization of passive and active ranges of motion, strength, reduction in pain, and an increase in the ability to integrate the utilization of adaptive techniques and equipment into activities of daily living with progressively less cueing from the therapist.

Determining Change in or Termination of Treatment

The level and speed with which the patient assumes or resumes active participation in life roles associated with work, leisure and/or self-care activities will help to guide changes or termination in treatment.

Case Study

Description

Mrs. M. is a 65-year-old widow who has been referred for outpatient treatment, presenting with a diagnosis of rheumatoid arthritis that has affected the joints in both hands. She lives alone in a newly built apartment building in the center of a large northeastern city. Her one bedroom apartment is accessible by elevator and is equipped with a bathroom grab bar next to the tub. The kitchen is modern and fully equipped with a refrigerator, microwave, and dishwasher. All kitchen appliances and handles are standard. Mrs. M. has always been productive and, until three years ago, when arthritis pain became more frequent and severe in both hands, she was an avid knitter. In addition, Mrs. M. has found it necessary to limit her writing, despite the fact that she enjoys writing notes to her grandchildren, and exchanging original recipes with her friends, the latter requiring her to pen recipes onto her personalized recipe cards. She has continued to cook and bake, despite her discomfort, in preparation for holiday meals, which she enjoys preparing for her two adult children and three grandchildren.

Long- and Short-Term Goals

The long-term goal of intervention for Mrs. M is to complete light meal preparation incorporating adaptive equipment and energy conservation techniques.

This goal will be reached in part through successfully achieving the short-term goals of demonstrating safe and proper use of selected adaptive cooking equipment independently (cutting board, jar opener, electric knife, rocker knife, large handled utensils) during simple cold meal preparation.

Therapist Goals and Strategies

The therapist's goals include:

1. Increase patient's knowledge regarding adaptive equipment.

2. Increase patient's ability to use selected adaptive equipment safely and appropriately.
3. Increase patient's awareness of resources for medical information, social support, community mobility (transportation), and sources for adaptive equipment/devices.

The therapist's strategies include:

1. Avoid manual muscle testing and passive ROM during acute exacerbation of arthritis symptoms (joint swelling, redness, pain).
2. Provide bilateral resting hand splints to prevent deformity and reduce pain.
3. Provide large handled fork, spoon and rocker knife to facilitate self feeding and reduce stress on joints.
4. As symptoms subside institute graded exercise program to maintain/increase upper extremity strength.
5. Provide written materials, direct verbal instruction, and modeling the use of assistive devices to increase patient's knowledge regarding concepts of energy conservation and joint protection (avoidance of excessive grip, pinch or ulnar deviation of the wrist).

Activity

Making Turkey Sandwiches

In preparation for this activity the therapist assembles the following adaptive equipment: an adapted cutting board which is fitted with a nails to stabilize large items, rubber or under-cabinet jar opener, electric knife, rocker knife, built-up handle knife, and rolling cart.

The patient uses the rolling cart to retrieve a turkey breast, butter, lettuce, and mayonnaise from the refrigerator and transport them to the counter. The patient retrieves the bread from the counter and the adaptive equipment listed from the drawers located at waist level. Use of the rolling cart and convenient location of bread and utensils represents effective use of energy conservation techniques. The patient is instructed to place the turkey breast on the adapted cutting board and use the electric knife to cut several slices. The step represents the integration of a piece of adaptive equipment (cutting board) with and energy conservation technique (electric knife usage). The patient uses the built up handled knife to butter the bread and uses the jar opener to open the jar of mayonnaise. After spreading the mayonnaise with a large handled knife, the patient assembles the sandwich and cuts it using the rocker knife. These steps represent the use of adaptive equipment. The patient places the sandwich on light weight plates. The cart is used to return items to the refrigerator, counters and drawers and the patient is instructed to rinse dishes in warm water and gently squeeze a large sponge during and after the cleanup.

As the symptoms subside, the focus for Mrs. M's program shifts to instrumental activities of daily living (IADL). The therapist then collaborates with the client to identify and prioritize meaningful activities which will be incorporated into therapy. Energy conservation and joint protection strategies are taught to the client so that the strategies may be implemented presently and in the future as needed. This will require her to generalize concepts of energy conservation and joint conservation to meal preparation.

Treatment Objectives

Mrs. M. will be able to safely and successfully manipulate adapted foods and equipment in the preparation of a simple meal.

Resources

The Johns Hopkins White Papers, The Johns Hopkins Medical Institutions, Baltimore, MD

Arthritis Resource Guide, American Occupational Therapy Association

Internet Resources

About.com: Arthritis:
www.arthritis.about.com

AllAboutArthritis.com:
www.allaboutarthritis.com

American Association for Chronic Fatigue Syndrome:
www.aacfs.org

American Occupational Therapy Association:
www.aota.org

Americans with Disabilities Homepage:
www.usdoj.gov/crt/ada/adahom1.htm

Arthritis.com:
www.arthritis.com

Arthritis Foundation:
www.arthritis.org

Johns Hopkins:
www.HopkinsAfter50.com

Oregon Fibromyalgia Foundation:
www.myalgia.com

Scleroderma Foundation:
www.scleroderma.org

SeniorShops.com:
www.seniorshops.com

Spondylitis Association of America:
www.spondylitis.org

UC Berkeley WellnessLetter.com:
www.wellnessletter.com

Contact Numbers

National Arthritis Foundation:
800-283-7800

Spondylitis Association of America:
800-777-8189

Fibromyalgia Network:
800-853-2929

National Institute of Arthritis and Musculoskeletal and Skin Diseases & National Arthritis Musculoskeletal and Skin Diseases Information Clearinghouse:
301-495-4481

References

Hansen, A., & Atchison, B. (2000). *Conditions in occupational therapy: Effect on* occupational performance (2nd ed.). Philadelphia: Lippincott Williams & Wilkins.

Henry, A., & Kielhofner, G. (1989). The occupational performance history interview. Rockville, MD: American Occupational Therapy Association.

Hunter, J., Mackin, E., & Callahan, A. (Eds.). (2002). *Rehabilitation of the hand and upper extremity* (5th ed.). St. Louis, MO: C.V. Mosby.

Hunter, J., Schneider, L., Mackin,E., & Callahan, A. (1990). *Rehabilitation of the hand: Surgery and therapy* (3rd ed.). St. Louis, MO: C.V. Mosby.

Kielhofner, G. (1997). *Conceptual foundations of occupational therapy* (2nd ed.). Philadelphia: F. A. Davis Company.

Law, M., Baptiste, S., Carswell, H., McColl, M., Polatajko,H., & Pollock, N. (1994). *Canadian occupational performance measure* (2nd ed.). Toronto, Canada: Canadian Association of Occupational Therapy Publications.

Livneh, H., & Antonak, R. (1997). *Psychosocial adaptation to chronic illness and disability*. Gaithersburg, MD: Aspen Publishers, Inc.

Melvin, J., & Jensen, G. (Eds.). (1998). *Rheumatologic rehabilitation: Assessment and management.* Bethesda, MD: American Occupational Therapy Association, Inc.

Nalebuff, E. (1990). The rheumatic thumb. In J. Hunter, E. Mackin, & A. Callahan (Eds.). *Rehabilitation of the hand: Surgery and therapy* (3rd ed.). Philadelphia: C. V. Mosby.

Diabetes

22

Rosalyn Lipsitt, MHL, OTR/L

Synopsis of Clinical Condition

Prevalence and Etiology

Diabetes Mellitus is a disorder of the endocrine system. There are three types, all characterized by increased glucose in the bloodstream (hyperglycemia). This hyperglycemia is due to the body's inability to produce sufficient insulin, or the body's cells' inability to respond to available insulin.

Type I Diabetes

In the past, Type 1 Diabetes was called juvenile diabetes, however, individuals over age 40 have been known to contract this type, and, therefore, the term is less common today. Type I diabetes is known to appear suddenly before age 30. (Margolis & Saudek, 2002). This type is characterized as an autoimmune disease. Antibodies are produced that attack and damage the beta cells in the pancreas; the cells responsible for producing insulin. At first, beta cells may just be impaired, however, in less than a year, they are likely to produce little or no insulin, which results in the patient with diabetes having to regularly inject insulin. The exact etiology is unknown, however, it is believed that possible causes may be exposure to common viruses or other substances early in life, and genetics, although most patients with this type have no family history (National Institutes of Health, 1994).

Type II Diabetes

This type is the most common form of the disease and is known as non-insulin dependent diabetes mellitus (NIDDM). Type II diabetes usually develops in adults over the age of 40, most of whom are overweight. Those at greatest risk for this type are African Americans, Native Americans, and Hispanic Americans (Margolis & Saudek, 2002). In Type II diabetes, the pancreas usually produces insulin, however, receptors on cell surfaces, which interact with the insulin, are unable to create passageways for the insulin to enter the blood cells. Therefore, glucose builds up in the bloodstream, rather than being transported as fuel to other body structures. As a result, the body is forced to break down lipids and muscle tissue to create glucose for use by the body's cells. Possible causes for Type II diabetes are genetic, pancreatic diseases, surgical removal of the pancreas, tumors in endocrine organs, corticosteroid use in treatment of asthma and arthritis, or niacin for treatment of high cholesterol. Symptoms for this type result from poor utilization of glucose by the cells. It is important to note that not all patients experience every symptom, and some symptoms may occur in a very mild form.

Symptoms for Type II diabetes include:

- feeling ill
- thirst
- weight loss
- blurred vision
- frequent infections
- slow healing of skin lesions
- hunger
- fatigue
- numbness or tingling
- impotence

Gestational Diabetes

This type of diabetes develops or is discovered during pregnancy, usually appearing at 24 to 28 weeks gestation. With gestational diabetes, the placenta produces hormones which interfere with the body's response to insulin. It typically recedes at the conclusion of pregnancy, however, women with this diagnosis are at higher risk for developing diabetes later in life (Sammarco, 1991). Because symptoms are rare in these cases, screening for elevated blood sugar is routine and takes place between the 24th and 28th week of pregnancy. If tests are positive, the mother is instructed to maintain a low-calorie, low-sugar diet and begin a monitored exercise program. Blood sugar will be monitored throughout the pregnancy (Ferris, 1997). Poorly controlled diabetes before conception and during the first trimester of pregnancy can cause major birth defects in 5% to 10% of pregnancies and spontaneous abortions in 15% to 20% of pregnancies. During the second and third trimesters of pregnancy, poorly controlled diabetes may result in excessively large babies, which poses risks to both the mother and the child (National Diabetes Information Clearinghouse, 2000).

Complications: Acute

Acute complications from diabetes include:

1. Diabetic Ketoacidosis: (hyperglycemia). Previously described, this response requires immediate medical attention. Symptoms include abdominal pain, vomiting, rapid breathing, extreme fatigue, drowsiness, and sweet breath odor.
2. Hypoglycemia: (low blood sugar). This condition may occur when too much insulin is administered, there has been a delay in administering insulin, when the patient has missed a meal, or when the patient has been exercising without having eaten prior to exercise. The symptoms patients may experience are "crankiness," confusion, excessive perspiration, and hunger. For these symptoms, it is necessary to administer a sweetened drink, a high sugar snack, or glucose tablets or gels. In the event of loss of consciousness or seizure, it is vital to seek immediate emergency medical attention.

Complications: Non-Acute

Non-acute complications from diabetes include:

1. Retinopathy: (Microvascular disease)
2. Glaucoma and Cataracts

3. Nephropathy (Kidney disease)
4. Coronary Heart disease, High Blood Pressure and Stroke
5. Peripheral Vascular disease
6. Neuropathy (Nerve damage): Neuropathy is the most frequent complication of patients with Type II diabetes. Of those who have had diabetes for 25 years, there is a 50% prevalence of peripheral neuropathy exists (Zuberi & Miller, 2000). The three types of neuropathies include: peripheral, mononeuropathy, and autonomic neuropathy. Peripheral neuropathy is the most common, characterized by a progressive loss of function of the sensory nerves in the limbs. The patient may experience numbness, tingling, and pain in the bilateral extremities (Landry, 1990). Mononeuropathy leads to pain and weakness in areas supplied by a nerve or nerves whose blood supplies have been disrupted. These symptoms may improve gradually, without any treatment, however, nerve damage from peripheral neuropathy responds slowly, if at all with diabetic control. (NIH, 1994) (Saudek & Margolis, 2003).
7. Amputation: Diabetic foot problems, which arise from peripheral vascular disease, neuropathies, and slow healing of wounds and infections, sometimes lead to limb amputation.

Target Areas for Intervention

Occupational therapy intervention focuses on the assessment of sensation in the limbs and related performance in activities of daily living (ADL) and instrumental activities of daily living (IADL).

Contextual Considerations

Clinical

An initial interview is essential for obtaining information about the patient's physical and social environment, prior abilities with self-care and productive and leisure activities. It allows the therapist to establish rapport, form an initial impression regarding the patient's cognitive status, and affords the patient the opportunity to communicate personal concerns and perceptions regarding the illness.

In addition to the interview, functional assessments such as those described below are useful in evaluating a patient who exhibits the complications of diabetes which may interfere with safely conducting daily life activities. The *Occupational Performance History Interview* (OPHI) is a semi-structured interview which allows for a more in-depth observation of the individual, and a picture of the person's occupational history over time (Kielhofner, Mallinson, Crawford, et al., 1998). The *Functional Independence Measure*™(FIM) is a measure of disability and functionally assesses ADL communication and cognitive function. The patient is rated on 18 critical tasks, on a 7-point scale, from independent to dependent (Uniform Data System for Medical Rehabilitation, 1993). The Semmes-Weinstein Calibrated Monofilament Test is used to determine the extent of neuropathies in the hands or to determine if any sensory loss in the hands exists. The various microfilaments measure degrees of light touch. Information from this instrument is important so that safety issues may be addressed with the patient when planning ADL or leisure activities. Inability to accurately judge sensations of sharp and dull may be dangerous (Semmes, 1960). Other sensory testing should include the ability to feel temperature, tactile localization, stereognosis and two-point discrimination. Manual muscle testing, in the absence of acute arthritis or other contraindications, is important in determining an exercise program or other functional activities.

Family

The dietary requirements of persons with diabetes may impact the household. Families must be sensitive to these requirements when making food and menu choices. Medication and dietary requirements may necessitate adaptations in social activities. Spouses may require education regarding the effects of diabetes on sexual intimacy. Environmental adaptations and adaptive utensils may be required for the person with diabetes, depending on the extent of complications that are present such as visual and other sensory deficits as well as mobility restrictions due to amputations. Life insurance is particularly costly for persons with diabetes and their families. The American Diabetes Association provides information on policies designed to accommodate this population.

Practice Settings

Treatment of an individual with diabetes involves a team of professionals: diabetes nurse educators, endocrinologists, primary care physicians, registered dieticians, exercise physiologists, mental health professionals, ophthalmologists, podiatrists, occupational therapists, and physical therapists (Saudek & Margolis, 2003). Occupational therapists (OT) most likely treat individuals with diabetes who have undergone surgery for amputation, or hospitalization in a rehab setting for other reasons. In addition to the rehab setting, the OT may encounter a patient with diabetes in a community setting, nursing home, or home care.

Sociopolitical

The major sociopolitical issue related to patients diagnosed with diabetes is medical insurance coverage. Individuals with diabetes incur many expenses related to medications, testing equipment, supplies, and shoe gear. Medicare coverage is as follows:

Table 22.1
Medicare Coverage for Patients with Diabetes

Supplies/Services	Individuals Covered Under Medicare
Self-testing equipment and supplies	Individuals with diabetes who have Medicare coverage. Limits on supplies and how often purchased. Not restricted to insulin users. Medicare pays 80% of the cost of test strips.
Depth-inlay shoes **Custom-molded shoes**	
Shoe inserts	Individuals with diabetes who qualify under Medicare Part B must have one or more of these conditions in one or both feet: ■ history of partial or complete foot amputation. ■ history of previous foot ulcers.

(Continued)

Table 22.1 (*Continued*)

Supplies/Services	Individuals Covered Under Medicare
	■ history of callus that could lead to ulcers
	■ peripheral neuropathy with signs of problems with calluses
	■ poor circulation
	■ foot deformity
	Individuals being treated under a comprehensive diabetes care plan and need therapeutic shoes and/or inserts because of diabetes.
Medical nutrition therapy services	Individuals covered by Medicare when referred by a physician
	Patients pay 20% of Medicare-approved amount after the yearly Part B deductible.
Flu and Pneumoccocal Vaccines	For individuals with diabetes under Medicare
	■ flu shot once a year
	■ pneumonia vaccine
Glaucoma Screening	For individuals with diabetes once every 12 months under Medicare. Also available for anyone at high risk for glaucoma or with a family history for glaucoma. Patient pays 20% of the Medicare approved amount after the yearly Part B deductible (www.medicare.gov).

Lifestyle/Lifespan

Lifelong adjustments in self-care habits include glucose monitoring, administration of insulin, weight management/dietary restrictions, and skin management. Community mobility may be impacted in many states that require a doctor's certification confirming the ability of the individual with diabetes to be a safe driver. Coping issues related to possible role loss, managing chronic illness and other lifestyle changes may place individuals with diabetes at risk for depression. Diabetes may have an impact on vocational choices and the work environment. Persons with diabetes may require work place accommodations in the form of flexible scheduling to allow for meals and medication.

The American Diabetes Association provides advocacy and an attorney's network for cases of employment discrimination.

Clinical Decision Making Process

Defining Focus for Intervention

The focus of an occupational therapy program may be preventative, restorative, or a combination of both. Working in collaboration with the nurse, diabetes educator, or dietician, the OT plans patient education related to diet. The OT will plan and set up a cooking activity, with one or more patients, to cook appropriate meals or snacks, while at the same time addressing safety in the kitchen and safe functional mobility for those with walkers, prostheses, or wheelchairs. The OT will address proper stump management in the case of amputation, as well as foot care for all patients with diabetes. Patients are issued long handled mirrors in order to perform daily skin inspections of a residual limb and unaffected foot, and are educated to notice any sores or abrasions and to report these to their physicians. The OT will assist the patient with any issues related to his or her work environment or work schedule. Organizational skills may need to be improved in order to accommodate glucose testing and self-medication into the workday. The therapist will also educate the patient regarding energy conservation, if needed. In addition, patients with low vision may need adapted workplace environments. Safety education in light of sensory deficits is an important OT intervention. Patients with diabetes must be educated about wearing shoes at all times, both indoors and out, due to decreased sensation in the feet. Patients are also advised to test bath water with their elbows, or have a family member assist with this task, to avoid scalding of the hands and feet. Individuals with compromised sensory systems are also advised to avoid using sharp objects during leisure activities or in the kitchen. The OT will offer the patient alternatives for kitchen tasks, as well as explore safe leisure activities.

OTs will also address patients' concerns and anxieties about the condition itself. Many patients with chronic or progressive illness may experience anxiety and depression. Proper education regarding self-care and safety, and assistive devices serve to relieve many concerns. However, the OT will need to be aware of supportive services in the community, such as volunteers, paratransit, and support groups, in order to address patients' psychosocial issues.

Establishing Goals for Intervention

Occupational therapy goals for persons who present with diabetes are determined by several factors including the physician's referral, the setting, the results of the initial evaluations, and the insurance coverage defining the length of treatment. Informed by these factors, the occupational therapist analyzes data collected from interview and assessments and collaborates with the patient in the establishment and prioritization of long- and short-term goals for treatment.

Designing Theory-Based Intervention

It is important for the patient with diabetes to adapt to the chronic progressive nature of this condition. The Occupational Adaptation frame of reference assists the therapist in constructing an intervention process that facilitates internalized adaptation on the part of the patient (Schkade & Schultz, 1992). In order for the process to take place, the therapist must empower the patient to be his or her own advocate, and give the patient the tools to adapt to the chronic condition. This frame of reference is holistic, and its use ensures that the intervention is relevant to the patient's context.

Evaluating Progress

Because occupational therapy intervention for patients is largely guided by an adaptation model, progress is noted when the patient demonstrates consistency in incorporating adaptive strategies into daily activities. Examples of such progress would be evident in a patient who uses a skin inspection mirror as part of a morning self-care routine or who consistently plans and prepares meals that meet nutritional guidelines.

Determining Change in or Termination of Treatment

Termination of treatment would be recommended if either the allotted time for therapy had been reached, or therapy goals had been attained. Goals may be modified if the patient does not show signs of improvement or movement toward goals.

Case Study

Description

Rose is a 73-year-old, cognitively intact widow, with a past medical history of CVA and insulin-dependent diabetes mellitus. During her routinely scheduled doctor visit, Rose related that she was feeling "weakness in her arms and legs" and found herself "fumbling more" as she handled smooth objects. She felt that the combination of the weakness and decreased dexterity was compromising her ability to safely complete activities of daily living. The doctor scheduled a series of neurological tests for Rose to determine the etiology of her symptoms. It was determined that the decrease in strength was a result of deconditioning secondary to a sedentary lifestyle following the stroke and the decrease in fine motor function was the result of a peripheral neuropathy. Rose was referred to a skilled nursing facility for a short stay to participate in a rehabilitation program.

Rose has been living in a two-story home with her single daughter for three years, since she was discharged from the hospital following a stroke. Prior to this admission, Rose was independent with ADLs, light meal preparation, and light household tasks. She was able to self-monitor her glucose levels and administer insulin. She did not drive. Rose's daughter, Gail, is 50 years old and works full-time as an administrative assistant in a large insurance company. Once a year, Gail takes Rose on a one week vacation, however, most of the time, Rose is alone in the house watching T.V., playing solitaire, or talking on the phone with friends. She enjoys needlepoint, but has found it increasingly difficult to do.

The occupational therapy initial evaluation included an interview to determine the details of the patient's physical and social environment, her productive activities, her overall cognitive ability, her experience of the recent setback, and her priorities for treatment. An Occupational Performance History Interview was also conducted. Manual muscle testing was applied to determine the extent of weakness in the extremities and a functional assessment of self-care tasks to observe the degree of functional independence and need for assistive devices. Sensation testing was performed to assess any sensory deficits in the patient's hands. The initial evaluation revealed a slight decline in Rose's upper extremity strength, 3+/5 and 4/5 for the lower extremities. She required setup to minimum assistance with morning self-care tasks. She exhibited diminished sensation to Semmes test for light touch, also, sharp/dull, and hot/cold in both hands due to peripheral neuropathy.

Results of Rose's initial evaluation were discussed with her. In addition, possible interventions for ameliorating some of her declining abilities were offered. Collaboration with the patient resulted in setting priorities for treatment. During the course of the discussion, Rose emphasized the importance of her maintaining independence with self-care. Because she valued her sense of independence, she was agreeable to accepting assistive devices for dressing and bathing while participating in functional activities designed to gradually build strength. Equally important to Rose was exploration of leisure activities for the purpose of finding a satisfying occupation in which to engage during long hours at home while her daughter was at work. Rose was a creative person and was interested in discovering an outlet for her creativity. Ultimately, goals and interventions for Rose focused on ADLs and strengthening and leisure activities.

Long- and Short-Term Goals

The long-term goal of intervention for Rose is to demonstrate the ability to incorporate principles of safety awareness for sensory deficits into all ADLs, IADLs, and leisure activities.

This goal will be reached in part through successfully achieving the short-term goal of demonstrating the ability to incorporate safety awareness strategies into leisure activities.

Therapist Goals and Strategies

The therapist's goals include:

To provide education and demonstration of adaptive equipment and strategies which will promote safety awareness of sensory deficits during ADL/IADL and leisure activities.

The therapist's strategies include:

1. Educate patient in foot and nail care.
2. Reinforce importance of keeping skin protected and clean.
3. Provide assistive devices such as skin inspection mirror, button hooks, and zipper pulls.
4. Suggest the use of shoes with Velcro™ closures.
5. Advise patient to seek assistance with toe and finger nail care.
6. Demonstrate how to compensate for decreased temperature sensation in fingers with techniques such as testing water in sink or tub with elbows.
7. Provide simulations of daily activities in which the patient will have the opportunity to develop safe methods for approaching daily living activities. The therapist will provide intermittent correction or verbal cues as reminders, as needed.

Activity

Rubber Stamps

Rose was introduced to the craft of rubber stamping, which provided a creative and safe hobby; one that did not require fine motor skill or the use of sharp tools. Rubber stamps are available in different sizes and in myriad designs, ranging from children's themes to designs that would appeal to adults, such as flowers, border designs, and decorative alphabets. Inkpads are also available in many colors and sizes. The stamp is pressed onto the inkpad and then applied to paper, cardboard, or any surface for decoration. The design may be colored in or left as is.

In addressing Rose's goals, a large piece of shelf paper, approximately 20 × 20 inches was mounted on a slant board, in front of her and tilted away from her at approximately 120 degrees. Stamps were placed in front of her, while the ink pad was placed at midline. With the activity placed in this configuration, Rose not only enjoyed the leisure activity of creating a decorative piece of wrapping paper, but was also positioned so that shoulder flexion and elbow extension would be incorporated into the activity. Use of bilateral wrist weights could be incorporated into the activity to build upper extremity strength and endurance.

Block printing is chosen as a leisure activity that might substitute for the needlepoint that Rose had to abandon because of diminished sensation and vision. Block printing is safe for a person with diabetes because it does not require sharp objects that pose a danger to persons with peripheral neuropathies and low vision and will help to increase upper extremity strength. Since Rose is artistic and creative, block printing is a good choice.

Treatment Objectives

To increase the patient's awareness of how a particular activity may satisfy the need to be creative in a safe manner and also support the patient's need to maintain upper extremity strength and coordination.

Resources

American Association of Diabetes Educators (AADE):
www.aadenet.org

American Diabetes Association (ADA):
www.diabetes.org

Children with Diabetes:
www.childrenwithdiabetes.com

International Society for Pediatric and Adolescent Diabetes (ISPAD):
www.ispad.org

International Diabetes Center (IDC):
www.parknicollet.com/diabetes/

Medicare website:
www.medicare.gov

PRODoctors Guide to Diabetes on the Internet:
www.docguide.com

Contact Numbers

American Association of Diabetes Educators (AADE):
1-800-338-3633

American Diabetes Association (ADA):
1-800-232-3472

American Dietetic Association:
1-800-366-1655

American Dietetic Association:
1-800-366-1655

International Diabetes Center (IDC):
1-888-825-6315

References

Ferris, T. (1997). Gestational diabetes. In A. Fauci (Ed). *Harrison's principles of internal medicine.* New York: McGraw Hill.

Kielhofner, G., Mallinson, T., Crawford, E., Nowak, M., Rigby, M., Henry, A., & Walens, D. (1998). *A user's manual for the occupational performance history interview, version 2.* Chicago: Model of Human Occupation Clearinghouse, University of Illinois.

Landry, M. (1990). Peripheral nerve disorders. In L. Levy & V. Hetherington (Eds.). *Principles and practice of podiatric medicine.* New York: Churchill Livingstone.

Margolis, S., & Saudek, C. (2002). *Diabetes.* New York: Medletter Associates, Inc.

National Diabetes Information Clearinghouse, National Institutes of Health (1995). Diabetes overview.

National Institute of Diabetes and Digestive and Kidney Diseases (2000). *National diabetes statistics fact sheet.* Bethesda, MD: U.S. Department of Health and Human Services, National Institutes of Health.

National Institutes of Health, U. S. Department of Health and Human Services (1994). *Insulin-dependent diabetes.*

Sammarco, G. (1991). *The foot in diabetes.* Philadelphia: Lea & Febiger.

Saudek, C. and Margolis, S. (2003). *Diabetes.* New York: Medletter Associates, Incorporated.

Schkade, J. and Schultz, S. (1992). Occupational adaptation: Toward a holistic approach to contemporary practice. Part 1. *American Journal of Occupational Therapy, 46,* 917–925.

Semmes, J. (1960). Somatosensory changes after penetrating brain wounds in man. Cambridge, MA: Harvard University Press.

Uniform Data System for Medical Rehabilitation (UDSMR) (1993). *Guide for the uniform data set for medical rehabilitation (adult FIM), version 4.0.* Buffalo, NY: UB Foundation Activities.

Zuberi, L., & Miller, J. (2000). Metabolic and endocrine disorders. In S. Mandel & J. Willis (Eds.). *Handbook of lower extremity neurology.* Philadelphia: Churchill Livingstone.

Fall Related Injuries

23

Michelle Schleicher, MS, OTR/L

Synopsis of Clinical Condition

Prevalence and Etiology

Falls constitute the major cause of accidental and premature death, physical injury, immobility, psychosocial dysfunction, and nursing home placement in older adults. Sixty percent of falls occur at home, 30% occur in public places, and 10% occur in health care institutions. Of those older adults hospitalized due to a fall, one half will die one year later, usually as a result of secondary problems like pneumonia or congestive heart failure (CHF). The likelihood of falling rises steadily after age 75, peaks between age 80 and 84, then decreases after age 85 (likely due to a decline in activity at this age). Women are three times more likely to fall than men (Brummel-Smith, 1990).

It is important to remember that the true extent of falls in the elderly may be underestimated—only those who sustain an injury or require medical attention usually report the fall. Some do not report a fall for fear of nursing home placement or restriction of their activities.

Ten percent of falls in older adults result in non-fracture injuries such as head trauma, hematoma, joint dislocations, and muscle sprains. Five percent of falls each year result in fractures, the most common of which are of the forearm and hip. Approximately 200,000 hip fractures occur per year in the United States and 84% of these occur in persons over the age of 65. Some hip fractures may be spontaneous and secondary to osteopenia. It is often unclear as to whether a fall is the cause or the result of a hip fracture or both.

Common Characteristics and Symptoms

In persons over age 65, falls typically happen during routine or common activities such as walking, climbing stairs, transferring on /off chair and beds, bathing in bathtubs, or reaching or bending for objects. Falls occur when the body's mechanisms for compensation fail. This failure can be attributed to multiple intrinsic or extrinsic factors, including normal age-related physiologic changes such as vision, balance and musculoskeletal diseases, and changes in blood pressure and medications.

Vision changes can include alterations in visual acuity, contrast sensitivity, accommodation, visual fields, visual threshold, color perception, glare recovery, and depth perception. The body's ability to maintain balance is largely dependent on feedback from the vestibular, visual, and proprioceptive systems, and vestibular righting responses decrease with age. If any of these systems is not performing optimally, it will increase one's risk for falls. Age related changes to the musculoskeletal system include muscular atrophy, calcification of tendons and ligaments, flattening of discs between vertebrae, and increase curvature of the spine. All of these factors can attribute to decreased walking speed and decreased step length in the elderly.

The baroreflex activity is a mechanism of the cardiovascular system which regulates systemic blood pressure. Age related changes in this mechanism may diminish the adjustability of the heart rate to postural changes or to the hypotensive effects of medications. Older adults can often complain of a sense of "dizziness" when they sit up from a lying down position.

Various disease processes can put an older adult at risk for falls. Diseases to the visual system such as cataracts, macular degeneration, and glaucoma can interfere with safe mobility. Neurological diseases such as neuropathy, stroke, dementia, and Parkinson's Disease may alter proprioception, gait, and decrease spatial awareness. Diseases of the cardiovascular system may cause abnormalities in blood pressure regulation. Diseases of the bone (e.g. osteoarthritis) or to the muscle (e.g. polymyalgia rheumatica, hypokalemia) will cause muscle weakness. Psychological diseases such as depression can impair concentration and judgement and result in misperception of environmental hazards. The medications used to treat these disease processes and related conditions may increase an older adult's risk for falls. Drugs such as sedatives, antipsychotics, diuretics, and antihypertensives interfere with postural control, cerebral perfusion, and cognitive function and may increase the risk for falls.

Most falls sustained by older adults occur in the home, especially in the bedroom, bathroom, or stairway. Falls can occur when transferring from beds, chairs, or toilets that are either too high or too low, when walking in poorly lit or slippery areas, or tripping over low lying objects or floor coverings. Falls on stairways may be due to a lack of handrail support. In hospital and nursing home settings, falls may be attributed to similar environmental hazards as well as the improper use or fit of assistive devices and the use of physical restraints.

The most obvious sign/symptom that an older adult has fallen is the evidence of injury. Some older adults may report falls to a health professional, but for those who do not or who have not sustained an injury, the identification of risk factors best identifies characteristic signs and symptoms. These signs and symptoms can include age (fall risk increases with age), gender (women are more likely to fall than men), general complaints of dizziness, decrease in vision, an increase in confusion, or observed unsteadiness in gait patterns. Another characteristic sign of falls in the elderly is a gradual limitation in daily activities brought on voluntarily due to a fear of falling. For those who have sustained an injury or have admitted to a fall, investigation into the cause is essential for future prevention. It is important to ask the older adult to describe the circumstances leading up to the fall, how he or she felt at the time of the fall, and examine any intrinsic or extrinsic factors that may have contributed to the fall. Older individuals who have sustained a fall related injury are likely to fall again and they may begin to limit activity because of a fear of falling. This behavior can lead to decreased mobility and increased risk of falling and death by falling.

Target Areas for Intervention

The focus of occupational therapy for fall related injuries depends on the environment in which the individual is encountered. In community-based and home environments, individuals who have sustained a fall without injury or who are at high risk of injury from a fall can benefit from fall prevention education, and environmental assessment and adaptation. In outpatient or inpatient settings, intervention should focus on an examination of intrinsic and extrinsic causes for the fall and the physical and psychosocial ramifications of the fall. Ultimately, occupational therapists need to identify what roles and occupations are important to the older individual, what inherent risk for falls lies within these areas, and what interventions can be provided in order to allow them to function in their environment as safely as possible with the least amount of risk.

Secondary conditions may arise as a result of falls that can include fear of falling, immobility, deep vein thromboses, decubitus ulcers, urinary tract infections, hypostatic pneumonia, muscle atrophy, joint contractures, depression, and even death. Injuries that may appear to be or are reported to be fall related may be the results of elder abuse (Hopkins & Smith, 1993); Tideiksaar, 1994).

Contextual Considerations

Clinical

The clinical evaluation of a patient who has sustained an injury from a fall should include a thorough chart review and medical history, fall history, social history, physical assessment (including the visual/sensory systems), cognitive assessment, functional assessment, and environmental assessment.

The chart review and medical history should focus on any age related physiological changes and disease processes as well as medications that could have attributed to the fall. A fall history should include the person's recollection of recent falls (within 1–2 years), the location of the fall, and any symptoms he or she may have been feeling.

The social history should include a description of the home environment, prior level of functioning, use of durable medical equipment or assistive devices, and whether the person lives alone or with others. It may be necessary to verify this information with family members in the event the individual is not a reliable historian.

The physical assessment should include a musculoskeletal assessment (ROM, MMT) and a mobility assessment (including an assessment of gait, balance, and the ability to change position). The physical therapist is an excellent resource in determining issues relating to gait and postural stability. A thorough physical assessment may have to be ongoing, depending on the nature and severity of an injury, as the individual may be in acute pain or have limitations in their weightbearing capabilities.

Several assessment tools can be helpful in assessing the area of mobility in older adults. The *Tinetti Balance and Assessment Tool*, the *Tinetti Fall Risk Assessment*, the *Berg Functional Balance Test*, the *Functional Reach Test*, the *Timed 'Get Up and Go' Test*, and the *Duke Mobility Skills Profile* are all easily administered assessments for gait and postural stability.

The visual/perceptual assessment should include general information on visual acuity, proprioception, spatial awareness, and figure ground determination. Many of these areas can be screened through observation of the older adult during functional activity and if a problem is noted, examined more thoroughly via tools such as the *Motor-Free Visual Perceptual Test* (MVPT) or the *Visual Motor Index* (VMI). A consult to an opthamologist may also be indicated.

Similarly, a cognitive assessment can begin while the individual is completing basic activities of daily living (ADLs). Areas such as safety awareness, judgement, and problem solving can be observed and more formally assessed if the need arises. The *Mini-Mental State Exam* is a quick, easily administered screening tool to identify the possibility of cognitive impairment.

Of equal importance is the older adult's psychosocial functioning after having sustained a fall related injury. The *Geriatric Depression Scale* is a basic tool designed to quickly assess an older person's emotional/psychological status. The *Activities-specific Balance Confidence Scale* (ABC Scale) is a useful tool in assessing an older adult's (particularly community-dwelling) fear of falling. A psychiatric consult may also prove beneficial.

An environmental assessment in the person's home or present living condition may be arranged at any time along the individual's continuum of care. Typically, it is beneficial to assess the home as early as possible so as to provide the most appropriate treatment plan and recommendations. Frequently, this assessment is done when the individual is preparing for discharge from an inpatient setting. The occupational therapist can accompany the patient to his or her home where he or she can demonstrate safety in mobility and in managing activities of daily living. Recommendations are offered for removal of environmental hazards and possible changes in order to make the older adult as safe and independent as possible. In addition, an environmental assessment can serve as an excellent preventative measure for those older adults at risk for falls.

Family

It is important to have a good understanding of the older adult's family dynamics and support system. Most often, an individual who has suffered a fall related injury will require some level of support upon returning home. If the individual is unable to return home alone, it becomes critical to understand the family's values, priorities, and cultural preferences. A family's ability or inability to provide assistance/supervision to the older adult can sometimes mean the difference between a person's returning home and institutionalization. Also, families may consider cultural and financial issues when making decisions regarding the disposition of a loved one.

If possible, it is advisable that the occupational therapist involves the family in the older adult's care and discharge planning as early as possible. It is imperative that the occupational therapist remains as objective as possible when making professional recommendations relating to the safety and well being of the older adult who has fallen and possibly sustained an injury. The occupational therapist should assist the patient and family in discussing all alternatives to care and involve the social worker and discharge planner to discuss financial considerations and community assistance.

The occupational therapist should be educated on reimbursement issues relating to lengths of stay, durable medical equipment, assistive devices, and home care as well as financial alternatives to assist the older adult and/or family members in providing the equipment and/or assistance needed. A social worker may also be able to assist in these matters.

Family training might be necessary in order to educate the older adult's caregivers on how to assist their loved one at home safely. It is equally important to educate the family on fall prevention in order to keep their older family members living safely and independently as long as possible.

Practice Setting

Depending on the severity of the fall related injury, older adults can be treated by an occupational therapist in various settings. Education and intervention related to fall prevention can occur in wellness community settings as well as home care and outpatient settings. An individual who has fallen at home and sustained a minor injury such as a hematoma or wrist fracture may receive occupational therapy intervention on an outpatient basis or through home care. The older adult who has sustained a more moderate to severe injury (e.g. hip fracture, head injury) will receive occupational therapy services in a skilled nursing facility or an inpatient rehabilitation setting. Upon discharge, home-based occupational therapy services and outpatient services may be recommended. In long-term care settings, the older adult who has fallen may briefly receive acute care intervention for his or her injuries and then return to the long-term care facility for further occupational therapy intervention.

Sociopolitical

The Balanced Budget Act (BBA) of 1997 significantly affected reimbursement of rehabilitative services to older adults with Medicare coverage. The BBA impacted every segment of the health care industry, including hospitals, home health services, skilled nursing facilities (SNFs), comprehensive outpatient rehabilitation facilities (CORFs), and physician's offices, all of which can potentially offer rehab services to the elderly who have sustained a fall related injury. Of most significance is the imposition of an annual cap of $1500 per beneficiary for services that rehab agencies, CORFs, SNFs and physician's offices ($1500 for PT and SLP services and $1500 for OT services) provide. This annual cap may prevent some older adults from receiving the necessary rehabilitation services status post a fracture from a fall.

Of other sociopolitical concern is an older adult's access to adequate health care. The older adult with little social support and decreased mobility may not have access to proper health care facilities. In many inner cities, older adults may utilize the emergency room as their primary means of medical attention. Fall prevention and/or investigations into frequent falls are not always feasible in an emergency room setting.

Lifestyle/Lifespan

The impact of a fall related injury on an older adult's lifestyle depends on a number of factors: his or her previous level of independence, the severity of the injury, the recovery from the injury (both physically and psychosocially), and available support system or resources.

Frequently, an older adult who has sustained a fall related injury that requires hospitalization will suffer some loss of independence initially. He or she may need to rely on family or community organizations at least temporarily until further recovery and adjustment occurs. The older adult who has recovered well from a fall related injury may recognize the benefit of the support and resources provided and may choose to continue with them in order to maintain safety and lessen his or her fall risk for the future.

For the older adult who suffers a significant loss of independence due to a fall related injury, the adjustment to a change in lifestyle may be drastic. If the financial means and/or family support is not available to provide assistance in the home, he or she may have to consider alternatives to returning home such as assisted living or long-term care placement. Although some older adults may adjust well to this alternative, most find it to be a devastating realization.

Clinical Decision Making Process

Defining Focus for Intervention

The focus for OT intervention depends on a number of factors: the type and severity of the fall related injury and the setting in which intervention is provided. For example, for the older adult who may have sustained a wrist fracture from a fall in the bathtub and is being seen on an outpatient basis upon cast removal, the focus of intervention will be on gaining range of motion (ROM) and strength to complete the daily activities within his or her roles and occupations. Intervention related to the cause of the fall and fall prevention in the home and community may occur as a secondary focus to intervention.

If an older adult has sustained a hip fracture and is referred for OT services while in a skilled nursing facility (SNF), the focus of intervention will be defined by the individual's specific roles and occupations in the home and or community. Typically, basic self-care involving bathing, dressing, toileting, basic mobility, and IADLs are the focus of intervention in SNFs. Cognition may initially become the primary focus for OT intervention with the older adult who has suffered a hip fracture from a fall. A new onset of confusion/disorientation or difficulty following directions is not uncommon in an older adult who has recently been hospitalized. Time may need to be taken to fully assess and treat the individual's cognitive functioning before effective physical rehabilitation or education can begin. If psychosocial factors such as fear, anxiety, or depression threaten to hinder the physical recovery of an older adult who has sustained a hip fracture, these must become the primary focus of intervention. Therapeutic use of self is important in gaining trust and decreasing fear and anxiety in order to make the necessary physical gains. Education relating to home safety should be a constant theme throughout treatment intervention.

If a resident of a nursing home has fallen and has sustained a humeral fracture, the initial focus of occupational therapy should be an environmental assessment and/or caregiver education based on the cause of the fall. Depending on the severity of the injury and the individual's prior level of functioning, a secondary intervention may focus on resuming independence in areas of basic ADL and IADL.

Establishing Goals for Intervention

The therapist and patient must collaborate and determine the individual's previous roles and occupations in order to establish and prioritize goals for treatment. For example, the OT may approach the older individual who has sustained a fall related injury with a goal of modified independence with bathing and dressing in order to return home. The patient may choose to have assistance with these tasks at home in order to save energy to prepare snacks for her friends who meet to play cards three times a week.

It is also essential to consider the older adult's prior level of functioning when establishing goals. It may not be necessary for the individual to achieve independence in toileting when he or she has been incontinent for two years and receives assistance from a spouse. Or perhaps the individual has not cooked or cleaned in the last five years but orders out instead. Appropriate goals in this case would perhaps address functional mobility, walker safety, and the use of adaptive equipment to safely set up and clean up a meal.

Another important factor to consider when establishing goals for intervention is the patient's length of stay. In most settings, Medicare HMOs may significantly limit the number of visits an individual can receive OT services. The HMO may consider a goal of supervision to be adequate in order for the older adult status post hip fracture to return home. Although reimbursement issues should not dictate the OT's goals for intervention, they should be realistically considered.

Establishing goals for intervention involves thoughtful consideration of the older adult's prior level of functioning, his or her disposition, his or her goals, the family's goals and resources, and the influence of third party payors.

Designing Theory-Based Intervention

The biomechanical frame of reference is useful in working with persons who have fallen. In most falls resulting in injury, clear, measurable deficits relate to ROM, strength, and endurance. Intervention targets these areas in order to achieve functional outcomes. For instance, an individual may be working on improving standing tolerance to five minutes in order to be able to complete a simple meal preparation. A functional outcome that is meaningful to the patient will be motivating.

Another frame of reference used when treating an older adult who has fallen is the rehabilitation frame of reference. Frequently, a therapist may have to teach the patient to compensate for deficits that cannot be remediated as quickly as the inpatient process might allow. Therapists might find themselves approaching treatment intervention from both of these frames of reference, biomechanically (improving standing tolerance) or rehabilitatively (instructing on energy conservation techniques in the kitchen). As the needs of the patient, family support, financial resources, and reimbursement schedules vary, so may the approaches to occupational therapy intervention.

The occupational adaptation frame of reference is helpful in designing intervention and establishing goals for treatment of the fall related injury. Aging and the increased risk for falls can involve frequent adaptation to one's environment. As an occupational therapist treating an older adult who has fallen, it should be a goal to improve on the patient's internal adaptation process. Changes in their lifestyle because of a fall may be permanent, however, older adults can learn to adapt more readily and easily, making the process less challenging. This involves choosing activities that gradually challenge the patient while allowing the patient to achieve mastery over his or her environment.

Evaluating Progress

When working with the older adult who has suffered a fall related injury, progress may initially be determined by an improvement in basic mobility and self-care. However, once these initial hurdles are overcome, progress is measured by the individual's ability to internalize and utilize safety techniques such as reaching back for a chair before sitting or sitting for a few minutes before standing up from a lying down position. Progress in a home care situation might be evaluated by a family's or caregiver's successful modifications of the home environment to reduce the risk for falls, or acquiring the recommended bathtub equipment for an older individual living alone so he or she can safely transfer in/out of the tub. In a nursing home or long-term care setting, progress can be evaluated by successful interventions to the environment to reduce the risk for falls, restraint reduction or a routine caregiver use of fall prevention strategies.

Determining Change in or Termination of Treatment

Ultimately, the decision to terminate treatment is made when an individual has met all of his or her goals or is not able to meet the goals established in a reasonable time frame. It is important to involve the patient and family/caregiver in this decision making process. Perhaps new goals should be established or the existing goals downgraded to meet the needs of the individual. For example, an OT may find that after two weeks, the patient is simply not reaching a goal of supervision with lower body dressing despite multiple approaches and interventions. It may be necessary to discuss this with the patient and/or family, spend important time working towards another goal, or educate the family/caregiver in providing assistance.

A medical condition, impaired cognition, or emotional status may be hindering progress towards goals and discharge from OT services may be appropriate until the person is able to focus more effectively on OT intervention.

The type of setting in which one provides OT intervention may also determine when termination of treatment is warranted. For example, a previously independent older adult who has sustained a fall related injury may not want OT services to terminate until he or she is able to go food shopping independently. Unfortunately, an inpatient setting may not be the ideal setting to achieve this goal in a reasonable amount of time. What may be more appropriate is to discharge the individual from OT services with Meals on Wheels and continue pursuit of this goal via home care or on an outpatient basis.

Case Study

Description

Ms. J is an 88-year-old African American woman who sustained a left hip fracture after falling in her home while putting groceries away. She was admitted to the hospital and underwent an open reduction, internal fixation of her left hip. She was transferred to a skilled nursing facility for rehabilitation and referred for occupational therapy services.

A thorough chart review indicated a past medical history significant for hypertension, peripheral vascular disease, cerebrovascular accident, coronary artery disease, and chronic renal insufficiency. Her medications at the time of admission included Lopressor aspirin, Tylenol™ (regular and #3), Flonase™, and a multivitamin. Her orthopedic surgeon would only allow her to place partial weight onto her left leg when transferring, standing, or ambulating.

Ms. J lived on the first floor of a three-story house and walked independently with a rolling walker in the home. She managed all basic self-care and IADLs independently. She owned no other assistive devices or durable medical equipment. Her daughter lived on the third floor, but had medical issues of her own and was unable to provide any physical assistance to her mother. She did assist with grocery shopping and simple house cleaning. Prior to retiring, Ms. J worked as a real estate agent. She did not report any other leisure interests besides housework and listening to the radio.

Ms. J's recollection of her fall was, "I was reaching up to put something away and fell backwards." She did not report any previous falls at home or in the community. Her physicians did not clearly state the cause of her recent fall. She and her daughter anticipated that she would return home after her course of rehabilitation.

Upon initial assessment, Ms. J is observed to have considerable thoracic kyphosis, limiting cervical extension, and full upright posture in both sitting and standing. Her upper extremities are limited in range of motion, specifically in shoulder flexion and abduction, and has limited grasp in her right hand secondary to degenerative changes. Her overall upper body strength can be classified as 3+ out of 5.

She required complete assistance to go from a lying down to a sitting up position over the edge of the bed. Her unsupported sitting balance was poor. At the time of her initial assessment, she was unable to stand or attempt any weightbearing support through her legs secondary to pain and fear/anxiety.

If seated with support, Ms. J did demonstrate the ability to feed herself adequately given assistance with setup of her tray and the ability to complete basic grooming given setup of the necessary items. However, extensive assistance was required for all other self-care. She had a foley catheter inserted and was incontinent of bowel.

A visual screening indicated her visual acuity to be functional despite Ms. J having lost her glasses in the hospital. An ongoing assessment during treatment would later indicate impairments in spatial awareness and depth perception. No formal assessment was completed.

Cognitively, Ms. J was alert and oriented and was able to follow all directions concerning evaluation and treatment. Of most obvious concern during Ms. J's initial assessment was a vocalized fear with any kind of active or passive movement. She was fearful of moving her affected leg, fearful of attempting to sit unsupported on the bed, and later in treatment, fearful when attempting to transfer, stand, or ambulate. Her supported standing balance was poor, demonstrating a gross posterior lean. She scored a 1out of a maximum score of 65 on the Berg Test for Balance.

Interpretation of the data collected led to an initial treatment plan focusing on basic postural awareness (in both sitting and standing) and reduction of anxiety followed by participation in self-care activities. It was anticipated at the time of initial assessment, given her age and functional status, that she would not return to a modified independent level with her basic ADLs.

Throughout Ms. J's treatment, she required further hospitalizations for syncope, dehydration, and urinary tract infections and developed decubitus ulcers on the bottom of both heels, requiring treatments. She was not able to overcome her postural insecurity and fear of falling in order to return to being a functional ambulator or to care for herself safely. Her daughter was unable to care for her at home. Consequently, Ms. J became a resident of the nursing facility and requires extensive assistance for her activities of daily living. She has had difficulty adjusting to nursing home placement and is reluctant to engage in recreational activity outside of her room. She continues to express a fear of falling when provided care by her caregivers.

Long- and Short-Term Goals

The long-term goal of intervention for Mrs. J. is to complete basic self-care activities, household transfers and mobility with supervision.

These goals will be reached in part through successfully achieving the following short-term goals:

1. Mrs. J will transfer sit to stand from a toilet, chair, or bed with moderate - assistance.
2. Mrs. J will stand supported for two minutes with fair balance in order to assist in lower body dressing and toileting.

Therapist Goals and Strategies

The therapist's goals include:

1. Improve sit to stand transfer ability.
2. Improve standing tolerance and balance.
3. Reduce anxiety with postural changes in both sitting and standing.

The therapist's strategies include:

1. Conduct patient/caregiver education related to transfers.
2. Conduct patient/caregiver education in use of assistive devices and durable medical equipment.
3. Improve patient's postural awareness in both sitting and standing.
4. Conduct patient/caregiver education related to relaxation techniques.
5. Gradually increase length of time patient is standing and level of assistance provided.

Activity

Memory Game

A "Memory Game" of cards is placed in front of the patient at chair-height level. Two patients are seated unsupported side by side or across from one another. Each patient is asked to reach forward to turn over two cards to obtain a match. The surface can be changed to allow for increased forward or lateral flexion. When a match is obtained, each patient is asked to stand up to mark a slash under his or her name on a vertical surface.

In planning an activity for Mrs. J, it will be important to choose and structure an activity that incorporates multiple opportunities for her to practice moving from sit to stand and back using her rollator walker for support. Repetition of the sit to stand pattern will address her fear of changing position. Short periods of static standing should also be incorporated. Static standing will allow her to practice taking only partial weight on her healing hip using the walker for support. Mrs. J's ability to use her walker for standing will serve as a prerequisite for ambulation and functional mobility.

Treatment Objective

Ms. J will express less than 25% vocalizations relating to fear/anxiety when changing positions in either sitting or standing.

Resources

The following resources can be helpful for gathering clinical data:

Chart review

Present/Past

Medical history

Social history

Fall history

Physical assessment:

- ROM
- MMT

Visual/Perceptual assessment:

- MVPT
- VMI

Mobility assessment:

- Tinetti Balance and Assessment Tool
- Tinetti Fall Risk Assessment
- Berg Functional Balance Test
- Functional Reach Test
- Timed Get up & Go Test
- Duke Mobility Skills Profile

Cognitive/Psychosocial assessment:

- Mini Mental State Exam
- Geriatric Depression Scale
- Activities-specific Balance Confidence Scale (ABC Scale)

Environmental assessment

The following resources can be helpful for gathering family data:

Community/Cultural/Religious groups

Family/Support systems

The following are common practice settings:

Community/Wellness centers

Home care

Outpatient programs

Inpatient programs

- acute care
- SNF
- inpatient rehab
- transitional care
- long-term care

The following resources can be helpful for gathering sociopolitical data:

Balanced Budget Act of 1997

Medicare/Medicaid

Healthcare Accessibility

The following issues can be helpful in understanding and managing lifestyle/lifespan issues:

Fear of falling

Loss of independence

Frailty/Immobility

Home safety modification

Institutionalization

- Independent living
- Assisted living
- Long-term care

Internet Resources

American Association of Retired Persons (AARP):
www.aarp.org

American Occupation-al Therapy Association (AOTA):
www.aota.org

American Physical Therapy Asscociation (APTA):
www.apta.org

Centers for Disease Control (CDC):
www.cdc.com

Centers for Medicare and Medicaid Services (CMS):
www.cms.hhs.gov
www.medicare.gov

Department of Health and Human Services:
www.hhs.gov

National Institute on Aging email address:
niainfo@access.digex.net

Philadelphia Corporation for Aging:
www.pcaphl.org

Philadelphia Senior Center:
www.philaseniorcenter.com

Temple University:
www.temple.edu/older_adult/

References

Brummel-Smith, K. (1990). Falls and Instability in the Older Person. In B. Kemp, K. Brummel-Smith, & J. W. Ramsdell (Eds.), *Geriatric Rehabilitation* (pp.193–208). Austin, TX: Pro-Ed.

Hopkins, H. L., & Smith, H. D. (1993). *Willard and Spackman's occupational therapy* (8th ed.). Philadelphia: J. B. Lippincott Co.

Tideiksaar, R. (1994). Falls. In B. R. Bonder & M. B. Wagner (Eds.), *Functional Performance in Older Adults* (pp. 224–241). Philadelphia: FA Davis Company.

Cerebral Vascular Accident

24

Marlene J. Morgan, Ed.D., OTR/L

Synopsis of Clinical Condition

Prevalence and Etiology

The World Health Organizations define a cerebral vascular accident (CVA) or stroke as an acute neurological dysfunction of vascular origin that produces signs and symptoms corresponding to involvement of focal areas of the brain (World Health Organization, 1980). Cerebral vascular accident may result in a complex cluster of symptoms including motor paralysis, sensory disturbances, speech and language disorders, and intellectual and personality changes (World Health Organization, 1980).

Each year in the Unites States approximately 600,000 persons experience either a first or a recurrent stroke. This positions stroke as the third leading cause of death following heart disease and cancer. Seventy-two percent of persons who sustain a stroke are 65 years old or older. Stroke is a leading cause of serious long-term disability in the United States. Specifically, in stroke survivors: 48% experience hemiparesis; 22% are non-ambulatory; between 24 % and 53% experience difficulty with activities of daily living (ADL); 12% to 18% experience aphasia and 32% exhibit signs of depression (American Heart Association, 1999).

A cerebral vascular accident or stroke occurs when there is a failure to supply adequate blood and subsequent oxygen to the cells in the brain. Brain cells are susceptible to death when deprived of oxygen. There are two broad categories of stroke: hemorrhagic and ischemic. In a hemorrhagic stroke, a vessel ruptures causing leakage of blood into the surrounding structures. Hemorrhagic strokes account for 15% to 25% of strokes. Ischemic strokes are the result of emboli to the brain. Emboli, which cause blockages to the circulation in the brain, may originate in the heart or anywhere in the arterial circulation (Bartels, 1998). Risk factors for ischemic stroke include age, race, gender, heredity hypertension, diabetes, cardiac disease, smoking, obesity, stress, and a sedentary lifestyle (American Heart Association, 1999).

Common Characteristics and Symptoms

In a stroke, the neurological deficits persist longer than 24 hours. Some persons may experience intermittent signs and symptoms associated with stroke that last for a few minutes to 24 hours. These episodes are classified as transient ischemiic attacks (TIAs) (Bartels, 1998).

The specific presentation of the patient who has sustained a stroke depends on the artery involved. The anterior cerebral artery, the middle cerebral artery, and the posterior cerebral artery supply blood to the brain. Using diagnostic techniques such as computerized tomography (CT scan), and positron emission tomography (PET scan) allows the physician to determine which anatomic structures are involved (Bartels, 1998).

Interruption of the blood flow in the middle cerebral artery is the most common cause of CVA (Bartels, 1998). Characteristics of middle cerebral artery involvement include: hemiplegia on the contralateral side, aphasia if the lesion is on the dominant side, sensory deficits, and perceptual deficits if the lesion is in the non-dominant hemisphere. Interruption of blood flow in the anterior cerebral artery produces weakness in both the upper and lower extremity contralaterally. Typically, weakness in the lower extremity is more severe than weakness in the upper extremity. Related changes may include apraxia, incontinence of bowel and bladder, sensory loss, changes in intellectual function such as disorientation, and the re-emergence of primitive reflexes. Symptoms of interruption of blood flow in the posterior cerebral artery are more difficult to anticipate. This artery supplies blood to a number of important regions such as the upper brainstem, the temporal lobe, and the occipital lobe. Some patients with posterior cerebral artery lesions exhibit involuntary movement such as tremor. Memory loss, homonymous hemianopsia, and topographical disorientation may also be present (Bartels, 1998).

The complicated nature of stroke requires that the therapist be aware of complications and precautions that may accompany the primary diagnosis. Complications and precautions to be aware of include deep venous thrombosis, shoulder subluxation, impaired sensation, visual field deficits, and impaired communication. Deep venous thrombosis (DVT) is the formation of blood clots in the deep leg veins. They frequently form secondary to immobility. Physicians fear that the thrombosis may produce a pulmonary embolus. Pulmonary embolism is the most common cause of death in patients with CVA and are apt to occur thirty days after the incident. Management of DVT includes drug therapy, the use of compressive stockings, and movement (Roth, 1991).

Changes in tone and strength in the muscles of the shoulder girdle following stroke may result in a subluxation at the glenohumeral joint. Subluxation is a malalignment and instability of the glenohumeral joint. It typically results from a malalignment between the scapula and the trunk. Because the subluxed shoulder is unstable, it is important that it is handled and positioned carefully. Positioning with pillows, a lap tray, and taping are all suggested approaches to carefully handle a subluxed shoulder (Bartels, 1998).

Sensory impairment that occurs post stroke may result in the patient demonstrating decreased protective sensation. Limited awareness of and protective sensation in an affected extremity may subject the patient to the risk of injury. Patients and family members must be made aware of sensory impairments and be taught compensation techniques. Such compensation techniques may include using vision to monitor the affected arm and hand and/or using the sound side to test the temperature of the water before bathing or showering.

CVA may create visual field deficits. A patient with a visual field deficit receives limited or no information from a specific area of the visual field. Limited visual information creates an unsafe situation as the patient moves in and interacts with the environment. The patient and family must be made aware of the presence and implications of any visual field deficit. The patient may be taught to use head turning in combination with visual scanning to compensate for a visual field deficit. The patient and family may also be taught to modify the environment or activity by moving objects into the functioning visual field.

A stroke may impact a patient's ability to communicate. The most common post stroke communication impairment is aphasia. Aphasia is a language disorder in which there is a loss of language skills, slowed or slurred speech, impaired auditory comprehension, or difficulty retrieving words (Halper & Mogil, 1986). The occupational therapist may model for the family a system of communicating with an aphasic patient which includes using a patient tone of voice, and using short, simple sentences. Use of demonstrations and gestures may also aid understanding.

Target Areas for Intervention

Each patient who presents with a stroke will demonstrate an individual compliment of signs and symptoms. Additionally, a stroke will affect each patient's life roles and activities in a unique way. Despite individual presentations, OT intervention for a stroke survivor can be summarized into area of intervention focus:

- Improve motor control to support functional independence in ADL and IADL.
- Improve perceptual abilities to support functional independence in ADL and IADL.
- Improve cognitive abilities to support functional independence in ADL and IADL.
- Support psychosocial processes and adjustment to disability in support of independent ADL and IADL.

Contextual Considerations

Clinical

The occupational therapist collects information related to the patient's pre-morbid life roles and activities. This may be accomplished through an interview with the patient and/or family. The impact that the stroke has had on a patient's level of function in ADL and IADL can be measured using an assessment such as the Canadian Occupational Performance Measure (COPM), the *Functional Independence Measure*™ (FIM), or the Assessment of Motor and Process Skills (AMPS) (Keith, Granger, Hamilton, Sherwin, 1987; Law, et al., 1994; Fisher, 1995). The COPM, using an interview format, yields information about the patient's perspective of the impact of the stroke on his or her life by eliciting goals, information about his or her current level of performance, and his or her level of satisfaction with current performance. The FIM provides information on the patient's level of independence in basic ADLs on 18 items including self-care and mobility. The FIM provides scoring on a seven point scale which characterizes the amount of physical assistance, adaptive equipment and techniques, or cueing that is required to support performance. The AMPS provides information on the impact of motor and process skills on function.

Assessment of the patient's motor control is based on observation. The therapist assesses the presence of any abnormal reflexes during movement. Abnormal patterns of muscle tone are identified and compared to the typical pattern of deformity that is found in patients after stroke. Specifically, the therapist looks for evidence of neck flexion to the weak side, neck rotation to the sound side, scapular retraction, trunk flexion to the affected side, wrist flexion with ulnar deviation, finger flexion and adduction, elbow flexion, pelvic rotation up and back, hip extension adduction and internal rotation, ankle plantar flexion, foot inversion, and toe flexion and adduction.

Assessment of upper extremity status may include tests for range of motion (ROM), subluxation, sensation, coordination, and upper extremity function. Range of motion is assessed in both the affected and unaffected extremities through observation and/or goniometry. The presence of subluxation is tested for by first locating the head of the humerus in the glenoid fossa. The therapist attempts to insert one or two fingers in the space between the humeral head and the scapula. The number of fingers that the therapist is able to insert into the space describes presence of a subluxation.

A sensory test is completed to identify the pattern and degree of sensory awareness in the affected extremity. The therapist makes careful note of the areas in which protective sensation such as sharp/dull and hot/cold are absent or impaired. Coordination may be assessed formally through the Jebsen-Taylor Hand Function Test (Jebsen, R. et al., 1969) or through clinical observation. Upper extremity function, specifically the role that the affected extremity is able to play in bimanual tasks, can be assessed using the Functional Test for the Hemiplegic Extremity. The Functional Test for the Hemiplegic Extremity allows the therapist to evaluate the effectiveness of the affected extremity as a stabilizer, holder, or fine motor assist (Wilson, D., Baker, J., & Craddock, J., 1984).

The patient's perceptual status is assessed through a combination of functional observations and tests. During functional tasks such as dressing and cooking, the therapist observes for perceptual deficits, which may include body scheme disorders, disorders in spatial relations, apraxias, and agnosias. A patient demonstrating a body scheme disorder may have difficulty recognizing the relationship of his or her body parts. The patient may be unable to put his or her arm into the sleeve of a shirt without demonstration. Spatial relations disorders may limit the patient's ability to recognize recognize the characteristics of an object such as its position, form, or depth. A patient with distorted spatial relations may have difficulty finding a fork in a utensil drawer. Patients with apraxia demonstrate an inability to complete certain skilled movements even though the components such as muscle strength, sensation, and coordination are present. Finally, agnosia is an inability to recognize objects even though sensation is intact. The patient with agnosia may be unable to recognize his own clothes even though sight is intact. Formal tests such as the Motor Free Test of Visual Perception–revised (MVPT-R) may be used to assess specific perceptual skills (Colarusso, R. & Hammill, D., 1996).

Cognitive skills may be assessed using tests such as the Mini Mental Status Examination and the Lowenstein Occupational Therapy Cognitive Assessment (LOTCA; Katz, Itzkovich, Averbuch, Elazer, 1989). Such tests provide insight into higher level cognitive function. Results of formal tests provide valuable insights and a foundation for interpreting difficulty that the patient may be experiencing in ADLs or IADLs.

Psychological adjustment to disability is a critical area to assess. Psychological adjustment may affect the patient's willingness to participate in treatment as well as his or her interaction with family and friends. Occupational therapists may look to psychology or neuropsychology for guidance about how to address these issues. They may, however, administer tests such as the Beck Depression Inventory. The Beck Depression Inventory requires the patient to provide a self-rating of attitudes and behaviors related to depression (Beck, A. & Steer, R., 1987).

Assessments of home safety and accessibility are completed as discharge planning progresses. Clinical observation in combination with assessments such as the Kohlman

Evaluation of Living Skills (KELS) will alert the therapist to potential safety hazards at discharge (Kohlman-Thompson, 1993). Clinical information, test results, and interview data from the patient and family may point to the need for a home visit or a referral to a home care agency.

Family

Assessment of the family's reaction to the stroke is key. Since a stroke may have a major impact on the roles that the patient resumes, preparing for its effect on the family system is important. Family members may be called on to provide psychological support or direct physical care for the patient. It is critical that they understand the ramifications of the diagnosis to prepare them to interact with the patient ongoing post discharge. Since the majority of stroke survivors exhibit some degree of long-term effects from the insult, family members must be prepared for a potentially long period of adjustment.

Practice Setting

Occupational therapy may provide services to stroke survivors in a variety of treatment settings, including acute care hospitals, rehabilitation centers, outpatient facilities, home care, skilled nursing facilities, nursing homes, and specialized programs such as work hardening or driving. Because recovery from stroke may be slow and progressive, a single patient may receive care in more than one practice setting.

In acute care, the occupational therapy program focuses on early assessment, beginning treatment, and determining the subsequent level of care required to benefit the patient—rehabilitation unit, skilled nursing facility, nursing home, or home care.

A rehabilitation admission provides the patient with the opportunity to participate in a program designed to determine the motor, sensory, perceptual, cognitive, and psychological effects of the stroke and the impact that each has had on ADL and IADL function. It is during the rehabilitation stay that decisions are made as to whether deficits can be remedied, or if the patient will benefit from adaptive equipment and techniques. Inpatient rehabilitation requires that the patient be able to participate actively in three hours of combined therapy per day.

Stroke survivors who are making slow but steady progress may benefit from admission to a skilled nursing facility (SNF). In SNFs, the intensity of therapy is reduced allowing the patient to progress at a slower pace. Outpatient and home care programs provide opportunities for the stroke survivor to apply skills and techniques acquired in rehabilitation to a successful transition home. Specialty programs such as work hardening or driver retraining may be important components of a long-term rehabilitation strategy designed to manage independence in IADL.

Sociopolitical

Because the majority of stroke survivors are 65 years old or older, Medicare coverage and rules serve as a critical backdrop to much of the care in both inpatient and outpatient settings. Terms and limitations on services and equipment provided though Medicare and commercial insurers pose a challenge for health care providers, the patient, and family. The age of many stroke survivors makes them eligible for senior services such as senior centers, adult day care, and/or Meals on Wheels. These services may be factored into a comprehensive plan.

The Americans with Disabilities Act (ADA) insures community accessibility for stroke survivors. Additionally, for those patients returning to work, the ADA will insure reasonable accommodations to the workplace and job to facilitate the important worker role.

Many community-based support groups exist for stroke survivors and their families. These groups provide social, educational, recreational, and advocacy opportunities.

Lifestyle/Lifespan

Most persons who experience a stroke will have residual effects that impact their lives on an ongoing basis. The stroke may limit or change the roles that a person is able to play within the family. For example, a grandmother who provided care for grandchildren when her daughter was at work may be unable to continue in that role. Adapting to the limitations in activity imposed by the stroke may be a long process. The patient may experience challenges, and activities that were simple and comforting in the past may become difficult. For example, a stroke survivor who looked forward to making cookies twice a year with her church group may find that she is only able to participate in a limited way.

The cost of living with a long-term disability may be high and impact on the family's financial status and plans. In addition to the cost of medications, patients may be faced with the cost of additional therapy, adaptive equipment, and the cost of making home modifications for accessibility and safety.

A severe stroke may limit opportunities for a patient to return to work or seek employment in a related field. The extraction of such an important role from a person's life will create a void of time and activity that must be filled. After a stroke, a patient may experience residual motor, perceptual, or cognitive disability that makes driving unsafe. Many persons rely on driving, even short distances, for shopping, keeping appointments, and meeting friends. Inability to drive may result in increased dependence on others, increased fear of dependence, and social isolation.

Clinical Decision Making Process

Defining Focus for Intervention

The focus for OT intervention is guided primarily by a combination of the results of the functional assessments such as the COPM and the FIM. These assessments target areas of intervention that are most important to the patient. In the next stage of the process, the therapist carefully examines the results of specific assessments of motor control, perception, cognition, and psychosocial reaction. The relationship and impact of each of these areas to overall function is analyzed. Initial treatment will focus on those deficit areas which impact overall performance.

Practice area impacts the focus of OT intervention. During an acute hospitalization, the primary roles of OT intervention may be positioning the patient to prevent deformity and facilitate function. The therapist also completes an initial assessment. The assessment in acute care may be used to determine the best course of treatment after discharge: home, rehabilitation, outpatient, or skilled nursing facility. The length of stay in acute care for patients post stroke is very limited. This triage function is critical.

An inpatient rehabilitation stay for a patient post stroke is typically limited to several weeks. During this time, the focus is to work concurrently with the family and patient both to upgrade the patient's level of independence and to train the family to provide required care at home.

For more specialized settings such as work hardening or driver rehabilitation, the focus of the OT program is on the individual IADL.

Establishing Goals for Intervention

Establishing goals for a patient post stroke involves and ongoing process of assessment and re-assessment. In establishing goals for intervention, the therapist examines the options for improvement that are available. Initially, the therapist sets goals that will require the patient to demonstrate improvement in motor, sensory, perceptual, or cognitive areas. Such is the case when the therapist indicates that a patient's goal is be "independent in UE dressing." This indicates that the patient will develop the motor control and skills to complete the activity without equipment or assistance.

If the patient does not develop the required skills, the therapist then adjusts his or her thinking and amend the goals to focus on compensatory training. Such is the case when the therapist states that the patient will "complete UE dressing using one handed techniques sitting at the edge of the bed." The therapist may also amend the goal to focus on the use of adaptive equipment. In this case, the goal becomes the patient will "complete UE dressing using a button hook." In cases where the patient will require the assistance of another, goals are written to reflect the type and degree of cueing or physical assistance required.

The process of goal setting for this population is one that changes, as the prognosis for neurological recovery from the stroke becomes more apparent.

Designing Theory-Based Intervention

The complex nature of the signs and symptoms of a stroke in combination with the long recovery period requires that the OT give careful consideration to designing a treatment plan that meets the needs of the patient throughout. Because a stroke has the potential to impact so many areas of function, an integrated frame of reference such as the Model of Human Occupation (MOHO) can serve as an overarching frame. The MOHO requires the therapist to examine all aspects of the patient's life (i.e. values, habits, routines, and roles). It ensures that a comprehensive treatment plan is developed.

The focus for OT intervention, as noted earlier, includes attention to deficits in motor control, perceptual processing, cognitive processes, and issues of adjustment. Deficits in one or more of these areas may impact ADL and IADL. Each of these areas is best addressed by a different frame of reference.

Motor control deficits in patients post stroke may be addressed by the neurodeveolpmental (NDT), biomechanical, or rehabilitation frames of reference. During the initial period of recovery, the patient may be demonstrating abnormal reflexes or abnormal muscle tone. It is at this time when a neurodevelopmental frame of reference and techniques may be used. In the neurodeveolopemtal frame of reference, the focus is on inhibiting abnormal tone and movement and facilitating normal movement. As motor control improves and the patient's underlying motor control is normalized, the frame of reference may shift to biomechanical. Using the biomechanical frame of reference, the therapist can address problems of residual muscle weakness and limitations in range of motion and coordination. Should the patient fail to regain the motor control necessary for completing ADL and IADL, the rehabilitation frame of reference can guide the therapist in the choice of adaptive devices and techniques. Such an approach would include the use of an adapted cutting board to compensate for the limited use of the affected UE as a stabilizer.

Perceptual and cognitive deficits may be addressed using the cognitive and/or rehabilitation frames of reference. During the period of recovery immediately post stroke, a cognitive approach may be used to remediate specific perceptual or cognitive deficits. Such an approach may include graded training activities to improve memory or sequencing. Should the patient fail to regain the perceptual or cognitive skills necessary to participate in ADL and IADL safely and successfully, the rehabilitation frame of reference again can be used to guide the choice of adaptive equipment and strategies. One example may be the use of a memory book or planner to facilitate keeping appointments.

For issues related to psychosocial adjustment to disability the MOHO can be used to guide the selection of activities to reinforce motivation and engagement in activity.

Evaluating Progress

Evaluation of progress occurs throughout the recovery from stroke. The most comprehensive evaluation of progress is seen as the patient improves in functional measures such as the FIM and COPM. An increase in the FIM score implies more independent performance on the part of the patient and a decreased need for adaptive equipment, physical assistance or cueing. On the COPM a higher score indicates improved performance and satisfaction on the part of the patient.

For the components of the program addressing motor control, improvement in the neurodevelopmental frame of reference is noted as abnormal reflexes and patterns of movement are extinguished and the patient's movement becomes more normal. As motor control moves into the biomechanical frame of reference, improvement is noted in strength, range of motion, sensation, and coordination.

In the components of the program addressing perception and cognition, improvement is noted as the patient requires fewer verbal, tactile, or environmental cues to be successful. In the rehabilitation frame of reference, progress is noted as the patient demonstrates the ability to integrate adaptive equipment and devices into daily routines and generalize the use of equipment and techniques to new situations.

Determining Change in or Termination of Treatment

The thinking and decision making process regarding changes in or termination of treatment for this group of patients closely parallels that of goal setting. Initially a focus is on remediation of components and the integration of new skills to support ADL and IADL. An example of this approach is teaching the stroke patient to incorporate scapular protraction and elbow extension by positioning the affected UE between his knees and leaning forward during dressing. The expectation in this approach is that the control of UE spasticity will be developed and improve thereby supporting increased function at discharge.

If during the course of the treatment it becomes apparent that the remedial approach to developing skills is not working, the therapist should change the approach to include adaptive strategies, adaptive equipment, and family teaching.

The initial emphasis is to facilitate optimal neurological and functional recovery prior to teaching compensation or planning for ongoing family caregiving.

Case Study

Description

RCP is a 70-year-old female who had a left CVA one week ago affecting the middle cerebral artery (MCA). This resulted in a right hemiplegia. During her time in the acute care hospital, RCP was seen by OT. At that time her RUE (dominant) presented with low muscle tone. Additionally, RCP exhibited poor trunk control. RCP appeared alert and her orientation to approaching ADLs indicated that she may be having difficulty with visual spatial skills. This was evidenced by difficulty locating and positioning items on her tray during feeding. RCP needed physical assistance to complete all aspects of ADL. Physical therapy issued RCP a wheelchair. She required assistance to push it. These symptoms were consistent with the location of her lesion. OT established a positioning program to prevent deformity and facilitate function in the UE. OT further identified that RCP could benefit from admission to the rehabilitation unit.

Upon admission to the rehabilitation unit, RCP presented with a synergy pattern in her RUE. She positioned her RUE in a position of scapular retraction, adduction and internal rotation, elbow flexion, forearm pronation, and wrist and finger flexion. She was able to feed herself and had difficulty opening containers and cutting meat. RCP continued to require physical assistance for all other ADLs. The suspected visual spatial problems continued to persist. She had difficulty, among other things, with positioning her clothing correctly while dressing. RCP is single and lives in a two-story house with her sister. Her bedroom and bathroom are on the second floor. She is very motivated to be independent. Prior to admission, RCP was responsible for most of the cooking and housekeeping. She enjoys gardening and going to the local senior center to play bingo.

She has been referred for an initial two-week rehabilitation stay to increase independence in ADL, mobility, home management and adjustment to disability.

Long- and Short-Term Goals

The long-term goal of intervention for RCP is to be independent in upper extremity dressing.

This long-term goal will be reached in part through successfully achieving the short-term goal of completing UE dressing sitting at the edge of the bed, incorporating tone reduction strategies.

Therapist Goals and Strategies

The therapist's goals include:

1. Reduce spasticity in the affected RUE.
2. Facilitate the use of the RUE as a functional assist.
3. Facilitate safe sitting balance.
4. Facilitate functional mobility.
5. Teach the patient tone reduction strategies.
6. Improve ADL independence.

The therapist's strategies include:

1. Apply selected neurodevelopmental techniques to reduce spasticity and improve function.
2. Train to incorporate mobility aids (cane, walker, etc.) into ADL.
3. Train in use of selected adaptive devices to promote independence and participation in meaningful activities.

Activity

Planting Spring Bulbs in a Window Box

Prior to starting the activity, the therapist collects the following equipment and supplies: a small window box filled with soft soil, a bulb planter, an assortment of spring bulbs (such as miniature tulips and hyacinths), and a small stool. The planter box is positioned in front of RCP on the low stool. RCP sits at the edge of a mat or chair and straddles the planter box and stool. RCP places the bulb planter in her RUE. The bulbs are placed in a small container on a tray table to her left. To plant each bulb, RCP will grasp the bulb with her left hand, lean forward, and use the bulb planter to dig a hole. She will place the bulb in the hole with her left hand and cover the bulb with dirt. She will continue until each bulb has been planted.

This activity meets the requirements described above. Sitting and leaning will challenge RCP's dynamic sitting balance. Grasping and reaching for each bulb with her LUE will require trunk rotation. By leaning forward, she is encouraging scapular protraction and elbow extension. Digging the hole requires elbow extension and supination. Each of these aspects of the activity supports a neurodevelopmental approach. The visual demands of the task are low. Finally, the motor control required in this task mimics that which is required to integrate neurodevelopmental principles into upper extremity dressing.

In designing an activity for RCP, it is important to consider that she has two broadareas of deficit that appear to be impacting ADL—limited motor control and visual spatial perceptual problems. As the therapist designs a treatment session for RCP, he or she will complete an analysis of each activity that is being considered with a careful eye on the motor challenges of the activity as well as its visual spatial challenges. In structuring the treatment session, the therapist will design tasks that have high motor demands and limited visual spatial demands. The therapist will also design tasks which have high visual spatial demands and limited motor demands. The thinking behind this approach to activity analysis and creation becomes clear when RCP is reexamined. Because RCP is having difficulty with both motor control and visual spatial skills, she will be unable to successfully complete a task if that task is designed to provide a maximum challenge to her motor skills and visual spatial skills concurrently. Therefore, the therapist designs a series of activities that are incorporated into the treatment session which alternately challenge motor control and visual spatial skills. The goal for this sample activity is to provide RCP with an opportunity to improve her motor control.

Treatment Objective

The treatment objective for this session is to have RCP demonstrate the ability to complete self-inhibition techniques for her RUE.

Resources

The following resources can be helpful for gathering clinical data:

ADL status

IADL status

Cognition

Perception

Vision

Sensation

Muscle tone

ROM

Coordination

Psychological adjustment to disability

The following resources can be helpful for gathering family data:

Family interview to cover:

- adjustment to disability
- changing roles and family dynamics
- caregiving responsibilities

The following are common practice settings:

Acute care

Rehabilitation

Skilled nursing

Outpatient

Home care

Senior centers

Adult day care

The following resources can be helpful for gathering sociopolitical data:

Medicare

Commercial insurance companies

ADA

Stroke support groups

The following resources can be helpful in managing and understanding lifestyle/lifespan issues:

Role changes

Continued adjustment to disability

Cost of long-term disability to family finances

Potential for limited employment

Potential to have to give up driving

Change in worker role

Limited opportunity for socialization

Internet Resources

American Heart Association:
www.americanheartassociation.org

Stroke Association:
www.strokeassociation.org

American Occupational Therapy Association:
www.aota.org
4120 Montgomery Lane
P.O. Box 31220
Bethesda, MD 20824

References

American Heart Association (1999). *Heart and stroke statistical update.* Dallas, TX: American Heart Association.

Bartels, M. (1998). Pathophysiology and medical management of stroke. In G. Gillen & A. Burkhardt (Eds.). *Stroke Rehabilitation: A Functional Approach.* St. Louis, MO: Mosby.

Beck, A., & Steer, R. (1987). *Beck depression inventory manual* (Rev. ed.). New York: The Psychological Corporation.

Colarusso, R., & Hammill, D. (1996). *Motor-free visual perception test–revised.* Novato, CA: Academic Therapy Publications.

Fisher, A. (1995). *Assessment of motor and process skills.* Fort Collins, CO: Three Star Press.

Halper, A., & Mogil, S. (1986). Communication disorders: Diagnosis and treatment. In P. Kaplan, & B. Cerullo (Eds.), *Stroke Rehabilitation.* p. 12–13. Boston: Butterworth.

Jebsen, R.H., Taylor, N., Trieschmann, R.B., Trotter, M.J., & Howard, L.A. (1969). An objective and standardized test of hand function. *Archives of Physical Medicine and Rehabilitation, 50*(6), 311–319.

Katz, N., Itzkovich, M., Averbuch, S., & Elazer, B. (1989). Loenstein Occupational Therapy Cognitive Assessment (LOTCA) Battery for Brain-injured Patients: Reliability and Validity. *American Journal of Occupational Therapy, 43,* 184–192.

Keith, R., Granger, C., Hamilton, B., & Sherwin, F. (1987). The functional independence measure: A new tool for rehabilitation. In Eisenberg, M. & Grzesak, R. (Eds.) *Advances in clinical rehabilitation.* New York: Sprangier-Verlag.

Kohlman-Thompson, L. (1993). *The Kohlman evaluation of living skills* (3rd ed.). Bethesda, MD: American Occupational Therapy Association.

Law, M., Baptiste, S., Carswell, H., McColl, M., Polatajko, H., Pollack, N. (1994). *The Canadian occupational performance measure* (2nd ed.). Ottawa, Canada: CAOT Publications ACE.

Roth, E. (1991). Medical complication encountered in stroke rehabilitation. *Physical Medicine and Rehabilitation Clinics of North America, 2*(3), 563–577.

Uniform Data System for Medical Rehabilitation (UDSMK)(1993). Guide for the uniform data set for medical rehabilitation (adult FIM), version 4.0, Buffalo, NY: UB Foundation Activities.

Wilson, D., Baker, L., & Craddock, J.(1984). Functional test for the hemplegic upper extremity. *American Journal of Occupational Therapy, 38,* 159–164.

World Health Organization (1980). *International classification of impairments, disabilities, and handicaps.* Geneva, Switzerland: Author.

Dementia

25

Cindy Brillman, OTR/L

Synopsis of Clinical Condition

Prevalence and Etiology

According to the *Diagnostic and Statistical Manual of Mental Disorders IV* (*DSM–IV*), Dementia is a syndrome that may be caused or characterized by multiple cognitive deficits which include memory impairment. Dementia is a progressive, often irreversible disease, which impairs cognitive and functional abilities and results in a decrease in the ability to perform daily activities. The diagnosis of dementia usually includes aphasia, apraxia, agnosia, and disturbances in behavior regulation and social and occupational function. The incidence of dementia drastically increases with age. Every third person over 90 years of age suffers from moderate or severe dementia. It is not currently understood why people develop dementia. It is speculated that age, heredity, hormone replacement therapy, alcohol, and head injury, may be risk factors.

A number of diseases can cause the symptoms of dementia. The most common types of irreversible dementia include: Alzheimer's disease, Vascular (multi-infarct) dementia, Dementia with Lewy bodies, Fronto-temporal dementia (e.g., Pick's disease), Alcohol-related dementia (including Korsakoff's syndrome), and AIDS-related dementia. Medication-induced dementia and dementias due to hypothyroidism, B12 deficiency, and systemic infections are considered reversible dementias.

Common Characteristics and Symptoms

Half of those affected by dementia suffer from Alzheimer's disease. The number of Americans with Alzheimer's disease may rise to 14 million by 2050 (Alzheimer's Association, 1998). Senile Dementia of the Alzheimer Type (SDAT) is defined as a progressive neuropsychiatric disease of aging affecting brain matter and characterized by the inexorable loss of cognitive function and memory as well as affective and behavioral disturbances (Marcantonio, 2003). The most commonly known symptoms are confusion, memory loss, difficulty performing familiar tasks, problems with language, disorientation to time and place, poor or decreased judgment, problems with abstract thinking, misplacing things, changes in mood or behavior, changes in personality, and loss of initiative.

The progression rate of Alzheimer's disease varies widely. The duration of the disease may vary from 3 to 20 years. The areas of the brain that control memory and cognitive skills are first affected. Typically antidementia or psychotropic drugs are prescribed to improve disease symptoms. The most popular drugs presently used to treat Alzheimer's disease are cholinesterase inhibitors (Tacrine/Cognex®; Donepezil/Aricept®; Rivastigmine/Exelon®; Galantamine/Reminyl®); and vitamin E.

The individual course of the disease drastically varies with each individual. The disease is typically divided into three stages:

- Mild—Impairments of mental abilities as well as mood swings.
- Moderate—Behavioral disturbances increasingly develop.
- Severe—Physical problems are dominant in the advanced stage.

In the early stages, losses that are most noticeable are the loss or inability to complete complex tasks; for example, balancing a checkbook, planning an event or a meeting, or working at a demanding job. As the dementia progresses, and the neuropathological damage becomes more pervasive, a person may not recognize a spouse, understand how to use everyday objects such as utensils, or be able to recognize any type of hazard or emergency situation. Many persons with middle stage Alzheimer's become lost in familiar surroundings, experience hallucinations, and may need moderate to maximal assistance with personal hygiene. Cognitive degeneration, balance, and ambulation problems are exacerbated and eating difficulties, and bowel and bladder problems ensue. The late stage of the disease is marked by total dependence and inactivity.

Vascular dementia accounts for about 20% of all cases of dementia. Vascular disease occurs when blood vessels are damaged, and oxygen fails to get to the brain. Without the needed oxygen, the brain cells are likely to die leading to a series of mini strokes (infarcts) and possible vascular dementia. Vascular dementia and Alzheimer's disease frequently occur together. As a comorbid condition, vascular dementia may worsen the dementia of Alzheimer's disease.

With vascular dementia, the cognitive changes are likely to have a clear starting date. The symptoms usually progress slowly after each attack, suggesting that small strokes have been occurring. Since any area of the brain can be affected by the mini-strokes, the symptoms are varied and include severe depression, mood swings, and epilepsy, cognitive, or physical deficits. Some cognitive abilities may be relatively unaffected

Dementia with Lewy bodies is the third most common cause of dementia. Dementia with Lewy bodies is similar to Alzheimer's disease in that it is caused by the degeneration and death of nerve cells in the brain. An abnormal collection of protein, known as Lewy bodies, occur in the nerve cells of the brain.

The development of Dementia with Lewy bodies has been associated with the development of Parkinson's disease. People with Lewy body disease are very sensitive to some tranquillizers known as antipsychotic or neuroleptic drugs and their use should be avoided if at all possible. Dementia with Lewy body affects concentration, attention span, memory, proprioception, and the ability to estimate distances, reasoning, and language skills. Visual hallucinations can occur in Dementia with Lewy bodies.

Fronto-temporal dementia is one of the least common causes of dementia, and typically develops at forty to fifty years of age. The frontal lobe of the brain is particularly affected and a progressive decline in mental abilities occurs over a number of years. Damage to brain cells is more localized than in Alzheimer's disease and usually begins in the frontal lobe, which is the area that controls executive functioning, social skills, reasoning, judgment, and the ability to take initiative. Individuals with frontal lobe dementia often lack flexibility in thinking and are unable to carry a project through to completion. However, there are no lapses of memory as in Alzheimer's disease.

Failure of executive functions may increase safety risk since they may not be able to plan appropriate actions or inhibit inappropriate actions. Changes in personality, ability to concentrate, social skills, motivation, and reasoning are connected with this form of dementia. These symptoms are often confused with psychiatric disorders. Memory, language, and visual perception are usually not impaired for the first two years, yet as the disease progresses and spreads to other areas of the brain, they too may become affected.

Typically, the disorder affects females more than males. Mood and behavior may become fixed and difficult to change, making patients appear selfish and unfeeling. A person with frontal lobe dementia may appear to have difficulty in many areas of cognitive function. The ability to maintain attention and concentration and the ability to organize information are all affected with frontal lobe dementia. The psychological, social, family, and financial issues that affect individuals with frontal lobe dementia occur earlier in life, and therefore financial issues such as job security, or caring for a family become paramount. Driving is usually unsafe for persons with this diagnosis. As more is known about the disease, more policy changes may come into effect. Some residential care and adult day programs are recognizing the needs of the younger dementia patient and are beginning to offer services to meet their needs.

Alcohol-related dementia is associated with the abuse of alcohol. This population seems to be at risk of developing problems with their memory. Some have a specific problem of loss of short-term memory known as Korsakoff's syndrome, which develops because of vitamin B1 deficiency. Others develop a wider range of problems that resemble Alzheimer's disease.

HIV is the virus which leads to AIDS, and can also be a cause of dementia. AIDS-related dementia is a condition that is usually referred to as AIDS dementia complex (ADC). The virus has been found in the brain of people with HIV as early as two days after initial infection.

Target Areas for Intervention

Occupational therapy treatment focuses on slowing functional deterioration and retaining existing functional skills and safety. There are three components that should be incorporated into any treatment plan: work or task simplification, environmental modification/home modification and caregiver training.

Contextual Considerations

Clinical

Referrals for occupational therapy are frequently made after a physician has evaluated an individual. The clinical data that is collected by the occupational therapist provides baseline data that is essential for tracking the progression of the disease process. In addition to the cognitive changes, which are most often experienced with Alzheimer's disease, the normal physical and sensory changes that occur with the normal aging process must be factored into the evaluative process by the occupational therapist. These include decreased mobility, limited reach, reduced range of motion, diminished visual acuity, altered perception of colors, increased accommodation time, and diminished hearing. These physical and sensory changes can greatly exacerbate the cognitive problems associated with dementia.

The occupational therapy evaluation incorporates the following areas: upper and lower extremity range of motion and strength, balance, coordination, visual motor coordination, personal care, feeding, memory, attention span, frustration tolerance, ability to express needs, and follow directions. Functionality in these areas is directly related to functional independence in the activities of daily living (ADLs), as illustrated in the following chart.

Table 25.1
Functionality and ADLs

Affected system	Functional Loss	ADL loss
Sensory	Decreased ability to integrate stimuli from different sources	Difficulty in distinguishing stairs, thresholds
Sensory	Increased sensitivity to stimuli	Decreased enjoyment and/or awareness of environmental stimulants (smell of food, flowers, smoke, etc.)
Muscular and Nervous	Decreased strength	Decreased mobility, difficulty walking on uneven surfaces difficulty with mobility
Muscular and Nervous	Decreased speed of reactions	Slowed protective reactions when falling
Skeletal	Increased porosity of bone	Frequent fractures from falls
Cardiopulmonary	Decreased cardiac output, myocardial strength	Decreased endurance for daily activities
Cognitive	Decreased/diminished ability to organize and make decisions	Increased time needed to respond in emergency situations

The Allen Cognitive Level Screen (Allen, 1996), the Assessment of Motor and Process Skills (AMPS) (Fisher, 1995), the Functional Assessment Questionnaire (FAQ) (Pfeffer, R., Kurosaki, T., Harrah, C., et al.) and the Physical Self Maintenance Scale (PSMS)-(Lawton, M., & Brody, E., 1969) are examples of assessment tools that assist the therapist in determining functional ability. The Fulstein Mini-Mental State Exam (MMSE) (Folstein, M., Folstein, S., & McHugh, P., 1975) is an assessment that provides information regarding the level of orientation, memory, attention span, and communication. The Global Deterioration Scale (GDS) (Reisberg, B., Ferris, S., deLeon, M., & Crook, T., 1982), the Alzheimer's Disease Assessment Scale, Cognitive Subsection (ADAS–Cog) (Rosen, W., Mohs, R. & Davis, K., (1984), the Clinical Dementia Rating Scale (CDR) (Hugh, C., Borg, L. & Danziger, W., 1982), the Progressive Deterioration Scale (PDS), and the Global Deterioration Scale (GDS) assist in establishing the level and tracking the progression of the disease process.

Assessments are used to determine the focus or baseline of treatment and may also be necessary to substantiate insurance claims, facilitate placement, determine independent living status, support litigation, document need for a specific program, or establish competence on the job.

Family

Dementia affects the individual and the family. Spouses and/or adult children are the primary caregivers for individuals in the early and middle stages of dementia. As Alzheimer's disease progresses, the patient may require care 24 hours a day. The family and caregiver(s) must cope with the progressive deterioration of the person with Alzheimer's and often fall prey to depression and other health problems. Local chapters of the Alzheimer's Association have support groups (www.ahaf.org). Programs such as Alzheimer's Family Relief provides financial assistance when no other means are available. The American Health Assistance Foundation (AHAF) is a nonprofit, charitable organization that has dedicated over 30 years to funding research on age-related and degenerative diseases, educating the public about these diseases, and providing emergency financial assistance to Alzheimer's disease patients and their caregivers.

Occupational therapists can provide caretakers with strategies to facilitate home management of the patient including home safety checkouts, task simplification techniques and adaptation of the physical environment so that the person with Alzheimer's disease can maintain their mental abilities and carry out their daily lives safely and with dignity.

As the disease progresses, occupational therapists may assist caregivers in exploring other care setting options.

Practice Setting

Occupational therapists may see persons with Alzheimer's disease in a number of settings including the home environment, assisted living facilities, long-term care facility and adult day care settings. The home environment is the optimal choice at the early stages of the disease but transition to more comprehensive care settings is almost always necessary. Persons with Alzheimer's disease do best in familiar surroundings; minimizing frightening or confusing distractions is a key element when assisting a client in transitioning to new care environments. When a person with Alzheimer's disease is no longer safe at home, two other environments maybe considered: assisted living and long-term care facilities.

Sociopolitical

Assisted living facilities, in general, require private payment. There are some state programs and private insurance policies that allow payment for services performed in an assisted living facility.

Most individuals with Dementia or Alzheimer's disease are over 70 years old and qualify for Medicare coverage, or have chosen an "HMO" form of Medicare coverage as an option. Medicare and private insurance will cover occupational therapy evaluation and treatment of the person with Alzheimer's disease if documentation provides the following:

- History of prior treatment.
- Prior level of function (related to the condition being treated), and documentation showing that there was a decline or "change of status."
- Description of any "safety risks."
- Baseline objective documentation/tests.

- Goals delineating how long and how many visits it will take to achieve the stated goal.
- The amount, frequency and duration of the services must be reasonable under accepted standards of practice.
- Plan for the timely achievement of goals and/or a safe and effective caregiver program.
- The client's condition must be such that the services required can be safely and effectively performed only by an Occupational Therapist or a Certified Occupational Therapy assistant under the supervision of an Occupational Therapist.
- The services must be considered to be a specific and effective treatment for the client's condition.
- The progress notes must show documented functional improvement or a decrease in the level of safety risk.

People with Alzheimer's have the right to receive care without the use of physical or chemical restraints that are not needed to treat a medical condition. Care providers have an obligation to try alternatives to restraints, such as diversions for aggressive behavior or safe places to wander. Restraints should be used only if a patient is a danger to him/herself or to others. According to the Joint Commission on Accreditation of Health Care Organizations (JCAHO), an organization that evaluates and accredits health care organizations, studies have demonstrated that effective programming can eliminate the need for restraints.

Lifestyle/Lifespan

Persons with Alzheimer's disease will live an average of eight years and as many as 20 years after the onset of symptoms. The financial and emotional burdens to the patient and family have been noted above. As the disease progresses, caregivers become increasingly responsible for making decisions that effect the client's safety, dignity, comfort and quality of life.

Clinical Decision Making Process

Defining Focus for Intervention

In the home setting, the physical environment, performance of daily living activities such as cooking, use of tools, bathing, shaving, and smoking and available level of supervision should be evaluated as potential sources of danger and/or injury.

In the assisted living facility, where supervision and safety features are more consistent, the intervention focus shifts to task simplification, adaptive equipment and techniques, energy conservation, joint protection, and safety positioning for tasks such as dressing, eating, and personal hygiene. As functional ability deteriorates, and nursing home placement is warranted, wheelchair and bed safety are often the first goals to be addressed.

Although environmental safety is the primary focus for occupational therapy intervention in home-based and institutionally-based practice settings, occupational therapy practitioners have an important role in maximizing the overall functional ability of persons with cognitive impairments and educating their caregivers in providing a comfortable and safe living environment.

Establishing Goals for Intervention

The goals for intervention are dependent upon the practice setting and the stage of the disease. The following five categories represent common target areas for occupational therapy intervention:

1. Activities of daily living (ADL)
2. Instrumental activities of daily living (IADL) (e.g., shopping, cooking, financial management)
3. In-service training and instructions to the caregiver
4. Therapeutic or environmental adaptations
5. Play/leisure

Examples of goals or expected outcomes of home treatment are purposeful activities such as setting the table, folding laundry, and assisting with meal preparation. Treatment goals for independence or minimal assistance in bathing, dressing and grooming are reasonable expectations in the early stages of Alzheimer's disease.

Goals in assisted living environments usually focus on ADL activities and the promotion and achievement of success oriented tasks, which allow the individual to feel pride and a sense of accomplishment.

In both of these settings, the maintenance of a structured, daily routine is an important goal.

The goals in a nursing home setting will vary depending on the physical and/or cognitive deficits that have developed. Safety and fall prevention become paramount.

Designing Theory-Based Intervention

Although there are many frames of reference that are cogent to the treatment of patients with dementia, the Person-Environment Performance Framework (Chrisitian, 1991) is particularly applicable for the geriatric population with physical and cognitive deficits. The Person Performance Environment Framework (PPE) (Chrisitian, 1991) identifies individual and environmental factors that impact performance and assists the therapist in identifying three broad goal categories:

1. Person (Personality and Abilities and Skills)
2. Performance (Activities, Tasks, and Roles of Occupation)
3. Environment (Physical, Social, and Cultural Factors)

Evaluating Progress

Objective assessments, such as those mentioned earlier in this chapter, establish baseline functional levels against which progress is measured. Medicare regulations have established terminology to describe functional performance levels (maximum, moderate or minimum assistance). The occupational therapist documents improvements at each level and compares the current cognitive/physical level with prior levels of functioning. Progress can also be shown by documenting the consistency with which a task is performed successfully and/or the degree to which a concept is generalized to new situations.

Determining Change in or Termination of Treatment

If the individual is no longer making measurable functional progress in the scope, level, or consistency of performance, than discharge plans which include a maintenance or restorative program should be initiated. A maintenance or restorative program usually includes daily feeding programs, routine exercise, and the daily practice of coordination and self care skills.

Case Study

Description

Anna is an 80-year-old widow, who raised three daughters and was very proud of her homemaker role and her ability to deftly manage the family's finances during hard times. She presently has mild to moderate dementia, and has been referred for home care, while recuperating from a hip fracture, due to a recent fall. For the past four years, Anna has been living with her youngest daughter, Jane, who is single and works full-time as a nurse. Jane has been finding it increasingly difficult to care for Anna, due to Anna's increasing memory loss and agitation. Through an in-depth interview and observation, the OT discerned that the most difficult part of the day for Jane is the hour when she returns from work to relieve the hired caregiver, and begins preparing dinner. It is at this time of day when Anna becomes increasingly agitated, and follows Jane around the kitchen continually asking the same questions, "Where is my purse? Where is my money? I want my money!" This repetitive behavior is very stressful for Jane at that hour of the day, and has made caregiving increasingly difficult.

As part of Anna's treatment, the OT will address the caregiver's concern.

Long- and Short-Term Goals

The long-term goals include enabling the caregiver to create simple activities that help to mitigate Anna's agitated repetitive behaviors.

As a short-term goal, the caregiver will implement therapist designed activities to reduce Anna's agitated behaviors during mealtime preparation.

Therapist Goals and Strategies

The therapist's goals include:

1. Increase caregiver's awareness regarding resources related to safety issues, medical information, social support, and behavior management.

The therapist's strategies include:

1. Educate the caregiver about Alzheimer's disease and its common symptoms.
2. Instruct the caregiver in setting up a diversionary activity which will modify the patient's behavior.

Activity

Sorting Coins

Following a demonstration by the therapist, the caregiver will set up a sorting activity on a clean table for the patient. With the patient seated at the table, the caregiver will give Anna a purse with a zippered pouch containing 25 quarters, 25 nickels, and 25 pennies. The caregiver will instruct the patient, in simple language and through modeling, to place all the quarters in the red container, all the nickels in the blue container, and all the pennies in the clear container. This activity will allow Anna to be engaged in an activity during the time that her daughter is feeling most stressed. Although some may argue that the primary focus this activity and intervention is Anna's daughter, it is important to note that the caregiver training for this population is a reimbursable session.

This activity choice is based on:

1. Context of the patient: age, prior roles, culture, interests, meaningful activities, goals, home environment, caregiver's priorities.
2. Analysis of client factors and skills necessary to complete the coin-sorting activity.
3. Analysis of cognitive level of the patient.
4. Collaboration with the caregiver.

Treatment Objectives

The caregiver will set up the coin sorting activity following the demonstration by the OT.

The caregiver will instruct the patient's mother to sort the coins using simple, direct language as recommended by the OT.

Resources

Internet Resources

The Alzheimer's Association:
www.alz.org

Alzheimer's Center. WebMD.com:
www.my.webmd.com/condition_center/alz?z=3074_nsb_03

Alzheimer's Disease International (ADI):
www.alz.co.uk

The Alzheimer's Disease Education and Referral (ADEAR) Center:
www.alzheimers.org

Alzheimer's Disease. MayoClinic.com:
www.mayoclinic.com/findinformation/diseasesandconditions/invoke.cfm?id=DS00161

Alzheimer's Disease: Unraveling the Mystery. National Institute on Aging:
www.alzheimers.org/unraveling/index.htm

The Alzheimer Page. Washington University, St. Louis, Missouri:
www.biostat.wustl.edu/alzheimer

Dementia.com:
www.dementia.com/

Health Policy Sites - George Washington University:
www.gwu.edu/~ihpp/Hpolicy.html

References

Allen, C. (1996). *Allen cognitive level test manual.* Colchester, CT: S&S Worldwide.

Dejong, R., Osterlund, O., & Ray, G. (1989). Measurment of quality of life changes in patients with Alzheimer's disease. *Clinical Therapeutics, 11,* 545–554.

Fisher, A. (1997). *Assessment of motor and process skills* (2nd ed.). Fort Collins, CO: Three Star Press.

Folstein, M., Folstein, S., & McHugh, P. (1975). Mini-mental state: A practical method for grading the cognitive state of patients for the clinician. *Journal of Psychiatric Research, 12,* 189–198.

Hughs, C., Berg, L., & Danziger, W. (1982). A new clinical scale for the staging of demential. *British Journal of Psychiatry, 140,* 566–572.

Lawton, M., & Brody, E. (1969). Assessment of older people: Self maintaining and instrumental activities of daily living. *The Gerontologist, 9,* 179–186.

Pfeffer, R., Kurosaki, T., Harrah, C., Chance, J., & Filos, S. (1982). Measurement of functional activities of older adults in the community. *Journal of Geontology, 37,* 323–329.

Reisberg, B., Ferris, S., deLeon, M., & Crook, T. (1982). Global deteriortation scale. *American Journal of Psychiatry, 139,* 1136–1139.

Rosen, W., Mohs, R., & Davis, K. (1984). A new rating scale for Alzheimer's disease. *American Journal of Psychiatry, 14,* 1356–1364.